D1379174

Best Practice Occupational Therapy

for Children and Families in Community Settings

Second Edition

Best Practice Occupational Therapy

for Children and Families in Community Settings

Second Edition

Winnie Dunn, PhD, OTR, FAOTA
Author, Senior Mentor, Professor and Chair
Department of Occupational Therapy Education
University of Kansas
Kansas City, Kansas

SLACK
INCORPORATED

www.slackbooks.com

ISBN: 978-1-55642-961-3

Copyright © 2011 by SLACK Incorporated

Instructors: *Best Practice Occupational Therapy for Children and Families in Community Settings, Second Edition Instructor's Manual* is also available from SLACK Incorporated. Don't miss this important companion to *Best Practice Occupational Therapy for Children and Families in Community Settings, Second Edition*. To obtain the Instructor's Manual, please visit http://www.efacultylounge.com.

All rights reserved. No part of this book may be reproduced, stored in a retrieval system or transmitted in any form or by any means, electronic, mechanical, photocopying, recording or otherwise, without written permission from the publisher, except for brief quotations embodied in critical articles and reviews.

The procedures and practices described in this book should be implemented in a manner consistent with the professional standards set for the circumstances that apply in each specific situation. Every effort has been made to confirm the accuracy of the information presented and to correctly relate generally accepted practices. The authors, editor, and publisher cannot accept responsibility for errors or exclusions or for the outcome of the material presented herein. There is no expressed or implied warranty of this book or information imparted by it. Care has been taken to ensure that drug selection and dosages are in accordance with currently accepted/recommended practice. Due to continuing research, changes in government policy and regulations, and various effects of drug reactions and interactions, it is recommended that the reader carefully review all materials and literature provided for each drug, especially those that are new or not frequently used. Any review or mention of specific companies or products is not intended as an endorsement by the author or publisher.

SLACK Incorporated uses a review process to evaluate submitted material. Prior to publication, educators or clinicians provide important feedback on the content that we publish. We welcome feedback on this work.

Published by: SLACK Incorporated
6900 Grove Road
Thorofare, NJ 08086 USA
Telephone: 856-848-1000
Fax: 856-848-6091
www.slackbooks.com

Contact SLACK Incorporated for more information about other books in this field or about the availability of our books from distributors outside the United States.

Dunn, Winnie.
Best practice occupational therapy for children and families in community settings / Winnie Dunn. -- 2nd ed.
p. ; cm.
Rev. ed. of: Best practice occupational therapy. c2000.
Includes bibliographical references and index.
ISBN 978-1-55642-961-3 (alk. paper)
1. Occupational therapy for children--Standards. 2. Occupational therapy services--Standards. I. Dunn, Winnie. Best practice occupational therapy. II. Title.
[DNLM: 1. Child. 2. Developmental Disabilities--rehabilitation. 3. Community Mental Health Services. 4. Early Intervention (Education) 5. Occupational Therapy--methods. 6. Professional-Family Relations. WS 350.6]
RJ53.O25B47 2011
615.8'515083--dc22
2011000338

For permission to reprint material in another publication, contact SLACK Incorporated. Authorization to photocopy items for internal, personal, or academic use is granted by SLACK Incorporated provided that the appropriate fee is paid directly to Copyright Clearance Center. Prior to photocopying items, please contact the Copyright Clearance Center at 222 Rosewood Drive, Danvers, MA 01923 USA; phone: 978-750-8400; web site: www.copyright.com; email: info@copyright.com

Printed in the United States of America.

Last digit is print number: 10 9 8 7 6 5 4 3 2 1

Dedication

I dedicate this book to my sister Mary Ellen O'Hare.
"Educator" is woven into the fabric of her soul; every gesture, thought, comment, and action she creates is infused with insight to guide the path of everyone she encounters.
She doesn't "DO" it, she "IS" it.

CONTENTS

Instructors: *Best Practice Occupational Therapy for Children and Families in Community Settings, Second Edition Instructor's Manual* is also available from SLACK Incorporated. Don't miss this important companion to *Best Practice Occupational Therapy for Children and Families in Community Settings, Second Edition*. To obtain the Instructor's Manual, please visit http://www.efacultylounge.com.

ACKNOWLEDGMENTS

All my work is supported by complex scaffolding. Colleagues, family, and friends contribute to the process I use to complete my work. I am grateful to all the people in my life who tirelessly listen to my stories and my new ideas (some of which do not deserve the air I use to tell them!) and encourage me along the way. In fact, every act of support contributes to this book, because giving me space so I can write is one of the best gifts of all.

Of special note are those who explicitly provided help to get this book to press.

Jane Cox, Becky Nicholson, Ellen Pope, and Louann Rinner met with me every week as we hammered out what needs to be the next generation of Best Practices for our profession. We talked and debated and bantered; they read endless emails as I responded to colleagues and families asking for advice; they listened to my crazy ideas and plans; and out of all of it we created a coherent story to tell. You are the rudders for my boat, and I thank you.

The faculty, staff, and GTAs at the University of Kansas Occupational Therapy Education Department make sure everything is handled in our curricula, service, and research programs so I have the luxury of committing my ideas to paper. They encourage me every day to do this, and I am grateful.

My staff, Michael Ahlers, Candy Conner, Jennifer Tanquary, and Angie Ford, make sure that all the parts are in place so I can write. They also find obscure materials, clean things up, and stand at the ready no matter what needs to be done. Thanks!

Lauren Foster let me interrupt her to try out ideas, and Beth Antonacci organized all the bibliographies.

Beth Cada, Liz Maryama, Kristie Koenig, Mary Law, Wendy Coster, Nancy Pollock, and Deb Stewart, by being themselves, gave me courage to speak clearly about best practices and the high ground we are called to as occupational therapists; they have all had a profound influence on me as I worked on this material.

Mary Ellen O'Hare, Jessica Dunn, Jim Dunn, and Maureen Kelly have all engaged in lively banter with me about education so that I keep my grounding about the teachers' and learners' experiences.

Tim Wilson also listened tirelessly and with great enthusiasm, even though these are not his areas of interest.

Brien Cummings and John Bond from SLACK Incorporated encouraged me to stretch my ideas and creativity, and if they were afraid, they never let on.

About the Author

Winnie Dunn, PhD, OTR, FAOTA is Professor and Chair of the Department of Occupational Therapy Education at the University of Kansas. Dr. Dunn holds a bachelor's degree in occupational therapy and a Master of Science degree in special education-learning disabilities from the University of Missouri. She earned her doctorate in Applied Neuroscience from the University of Kansas.

She is a fellow of the American Occupational Therapy Association (AOTA), has received the Award of Merit for outstanding service contributions to the profession, is a member of the Academy of Research of the American Occupational Therapy Foundation (AOTF), has received the A. Jean Ayres Research Award for her outstanding contributions to knowledge development, and was the Eleanor Clarke Slagle Lecturer in 2001 for her significant contributions to "conceptual and evidence based neuroscience research and practice." She has served on the Commission on Practice, the Early Intervention, and School Based Practice Task forces of AOTA, has been the chair of the Research Development Committee of the AOTF, and has served on the National Board for Certification of Occupational Therapy (NBCOT).

Dr. Dunn has written extensively about service provision practices for children and families, with more than 100 articles and numerous books and book chapters to her credit. She also teaches internationally, serving as visiting professor in numerous programs around the world. Through her research, she has demonstrated the effectiveness of consultation and the use of theory to guide contextually relevant practice.

Her line of research about sensory processing in daily life has been very fruitful, producing the family of *Sensory Profile* assessments that identify distinct patterns of sensory processing in various groups of infants, toddlers, children, youth, adults, and older adults. These assessments are used internationally by professionals in many disciplines, and they have been translated into dozens of languages for use in research and practice programs. Most recently, she wrote a book for the public based on this research. *Living Sensationally: Understanding Your Senses* has been covered in international media and is currently translated into German and will soon be available in Hebrew.

Contributing Authors

Jane A. Cox, MS, OTR/L
Clinical Assistant Professor
Department of Occupational Therapy Education
University of Kansas
Kansas City, Kansas

Becky Nicholson, MEd, OTR
Clinical Assistant Professor
Department of Occupational Therapy Education
University of Kansas
Kansas City, Kansas

Ellen Pope, MEd, OTR
Clinical Assistant Professor
Department of Occupational Therapy Education
University of Kansas
Kansas City, Kansas

Louann Rinner, MS, OTR
LEND Training Director
Center for Child Health and Development
University of Kansas
Kansas City, Kansas

Introduction

Working on the new edition of this book has provided me with the opportunity to reflect on practice with children once again. I have been thinking about the interesting challenge of knowing what material to change and what material to keep the same. We examined what parts of each chapter reflected core principles of best practice, and therefore needed to remain, while also identifying new trends in practice that needed to be included as current methods for implementing core principles. We noticed that there were some forward-thinking ideas in both the previous editions; some of the ideas in the first edition that invited occupational therapists to expand their ideas of practice have become expectations of quality practice for this next edition.

In a way, we are called to be courageous when we decide to provide best practices rather than standard practices. We are agreeing to take some risks, to evaluate the effectiveness of our own work, to be willing to say "that was a good idea, but it wasn't the right idea for this situation," to believe that we can find the therapeutic opportunities inside a child's everyday experiences, and to trust that our core knowledge and new evidence will provide the tools to improve our practices. This second edition is your "how to" manual.

We certainly have role models for this pioneering spirit. Dr. A. Jean Ayres forged new knowledge on our behalf at a time when no one was thinking about the challenges she saw in children's lives. Her ideas were not easily accepted and took years to become a critical component of occupational therapy wisdom. She believed that her skilled observations had substance, and she was willing to find out about her hunches. Occupational therapy knowledge grows when all of us embrace this spirit of discovery and when we are willing to adapt our current practices as we know more about what is an effective practice.

We are inviting you to be nimble as you construct your ideas about practice and its possibilities. This new edition will provide you with scaffolding for being that best practice occupational therapist.

Chapter 1 introduces the concept of "best practice" and outlines the 5 core principles and philosophies of best practice.

Chapter 2 reviews all the laws and regulations that guide practices that serve children, families, and community practice settings.

Chapter 3 summarizes the clinical reasoning process in occupational therapy practice, with illustrations for serving children.

Chapter 4 summarizes key theoretical frameworks and practice models that guide practice with children, families, and community practice.

Chapter 5 provides a guide for the structure of best practices, including effective communication strategies and workload and management methods to support practice.

Chapter 6 outlines the assessment process to illustrate how to keep the child's life in focus while we explore what is supporting or interfering with participation.

Chapter 7 provides information on the structures that guide the intervention planning processes, including guidance from the laws and regulations, our roles on interdisciplinary teams, and solving common dilemmas in intervention planning.

Chapter 8 illustrates how to design interventions that reflect the best available evidence and are imbedded in the children's daily lives.

Chapter 9 provides a summary of cases with all the components put together, so that you can refer back to them as you encounter practice challenges of your own.

For all Web site links listed in this textbook, go to the main Web site, and then search for the document you are interested in. This strategy has 2 benefits. First, the links to the Web sites are not as likely to change, whereas links to specific documents can change with updates. Second, when you search at the primary Web site, you might also find other resources that are helpful to you.

Because we want to make it easy to implement the best practices outlined in the text, we are including copies of all the forms on the Web site www.slackbooks.com/bestpracticeforms so you can download and use them.

Collectively, my colleagues who contributed to this edition and I have nearly 1.5 centuries of experience serving children, families, and communities. We have served on local, state, and national interdisciplinary committees to design innovations and set standards for best practice. We have mentored hundreds of young therapists as they work with children, families, and communities. We have collaborated with our colleagues in other disciplines to improve systems and structures when they did not support children and families. We have also practiced in all the ways that may be outdated now (over decades that happens!), so we also know what it is like to confront, examine, embrace, and reject new ideas. This new edition will explore all of these experiences and show you how to navigate across your career to provide the best possible services for children, families, and communities.

Winnie Dunn, PhD, OTR, FAOTA

With conceptual and section contributions from my wise colleagues:
Ellen Pope, MEd, OTR; Becky Nicholson, MEd, OTR; Jane A. Cox, MS, OTR/L; and Louann Rinner, MS, OTR

Preface From the First Edition

How is it that a person comes to have strong beliefs about something? I suppose there are many ways. Sometimes it is our missteps that show us the edges, and the core of our beliefs; this is certainly true for me.

A very young mother taught me the importance of family-centered care. As I was serving her and her daughter, I determined that her daughter was ready to try self-feeding. The mother was quite reluctant about my suggestions and was not following my recommendations. The mother continued to feed her daughter.

I was quite put out by this mother's actions. I was giving her my best advice, the expertise that I spent many years learning, and the mother was being "passive-aggressive" with me by not following through. I spoke to others about this with frustration and disgust. Why would this mother neglect this opportunity to support her daughter's development?

It is fortunate for me (and for this mother and child) that I had a wise administrator at the time. He said "Winnie, why don't you go visit the mother in her home and see what you discover." I was not interested in investing that kind of time on this mother when she wouldn't even do what I had already told her to do. But each time I ranted and raved around the office, he would quietly suggest this same strategy over and over again until I felt pressure to comply.

So with little excitement, I scheduled a visit. I did have the insight to go close to a meal time since we were supposed to be working on feeding. It did not take long once I was immersed in this mother's life, to understand why I needed to be there. I needed to experience these two people's lives; only then could I know how to apply my knowledge and expertise in their service.

Although the mother had many appropriate toys around for her daughter, they were not interacting when I arrived. The daughter was sitting among the toys, but was not playing. This continued while the mother and I chatted. Then we began to move toward the kitchen for the meal, and everything changed. The mother and daughter began to interact with each other, using reciprocal eye contact and vocalizations; the mother played with her daughter, pulling the spoon in and out, and making her daughter move in anticipation toward the food.

In those moments, the clarity of my insight became so bright it was blinding me. I realized that with all her reluctance, comments, and behaviors, the mother had been trying to convey something very important. She somehow knew the essential nature of her intimacy with her daughter and only knew how to maintain this within the ritual of feeding time. I was so focused on my expertise that I failed to *listen*, observe, and derive meaning from her behaviors. My insight enabled me to see that she certainly could profit from my expertise, just not the part I was trying to wedge into her life. This mother and daughter needed me to teach them how to play together as an expanded form of intimacy.

It is for this mother and daughter and all the parents and children that have come into our professional lives since that defining moment that I am relentless about what constitutes best practice for children and families. Vulnerable children and families cannot afford the time it might take for service providers to discover the ideas in this book on their own. Perhaps having my best wisdom collected here will move us along to make these practices standard ways of working and provide the fertile ground for the next "best practices."

Winnie Dunn, PhD, OTR, FAOTA

Preface

One of the great things about growing older is that you accumulate a lot of experiences. If you are lucky, your brain sorts through these experiences, and you gain insights. One of the biggest things I have learned in the past decade is that "normal" is both ambiguous and overrated. Lorraine Ali, a journalist, wrote this in an article for *Newsweek Magazine:*

> *"...there is something unexamined in our thinking when we elevate the need for normalcy to a state of spiritual grace, and live under a constant anxiety that we fail to measure up to its demands..." [p. 50, Newsweek, September 17, 2007]*

I have often said that, with degrees in occupational therapy, special education, and neuroscience, I could find something wrong with everyone. Then, I wonder how all of us would feel if we had to focus our attention on those weaknesses all day; sounds pretty awful. Instead, most of us gain insight about our interests and talents and then tailor our personal and professional lives to take advantage of our interests and talents. We spend little or no time on our weak areas, and if we have to encounter them, we develop strategies to minimize their impact. For example, I hold the purses and jackets at the amusement park so I don't have to encounter the "assault" on my vestibular system on those rides. I recognize that others find the input quite invigorating—you keep getting back on the rides! I am glad we don't use the vestibular metric to decide who isn't normal.

What is normal anyway? Perhaps it is an abstract concept that we have created so we can say what abnormal might be. Perhaps it is a steady state within which things generally go smoothly. Perhaps it is an absence of "not normal" things. And who gets to decide what qualifies as normal? Do those of us who have a particular education get to say? Do professionals serving the public get to say? In any case, I have grown weary of the idea of normal because it seems the most interesting things happen in the places and with the people that might not be considered normal at all.

In the past decade, I have increasingly encountered people who would be classified by our current mechanisms as having a disability, yet who do not consider themselves disabled. Like everyone else, these individuals see their own interests and talents and choose to focus on them as they construct their lives. In an even more radical move, some recast their disability features as strengths! For example, the "narrow and restricted interests" of people with autism are being considered areas of special expertise used to build a career.

Think of something challenging that has created an affordance or opportunity you would not have had without the challenge. I had to work hard to learn, which taught me persistence and helped me see HOW people learn. Both persistence and understanding the process of learning have served me well in my career. If I had had an easy time learning, perhaps I wouldn't have understood how to teach someone new and difficult material. I still have challenges with visual figure ground perception, and so my home and office have compartments galore to narrow my search area; I have to rely on my family and colleagues to put things back into the same compartments though! Looking at me "objectively," someone might say I am clever, creative, or resourceful; from a "normalcy" perspective, I might be considered tedious, rigid, or too focused. I like the first list.

I am struck by how consistent core occupational therapy philosophy is with this new way of thinking. We want to make sure that people live satisfying lives, as judged by THEM, not us or society. If we make a complete commitment to this idea, what would we need to do differently? Perhaps we need to focus less on what's wrong and more on what's great about a person. Perhaps we need to even look at what would have been considered wrong in the past and think what is great about THAT, too. Perhaps we need to trust ourselves to see the therapeutic possibilities in every story and spend less energy on creating a therapeutic story for people we serve. Perhaps we need to be the primary champions of people's wholeness.

I don't mean we ignore information that informs our problem solving. There are diagnoses that help us understand the human process and how factors are likely to affect a person. And there are interventions that line up with a diagnosis (eg, a particular drug regimen). However, we also know that two people with the same diagnosis can have very different trajectories; their experience with the condition carves out their path. I want occupational therapists to be seen as making the path of possibility more visible and traversable.

That is what this second edition will help you to do. The core principles of *best practice* remind you every day to consider the wholeness, the possibility, and the unique gifts that each child and family and colleague has to offer. I want you to imagine what would change in your practice: if meetings discussed a child's gifts, contributions, and potential; if we prioritized finding ways to minimize the impact of a child's challenges so the child could participate successfully; if families heard what is the same about their children when compared to their peers or what is interesting about their children?

As these ideas catch on, how will you respond? And, what's normal got to do with it anyway?

Winnie Dunn, PhD, OTR, FAOTA

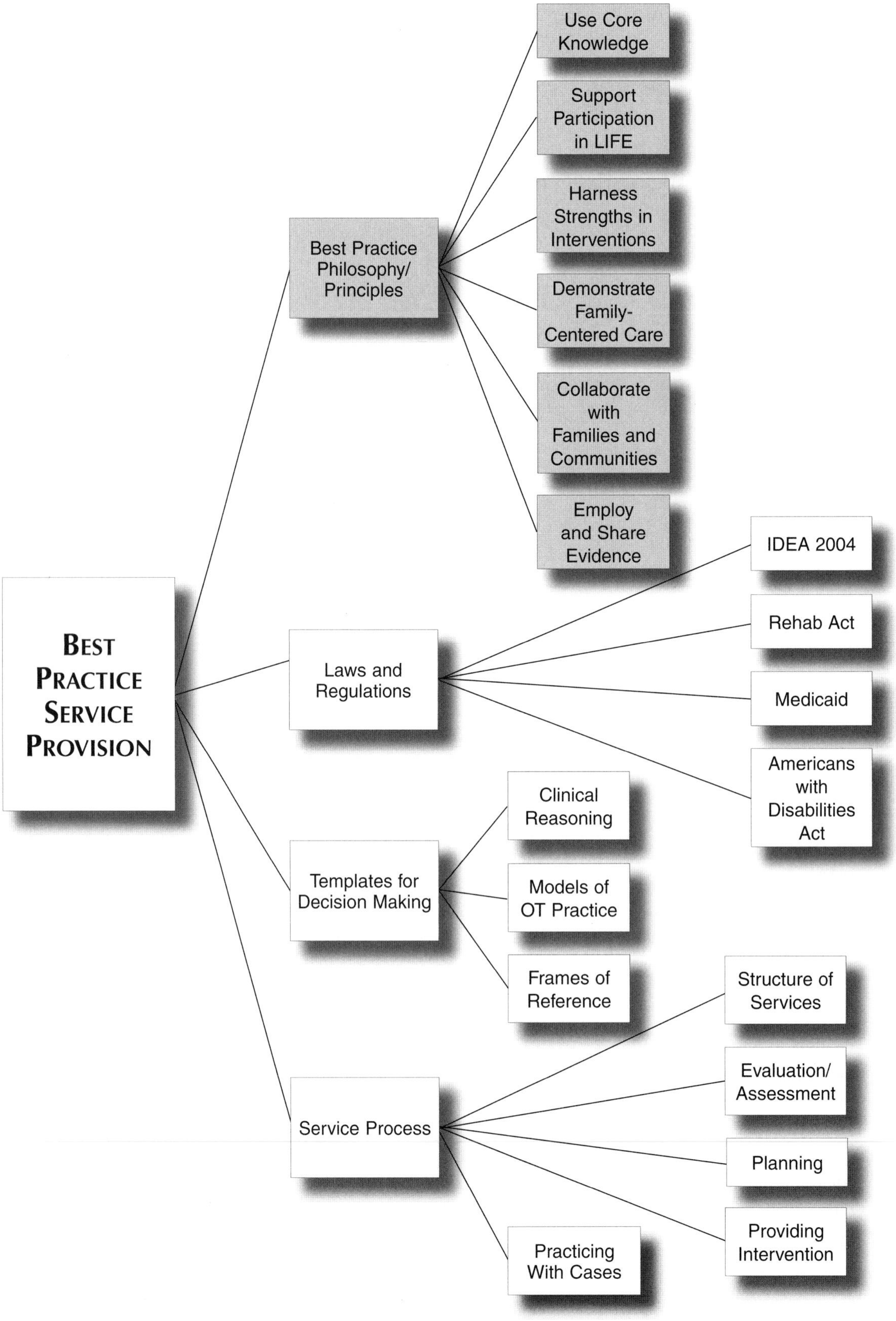
BEST PRACTICE SERVICE PROVISION
Best Practice Philosophy/ Principles
Use Core Knowledge
Support Participation in LIFE
Harness Strengths in Interventions
Demonstrate Family-Centered Care
Collaborate with Families and Communities
Employ and Share Evidence
Laws and Regulations
IDEA 2004
Rehab Act
Medicaid
Americans with Disabilities Act
Templates for Decision Making
Clinical Reasoning
Models of OT Practice
Frames of Reference
Service Process
Structure of Services
Evaluation/ Assessment
Planning
Providing Intervention
Practicing With Cases

CHAPTER 1

Best Practice Philosophy for Community Services for Children and Families

Providing services in community-based settings is vital to the best application of occupational therapy principles and beliefs because occupational therapy professionals are concerned with individuals' daily lives. Community settings present life as it is, suggesting both a simplicity and a complexity that creates a practice with potency that is unattainable elsewhere.

Best practices in early intervention, school-based, and transitional services demand that occupational therapy professionals not only act in accordance with the knowledge, principles, and philosophies of their own profession, but also with a larger set of beliefs in mind. These beliefs and philosophies have grown out of collective experiences across disciplines and among families, as everyone finds the best way to support children's growth when they have various challenges to their development and learning. Figure 1-1 outlines the principles and philosophy of best practice with an image to remind you about each principle as you study.

We will discuss these statements in the subsequent sections of this chapter and offer examples of how occupational therapists construct and implement services while using these principles to guide their practice.

Defining Best Practice

Throughout this book, we use the term *best practice* when referring to various actions of the occupational therapist. We use this term to invite therapists to conduct their professional business in a particular way. *Best practices are a professional's decisions and actions based on knowledge and evidence that reflect the most current and innovative ideas available.*

Many therapists, teams, and agencies engage in "standard practice," which is employing more traditional, routine, and established ways of providing services. In a traditional approach, professionals are more likely to take a deficit approach, emphasizing expert interventions to fix a problem. Therapists are more likely to select direct interventions, in which the person and therapist work individually in a place separate from the daily routines. This is a common paradigm for conducting professional business (i.e., the routines or protocols are known and good enough); it is simply not the paradigm we are reflecting in this book.

It is not the location of practice that determines whether one engages in best practice; therapists can work in traditional or nontraditional settings and

Dunn W. *Best Practice Occupational Therapy for Children and Families in Community Settings, Second Edition* (pp. 1-13)
© 2011 SLACK Incorporated.

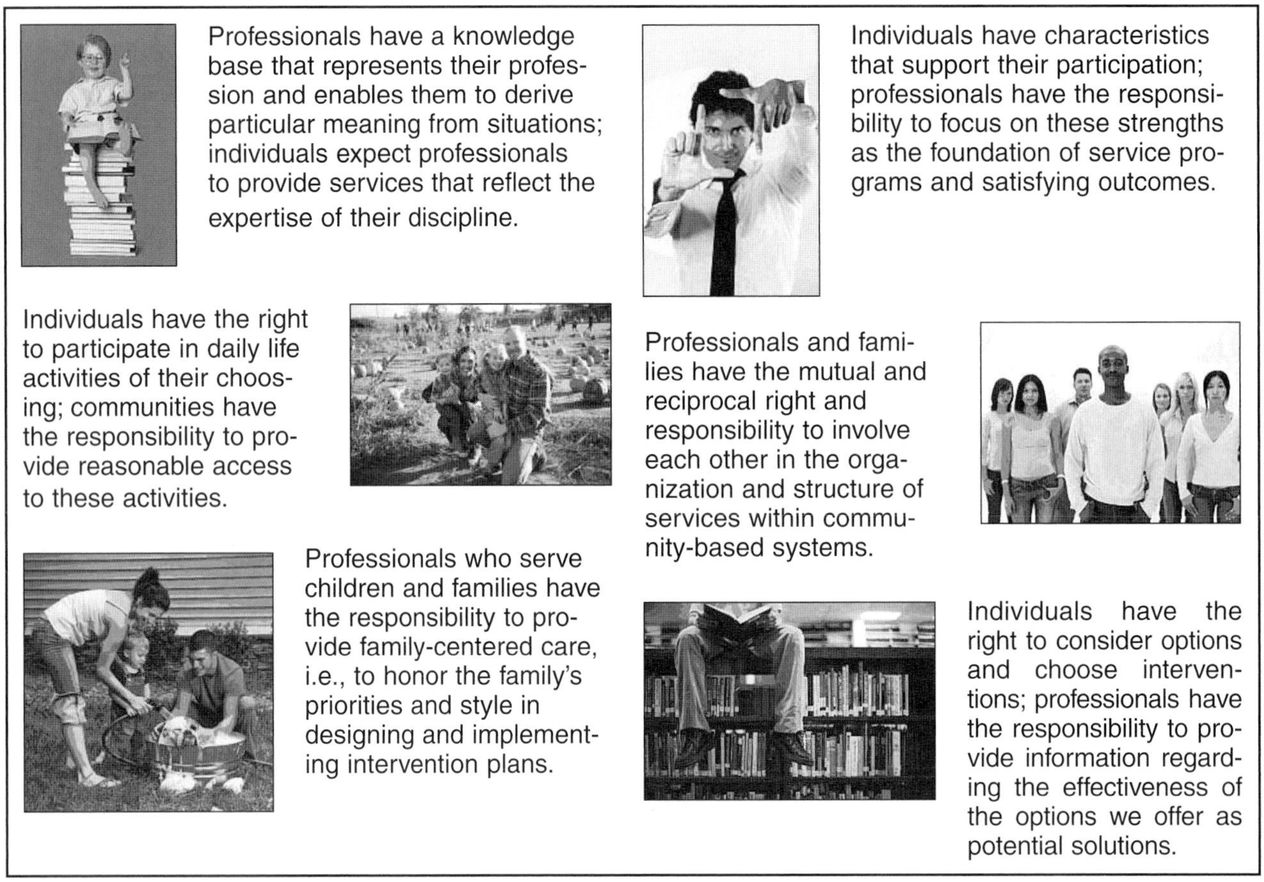

Professionals have a knowledge base that represents their profession and enables them to derive particular meaning from situations; individuals expect professionals to provide services that reflect the expertise of their discipline.
Individuals have characteristics that support their participation; professionals have the responsibility to focus on these strengths as the foundation of service programs and satisfying outcomes.
Individuals have the right to participate in daily life activities of their choosing; communities have the responsibility to provide reasonable access to these activities.
Professionals and families have the mutual and reciprocal right and responsibility to involve each other in the organization and structure of services within community-based systems.
Professionals who serve children and families have the responsibility to provide family-centered care, i.e., to honor the family's priorities and style in designing and implementing intervention plans.
Individuals have the right to consider options and choose interventions; professionals have the responsibility to provide information regarding the effectiveness of the options we offer as potential solutions.

Figure 1-1. Principles and philosophy of best practice.

use standard or best practices. Best practice is a way of thinking about problems in imaginative ways, applying knowledge creatively to solve participation problems, and taking responsibility for evaluating the effectiveness of the innovations to inform future practices.

Let's consider an example: A therapist wishes to serve preschool-aged children with disabilities. Using standard practice, this therapist might work in preschool programs within the school district that serve children with disabilities and include some peer models (sometimes called "reverse mainstreaming"). This therapist would set up routines or protocols for conducting occupational therapy assessments for the children with disabilities. The therapist would also participate with the team in designing intervention plans and provide direct therapy with selected children by working with them in the corner of the preschool room using special equipment when needed. When asked, the therapist would make suggestions about ways to support these children in the curriculum.

Using best practice, the therapist would work in community preschools that serve all the children in a neighborhood, including children with disabilities. The therapist would talk with teachers and parents about their concerns, observe and evaluate the skills of particular children with disabilities across settings (e.g., during snack time, free play, directed activity, or home via videotapes if necessary), and use this information in concert with records to identify supports and barriers to participation. The therapist would then work through service staff to implement strategies that support the children during their daily routines, test their effectiveness (both for the child and for the staff), and make adjustments as needed.

In both cases, occupational therapy expertise is being applied to both the children's and care provider's needs. The second example illustrates an emphasis on child-context interaction, a more integrated service pattern in which the therapist demonstrates responsiveness within the service system. In standard practice, there is a stronger focus on addressing the child's skill development. In best practice, we target our impact on a larger scale: we want to affect the child's everyday experiences, so the routines of the day are therapeutic, providing more opportunities for practice in the participation opportunities.

In standard practice, it is more common to see separate attention to the child and the context/system, while in best practice the therapist is more likely to "stand in the space" between the child and the context and consider the impact of each part (i.e., the child and the context) on the other. Best practice therapists are continuously seeking new ideas from evidence and dialogue in the profession; they are "early adopters" of new ideas and practices. Standard practice therapists are "late adopters" of new ideas and practices (i.e., they stay with demonstrated practices a longer time before changing routines) (Rogers, 2003).

Remember: What is best practice today evolves into standard practice in the future. This is how knowledge advances in our discipline. The standard practices of today were best practices of the past that have influenced practice. When someone continues his or her standard practices across too long a time, we would say that his or her practice is out of date and would not stand up to standard practice scrutiny. As your career unfolds, watch for these transitions, and recognize their contributions to our evolution as a discipline.

Best Practice Beliefs and Philosophies

Use Core Knowledge of the Profession

Professionals have a knowledge base that represents their profession and enables them to derive particular meaning from situations; individuals expect professionals to provide services that reflect the expertise of their discipline.

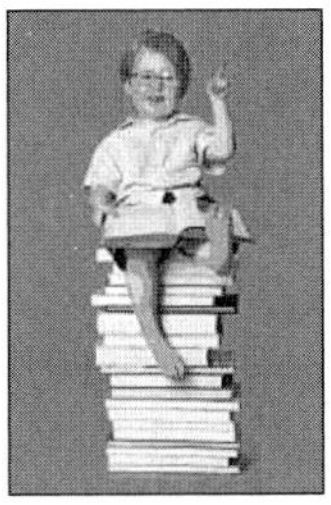

Each discipline embraces a body of knowledge that reflects that discipline's perspectives. The background knowledge includes related subjects to the discipline as well as the core concepts of the discipline. For occupational therapy, we bring knowledge about development, neuroscience, psychology, and disability conditions to the table along with our discipline's core concepts about occupation and participation. This background illustrates our perspective about the importance of participation and the meaning people derive from engaging in their everyday lives. Other disciplines combine knowledge to create another perspective.

When families engage with us related to their children's needs, they make an assumption that we are prepared with the background knowledge, have the perspective of occupational therapy, and are competent to apply that perspective (with its incumbent knowledge base) on behalf of their children. Our profession has mechanisms to ensure that entry-level professionals meet this expectation, such as the accreditation of educational programs, requirements for successful performance in school, certification from the National Board for Certification in Occupational Therapy (NBCOT), and state licensure or registration.

The materials in this text are designed to support you to learn how to apply the background knowledge you are acquiring to the practice challenges you face when serving children and families in community settings. You will need to refer to your other resources for the background knowledge (e.g., development books and notes, books, and articles on models of practice) to solve the practice challenges set before you in this book and that you will encounter in practice. Be prepared to access those resources because they will support your decisions in practice.

Support Participation

Individuals have the right to participate in daily life activities of their choosing; communities have the responsibility to provide reasonable access to these activities.

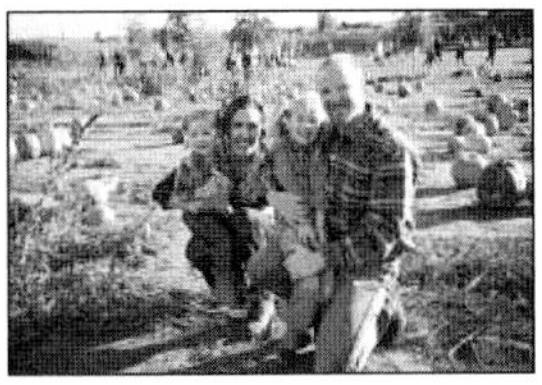

The Individuals with Disabilities Education Act (IDEA 2004), and all of its previous versions (e.g., originally called Public Law No. 94-142), Section 504

of the Rehabilitation Act, and the Americans with Disabilities Act from previous decades (see Chapter 2) outline a clear process of clarifying the ways that people obtain access to their environments for daily life. In the first half of the 20th century, our society focused on reducing the number of residents in large institutions (called deinstitutionalization). Now, we are more aware of the importance of self-determination for children and families; we understand that families can tell us what they need and want to do and how they like the rhythm of their life to unfold. Fitting into these parameters improves outcomes. There were many steps along the way.

As individuals who had various disabilities were more "present" in communities, the issues of how to involve them in living were on everyone's minds. The concept of "mainstreaming" was developed to address the need to provide access to natural environments for students in school. Public Law 94-142 stated that, to the extent possible, children with disabilities would be placed with other children in the "least restrictive environment" for activities throughout the day. Many teams began placing children with disabilities in art, music, and physical education classes with peers who did not have disabilities and called this "mainstreaming." The children continued to have the bulk of their academic days in separate special education classrooms.

During the 1970s and 1980s, professionals began to see that children might be successful in more activities and that professional expertise could be designed in new ways for children's benefit. The concept of mainstreaming evolved into "integrated" programming. This manner of combining programming invited best practice professionals to identify and implement creative ways to synthesize their knowledge; educational programs began to look very different for special education students. At this point, best practice involved a more collaborative effort on the professionals' parts, and children were spending more time with peers than in segregated classrooms. However, special education classrooms remained the home base for children with special education needs, and when children with disabilities were in regular education classrooms, they were still "separate" in the sense that they had different work, sat in the periphery, or had an aide right there with them. During this period, there was a lot of tension between the educators and the related service personnel (e.g., occupational therapists). There was pressure for therapists to participate in planning together rather than pull children out of their educational settings to provide therapy in isolation from the educational experience. Therapists were not as responsive as they needed to be during this period and continued to provide isolated services.

During the 1990s, the concept of daily life experiences and the "least restrictive environment" for children with disabilities reached a new level of intensity. The concept evolved to one called "inclusion," which urged professionals to do whatever it takes to make sure a child is successfully involved in the activities of peers in natural settings. The Americans with Disabilities Act also outlined the responsibility of community members to make the world accessible to people. During this period, families and people with disabilities also had a greater voice in our society, making this evolution possible.

In a sense, this latest version of the principle of involvement acknowledges several things. First, inclusion invites us to acknowledge that everyone has the right to have access to what they want and need to do. People also have the right to "self-determination," or the right to make choices that are goal-oriented and reflect their personal interests and priorities within the settings that are consistent with their choices.

Second, inclusion practices point out that disabilities are not the person's fault or responsibility any more than being short or tall. As a society, we have the opportunity to make some aspects of disability transparent, that is, to reduce or erase the impact of the disability on the person's performance and life options. When *all* bathroom stalls are big enough for a wheelchair, it will not matter how a person mobilizes to move about in the environment. Third, inclusion provides an opportunity for children without disabilities to experience the heterogeneity of the human experience, thus enabling them to keep disabilities in perspective (Salisbury & Dunst, 1997). When children grow up and learn together, disabilities are no more or less important or noticeable than other traits, such as "funniness," "shyness," or "thinness."

Inclusion practices are difficult to implement correctly. Just because a child is physically present in a regular education classroom does not mean the child is "included." Inclusion means that the child is immersed and involved in the culture and learning of that setting; this might not mean that all the children will learn the same things, but it does mean that all children will participate to the extent possible in learning tasks. For inclusion to be implemented properly, schools have to reconstruct themselves by shifting resources and conducting business differently. Teachers have not been prepared to conduct business this new way; special educators feel displaced when they do not have a "classroom" full of children. Aides have to learn to support the whole class and not just the child with the disability. Because occupational therapists are concerned with performance in daily life, they are the consummate professionals to take a leadership role in supporting inclusion practices. The American Occupational Therapy Association (AOTA) published an official paper stating our profession's firm commitment to inclusion practices and outlining our domain of concern related to this goal. Now, we are working with new legislation, including "No Child Left Behind" and IDEA 2004. Regulations and laws change quickly, so it is best to keep in touch with trends using quality internet sites. The Wrightslaw Web site (www.wrightslaw.com) provides resources for those of you who will work with children in the community.

In early intervention, the importance of supporting children in their daily routines cannot be over-emphasized. The Workgroup on Principles and Practices in Natural Environments (2008), part of the Office of Special Education Programs Technical Assistance Program, outlined best practices and emphasized the importance of selecting outcomes that are compatible with family interests and priorities and that are part of their everyday experiences (www.nectac.org/topics/families/families.asp). Using research as the basis for their decision making, this group identified 7 key principles for providing evidence-based early intervention services in natural environments:

1. Infants and toddlers learn best through everyday experiences and interactions with familiar people in familiar contexts.
2. All families, with the necessary support and resources, can enhance their children's learning and development.
3. The primary role of a service provider in early intervention is to work with and support family members and caregivers in children's lives.
4. The early intervention process, from initial contacts through transitions, must be dynamic and individualized to reflect the child's health and family members' preferences, learning styles, and cultural beliefs.
5. IFSP outcomes must be functional and based on children's and families' needs and family-identified priorities.
6. The family's priorities, needs, and interests are addressed most appropriately by a primary provider who represents and receives team and community support.
7. Interventions with young children and family members must be based on explicit principles, validated practices, best available research, and relevant laws and regulations.

The workgroup also provides explicit information about what these practices "look like" and "do not look like" so professionals and families can understand clearly what to expect in services. Review this material at the following Web site: www.nectac.org/topics/families/families.asp. We will discuss the application of their recommendations further in later chapters.

The International Classification of Functioning, Disability, and Health (ICF) outlines "health," "disability," "activity," "participation," and "social context" as more appropriate levels of concern for health policy and research (www.who.int/classifications/icf/en). Participation involves the interaction between the person and the context, with the desired outcome of living a satisfying life. I am confident that we will evolve as a society to the point that the human features we call disabilities today will just be human traits, nothing more and nothing less. Toward this outcome, Rick Guidotti, a photographer, published a photo essay in *Life* magazine (1998) showing the beauty of albinism. He shot young people in a glamorous venue, showing that what might have been considered a disability or limitation (e.g., lack of pigment) could be their signature feature of beauty that others might admire. Occupational therapists can also contribute forward-thinking perspectives to our society by finding ways for people to participate successfully and in satisfying ways.

Implement Family-Centered Care Principles

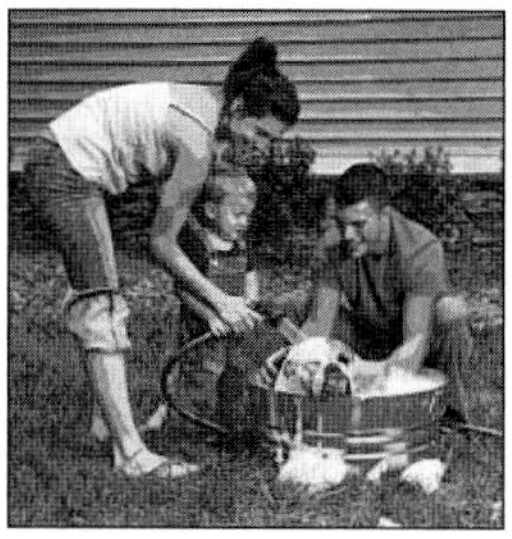

Professionals who serve children and families have the responsibility to provide family-centered care (i.e., to honor the family's priorities and style in designing and implementing intervention plans).

Family-centered care means that professionals value, encourage, and commit themselves to meaningful involvement of families in planning and implementation (Salisbury & Dunst, 1997). There has been a great evolution in our perspectives on family involvement in children's care. We now know that children whose parents participate in programming are more successful than children whose parents do not (e.g., Epstein, 1993).

Parents and other family members are the most consistent people in a child's life. Therefore, open communication is imperative among the various teams of professionals (e.g., the school team and the early intervention team) and the family. Family-centered care dictates that professionals value and therefore create a successful communication strategy (Salisbury & Dunst, 1997), including providing interpreters, avoiding jargon, and using positive nonverbal strategies (e.g., eye contact, active listening).

Salisbury and Dunst (1997) outline several major barriers to family-centered care. Sometimes, professionals are insensitive to the unique features of families and therefore interpret them as negative, difficult, or adversarial. For example, professionals might interpret a mother who has difficulty scheduling a time to come to school for a meeting as "noncompliant," without considering factors that underlie this behavior (e.g., that she has two jobs to support her family and their schedules conflict with typical school hours). In best practice, we use family-centered care values, and therefore we recognize and respect the mother for being resourceful as she cares for her children.

For every parent and family, there will be a preferred and optimal way to communicate; the professionals who practice family-centered care will take the time to identify these strategies and implement them in the interest of supporting the family's development as informed advocates for their child. Some families will want to meet more often, while others will request other ways to stay informed (e.g., e-mail, texts, phone messages and conversations, notes, videotapes).

Another barrier occurs when professionals consider the parents less informed, insightful, or intelligent than the professionals. Regardless of their backgrounds, parents are the most knowledgeable about their own children. Practices such as constructing plans prior to the parents' involvement and disregarding the parents' observations (particularly when they are in conflict with the professionals' findings) indicate lack of respect for parents as equal partners in the endeavor of serving their children and violate family-centered care principles. In fact, scholars have reported that parents are accurate assessors of their children's abilities and report information that the professionals cannot obtain through other means (e.g., Bricker & Squires, 1989; Dunn, 1999). For example, a parent might tell the team that the child eats successfully at home, when the team has reported difficulty with eating at school. Without family-centered care values, the professionals might dismiss the parents' comments as incorrect. From a family-centered care perspective, the professionals would invite the parents to describe eating at home so the team can identify how they have been successful (they might even have a video the team can view) and how eating at home and school differ so they can implement more successful interventions at school as well (Dunn, 1999).

A related issue in family-centered care is the use of "person-first language." *Person-first language is the use of the person's name rather than other references such as the disability or disorder to identify the person.* We say "Chris needs a supported chair," rather than "the cerebral palsied (CP) child needs a supported chair." Or, we say "When a child who has cerebral palsy needs to work at the table, we might design a supported chair," rather than "a CP child needs a supported chair to work at the table." In best practice, we are vigilant about using person-first language because it is an ongoing way to demonstrate our respect for the child as a human being *first*, regardless of whatever other characteristics might be relevant to the problem we are addressing. Kathie Snow has written extensively about this topic; visit her Web site for lots of examples and explanations about person-first language: www.disabilityisnatural.com/free-articles.

In occupational therapy, there are many times when it is not even necessary to state the disability or disorder; our focus is on participation in daily life, so this needs to be our emphasis. Our knowledge about disorders is background for our problem-solving (i.e., scientific reasoning, see Chapter 3). We are not "curing" the disorder; we are addressing the participation need. Therefore, in best practice occupational therapy, professionals discuss the child and family in relation to what they want and need to do (e.g., "Chris wants to work with his peers at the table during social studies"). It does not matter (except for our internal clinical reasoning processes to determine the best intervention) whether Chris has CP, a brain injury, muscular dystrophy, or attention deficit hyperactivity disorder; what matters is our ability to use our expertise to accomplish this desired performance outcome.

Employ a Strengths-Based Approach

Individuals have characteristics that support their participation; professionals have the responsibility to focus on these strengths as the foundation of service programs and satisfying outcomes.

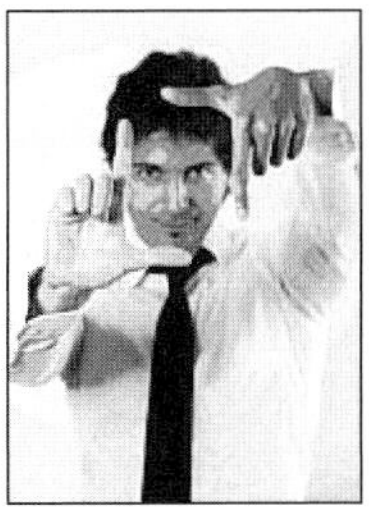

Professions and programs develop based on needs; historically, we identify needs because something is lacking, such as "I need some water," or "Carrie needs better handwriting." There certainly is a place for finding out what is interfering with participation (i.e., what the "need" is). However, what has happened is that, in doing the detective work to identify needs, professionals have gotten caught up in the empty places and have forgotten to consider what is working! This is the reason that we must emphasize a strengths-based approach to care.

There is growing discontent with this "deficit focus." More and more, people who already have an identified condition do not wish to be considered disabled. Aimee Mullins set NCAA records in the 100 meter, 200 meter, and long jump in 1996; she also happens to be missing the lower parts of her legs. She does not consider herself disabled and is offended by the meaning of this term being applied to her (see box). In a lecture she gave about changing our perspectives (www.ted.com: The Opportunity of Adversity, Feb. 23, 2010), she says that we must be careful with our words:

It is not about the words, it is what we believe about the people when we name them with these words. It is about the values behind the words, and how we construct those values. Our language affects our thinking and how we view the world and... other people.... Those thesaurus entries are not allowing us to evolve into the reality that we all want: the possibility of an individual to see themselves as capable.

DISABLED

Synonyms: Crippled, helpless, useless, wounded, mangled, lame, mutilated, weakened, paralyzed, handicapped, hurt, weak, unhealthy.

Antonyms: Healthy, strong, capable, whole, wholesome.

She suggests that focusing on the disability might actually be the most damaging part of our services process because it limits people's views of themselves. She calls on us to see the potency and capacity of people, inviting them to conceive their best "selves." She urges us to take a "strengths" perspective. She also points out that we must embrace the fact that we are changed by challenges, that they are not obstacles to overcome, but part of how we develop our clear sense of ourselves as viable human beings.

People who have Autism Spectrum Disorders (ASD) and their families feel the same way as Aimee Mullins. Davidson & Henderson (2010) reviewed the writings of people with ASD as they write about their own sensory experiences. They found that these authors want to have their distinctiveness recognized, and not as disabilities or a deviance from "typical." They do not believe their differences need to be corrected; rather, they believe that their differences are part of the greater "spectrum" of human experiences. Parents of children with ASD see the value of their children's perspectives. For example, Grinker (2007) talks about his daughter's perspective as one that makes him look at the world differently, too. He goes on to comment that there are parts of our society that people with intense interests are better suited for than anyone else. Thorkil Sonne (http://specialisterne.com) founded Specialisterne, a company that provides specialist consultants for business. He hires people with ASD, seeing them as "natural born specialists," to serve in these consultative roles. Like Dr. Grinker, Sonne sees all the strengths and potential. A young man named Jeremy sums up his perspective in a commencement speech: you can view it at www.youtube.com/watch?v=O8cEtand01w.

Dunst (2000) describes a strengths-based model as one in which the professionals recognize the assets and talents of children, family members, teachers, etc., and use this information to design programs that expand competencies and participation. In his model, child learning opportunities, family and community supports and resources, and parenting supports are the key features that support the child's learning and development. Judge (1998) studied families that had young children with disabilities and found that social supports and the family's ability to maintain a positive attitude were critical factors in promoting and maintaining the family. She recommends that professionals harness the social supports around a child and family to obtain the best outcomes.

Implementing a strengths-based approach can be challenging within systems that are currently geared to detect weaknesses, impairments, pathology, and disability. Taking a strengths-based approach means that we incorporate questions into each phase of the professional process that bring strengths to light. During interviews, observations, and initial meetings, we ask questions like "What does he do well?", "What is great about her?", "What is your favorite family activity together?", "What settings are easiest for you and your child?" Just asking these questions opens the door to taking a strengths approach because you are informing others that you want to know what is good, and you are giving people permission to talk about something other than what concerns them. During evaluation, we observe during a successful time of the day; during planning, we consider how to expand these successful times as part of intervention planning.

Of course, a strengths-based approach does NOT mean that we ignore or fail to identify possible barriers to participation. We learn the barriers along the way, too. However, in a strengths-based approach, we do not emphasize the interfering conditions. We might even ask ourselves "what might be helpful about what I currently view as a barrier?" For example, Baranek and colleagues (2002) found that children with Fragile X syndrome who had an aversion to touch tended to have greater independence in self-care. The researchers reported this was a surprising finding; when we consider the situation, perhaps these boys became more independent because they did not want additional touch from others "helping" them with self-care.

In a strengths-based approach, professionals consider how to harness strengths first as they begin to plan a program of supports with a family, a school team, etc. If a teacher already has management strategies in place that will be in a target student's best interests, we would discuss with that teacher how to apply those strategies in the target student's case. If an adolescent seems absorbed in a topic (e.g., the ice age, wrestling), we would use that interest to build some learning and recreational activities, rather than seeing that topic as a dysfunctional fixation. When a family likes camping, we think of strategies to apply to camping (e.g., setting up a tent provides opportunities for strength, coordination, and cooperative work). We include parents, siblings, teachers, and other important supports to the child in a strengths-based approach. We need to know what everyone's strengths are so we can build satisfying interactions among all of the child's supports throughout the day.

Think how it would feel for someone to evaluate you, find your weakest skills, and then plan your life to address those skills all day long. This is not a pleasant thought, is it? We do not intend to create this feeling in a traditional "deficit-based" approach, but by focusing on what is wrong, all our energy bears down on these weak facets. All of us create our own lives based on our personal interests and our own strengths (e.g., what we are good at, what we really are interested in doing, what gives us satisfaction, or what suits our temperament). A strengths-based approach does the same thing for those we serve.

Collaborate to Support Families

Professionals and families have the mutual and reciprocal right and responsibility to involve each other in the organization and structure of services within community-based systems.

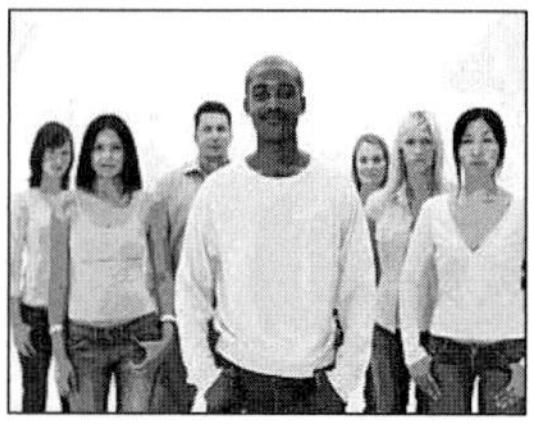

Team Collaborations

There are many team structures and processes (see Chapter 4), but all teams have the goal of combining expertise and perspectives for the benefit of a child and family. In early intervention programs, interdisciplinary teams always include families and can include educators, speech pathologists, dietitians, and social workers in addition to occupational therapists. School districts develop planning teams based on the regulations in IDEA 1997; these teams must include representatives from certain disciplines (i.e., psychology, speech therapy, and special education) and positions (i.e., parent of a child with an educational handicap). Occupational therapists are considered "related service" professionals; we will discuss this role further in future chapters.

Systems can involve other specialists or interested parties as needed to address the child's needs effectively. In some states, physician involvement in occupational therapy programs is mandatory under licensure statutes. It is appropriate for core team members to solicit input and feedback from specialists who might have insights to enhance the team planning processes. Core team members can use phone calls, copies of written documentation (including evaluations and notes), and e-mail conversations to obtain current information. When employing best practice, these specialists are considered equal partners in the team planning process for community programming; it is always the team's responsibility together to make decisions about the best course of action.

Parents are vital members of the teams that serve children. Parental concerns, goals, and resources (Dickman, 1985; Featherstone, 1980; Zins, Graden, & Ponti, 1988) are critical to the child's involvement in an intervention program. Additionally, federal mandates dictate that parents have the legal right to be an integral part of the planning teams for their children. The team can also include other family members and care providers if the parents believe it is important to planning. For example, siblings may want or need to participate in aspects of the child's at-home care and management (Muhlenhaupt, 1991). Certain family traditions or situations may necessitate that extended family members are the child's primary caregivers. Children with acute or chronic medical conditions may have nurses or other health-care workers who attend to their needs at home or school. These people have the potential to play an important role in planning and implementing the child's therapeutic and educational programs (Muhlenhaupt, 1991).

Interagency Collaborations

When serving families as part of the community, professionals must find effective strategies for communicating among each other on behalf of the child and family. Particularly when serving children with complex disabilities, communication is critical because these families will need service supports from a range of agencies. For example, a child with muscular dystrophy will need support from the physician, clinics that monitor the disease process and use of adaptive devices, community support groups (e.g., for family interactions and gatherings such as summer camps), school personnel, and pharmacists as part of comprehensive care. Interagency collaboration, then, is the mechanism that professionals create in a particular community to engage with each other in service to a family.

Occupational therapists are key members of the teams in any number of the community agencies that serve children and families and, therefore, have an important role to play in interagency collaboration. Therapists can participate in the formal mechanisms of communication across agencies, but sometimes the more informal networks of communication are equally or even more important to overall collaborative efforts. The relationships among the actual service providers can sometimes be more powerful than formal agreements that focus on procedures. For example, families need the school-based occupational therapist and the children's hospital occupational therapist to collaborate so that their efforts are in concert with each other and families get consistent information about how to support their child at home, school, and in the community. This relationship is more important to the family than whether the school and hospital have formal mechanisms for communication.

Quality interagency collaboration also requires members of the service teams to understand how and when to make referrals to each other. Each agency and each professional within a particular agency must have a clear awareness of the mission and purpose of the agency, which enables them to know what areas of service are inside and outside their purview as a community service agency. Additionally, each professional must recognize her or his own skills so that it is clear when to solicit another colleague within the same discipline or from another discipline to support the child and family. It is critical to successful interdisciplinary collaboration on behalf of families that professionals recognize the limits of their own and their agencies' capabilities. Families deserve the best services available in a community; making referrals to the most skilled community members demonstrates respect for families.

For example, if a school-based therapist determines that a child needs a resting hand splint based on the father's comments and her own observations, it is best for the school therapist to refer the family to a rehabilitation therapist who can make the splint efficiently for the family (e.g., the rehabilitation therapist has the tools and supplies and constructs splints more regularly). Although splint construction is theoretically in the skill domain of all occupational therapists, it is not typically in the scope of public school practice. Therefore, it is most appropriate for the school therapist to make the referral.

The Frank Porter Graham Child Development Institute conducted a study of interagency collaboration around their state of North Carolina (2001). The "Smart Start Partnerships" reported that there were significant obstacles to interagency communication on behalf of families, but, with persistent efforts, more respondents reported "minimal service gaps," "less duplication of services," "more convenient locations," and "more providers aware of other service options" after a 3 year period of working on interagency collaboration. (Go to their Web site to learn more at www.nectac.org/topics/families/families.asp.)

Supporting Transitions in Programming and Agencies

A transition is a change from one situation to another. Occupational therapists participate in and support a number of transitions when serving children and families. The most frequent types of transitions are those that a child and family make as the child grows and therefore becomes eligible for a different service system or agency. For example, infants at risk transition from hospital care to home and follow-along care. Preschoolers transition from early childhood and day-care programs to public schools. Adolescents transition to middle school and high school, and young adults transition to work and community living. Children and families can also transition from clinical therapy services to educationally related services. Occupational therapists are involved with the service systems at all of these pre- and post-transition sites and so will be intimately involved with the transition processes.

When participating in transitions, occupational therapists contribute in a number of ways. A therapist who serves in a pre-transition site has the responsibility to clearly document the child's interests, current levels of performance, adaptations, and supports that facilitate performance, other interventions that have been successful (and unsuccessful), and recommendations about goals and services for the future. A therapist who serves in a post-transition site has the responsibility to review materials about the child and prepare follow-up questions that will provide clarity for planning.

Both therapists have a shared responsibility to collaborate with each other to ensure a smooth transition. It is of utmost importance for the therapists to recognize the differences in their respective service systems and how each of these systems serves the children and their families. For example, when children transition from preschool services to the public schools, there are a number of issues to incorporate into planning and discussions with the families. Preschool services are frequently constructed to provide intense developmental interventions; the curriculum is developmentally oriented, and the therapy contributions have the same orientation. Professionals serve children in smaller groups or individually during the preschool years because this is developmentally appropriate for their cognitive abilities. As children move into the public schools, the focus is increasingly on cognitive and social development; children spend the whole day at school and work in larger groups, and the team works to incorporate the children's areas of therapeutic needs into the routines of this new kind of day.

Therapists providing best practice services make sure that families understand the meaning and importance of this transition; children who can function successfully in this more advanced environment are making the progress they need to make for independence in adulthood. Children who need the same level of support in elementary school as they did in preschool have not profited from the preschool services. Therapists supporting this transition will collaborate to design the next setting plans and will communicate their optimism about the transition together. The preschool therapist will communicate enthusiasm about the child's growth and opportunities at school; both therapists can discuss how services are reformulated to support the child in public school with peers. This supports family-centered care as part of best practice.

Employ Effective Practices

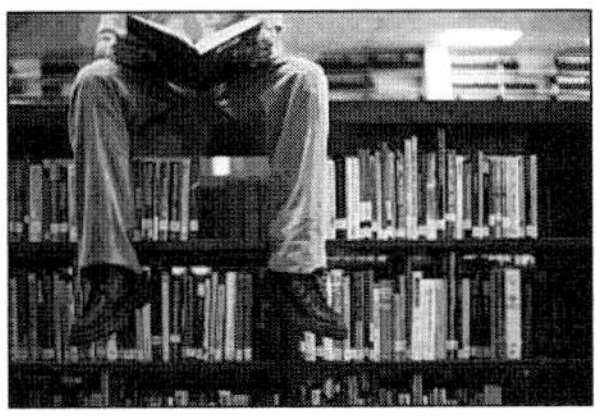

Individuals have the right to consider options and choose interventions; professionals have the responsibility to provide information regarding the effectiveness of the options we offer as potential solutions.

There has been an increasing call in professional circles for practice decisions and actions to be based on the evidence available about those practices (e.g., Jette, 1995; Lloyd-Smith, 1997; Sackett et al., 1991), rather than only on the background and experiences of a particular professional. Wennberg (1990) reported on several studies in which there was large variability in health-care practices of experienced professionals, suggesting a need for guidelines to ensure the best quality care for everyone. Professionals agree that it is important to distinguish between effective and ineffective practices, but there has not always been agreement about how to accomplish this goal. Additionally, as families have become more informed about their rights and responsibilities, they have wanted to make informed decisions about the care they will receive.

For professions to determine which practices are effective, scholars and practitioners must participate together in research that discloses the impact of intervention practices on salient outcomes for the service recipient. Once we have data about particular interventions, professionals who employ best practice use this knowledge for two purposes. First, professionals use the knowledge gained from research to advance their problem-solving capabilities for practice decision making. Second, professionals relate effectiveness findings to families and other service recipients so they understand the potential risks and benefits of service options.

When professionals use outcomes of research to guide their practices, we call this evidence-based practice. Evidence-based practice is a systematic process of locating, evaluating, synthesizing, and incorporating research findings into one's internal resources to advance problem-solving and decision-making in practice (Rosenberg & Donald, 1995). Evidence is becoming a central feature of practice as payers and consumers demand verification for the practices they finance and select for themselves. Best practice requires professionals to engage in evidence-based practice (Dunn, 2008).

There are several challenges to engaging in evidence-based practice. First, sometimes, there is a scarcity of research literature that demonstrates the effectiveness of our practices. Occupational therapy is a relatively young field, and its history as an applied science (therefore creating a research base) is even shorter. The studies available are typically on very small samples and address discreet problems that certainly do not represent the scope of occupational therapy practice. We need more studies that are rigorous enough to reveal insights for practice.

This leads to the second challenge; some of the criteria that have been established for an acceptable study would eliminate valuable data from consideration.

The "randomized clinical trial" (RCT) is the gold standard for studies that inform practice decisions (Sackett et al., 1996). An RCT requires random assignment and experimental and control groups with matched samples of subjects (Holm, 2000). There are many other types of studies that can inform practice, and we need to recognize what these studies can inform us about and how to use the findings to advance knowledge for practice. Holm's Eleanor Clarke Slagle lectureship outlines the criteria for evidence-based practice very clearly (2000).

Finally, even with the outcomes research available, it is difficult for those in practice to locate it and translate it into meaningful information for practice decision-making. There are studies from both occupational therapy and other disciplines that can inform occupational therapy practice. We must consider it a priority for our profession to organize and synthesize knowledge from this range of studies in a way that makes it easy for those in practice to gain access, interpret properly, and inform themselves and their families about the meaning of the findings for their service options. Dunn (2008) provides guidance about how to interpret interdisciplinary research to support practice.

Best practice means that we take the time to find out about the effectiveness of our intervention options for a particular child and family. We do not pass on "folklore" (i.e., suggest an intervention because our teacher or supervisor told us about it or we saw another therapist trying it). We only consider options that we understand and can articulate a rationale for; if something is a newer, more experimental intervention option, we inform the family and include an extensive plan for data collection to determine the impact of the new or experimental intervention on the child. If the newer intervention (or any intervention for that matter) does not show effectiveness for the desired participation, we stop using it and design another option. We never continue an intervention based on beliefs without evidence, even if that evidence is from our data collection on this child only. Evidence-based practice requires us to step back from our lived experience with a child and family and evaluate the impact of our work on the desired participation outcome. In this book, we will demonstrate strategies for applying evidence in best practice scenarios.

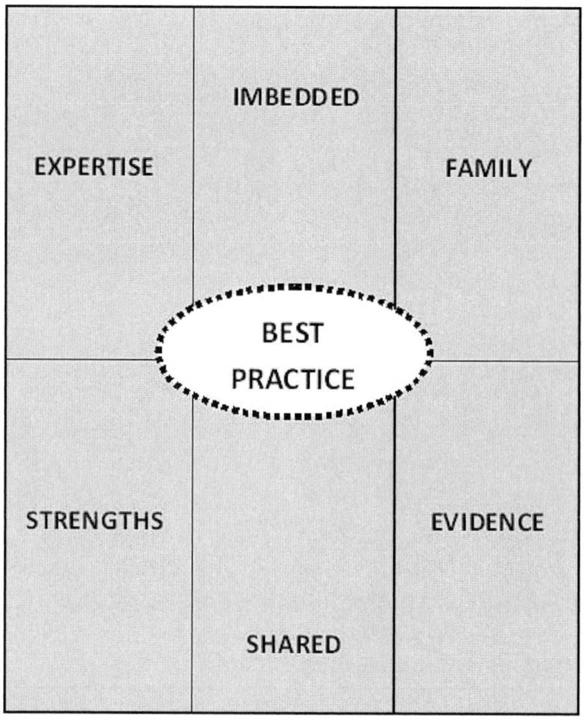

Figure 1-2. Principles of best practice philosophy.

Summary

Providing best practices means we employ particular principles (Figures 1-1 and 1-2) when approaching, designing, implementing, and evaluating our work. Although the particular strategies will change across time, the core principles that guide us remain the same:

- Our actions reflect the knowledge and expertise of occupational therapy.
- We provide services within children's daily routines, activities, and settings.
- Families' interests and priorities are the center of our decision-making.
- We collaborate with families and colleagues from other disciplines to design integrated services.
- We provide interventions based on the best available evidence.

In the remaining chapters, we will explore how to implement these principles in everyday practice with children, families, and schools.

References

Baranek, G. T., Chin, Y., Hess, L., Yankee, J., Hatton, D., & Hooper, S. (2002). Sensory processing correlates of occupational performance in children with fragile X syndrome: preliminary findings. *American Journal of Occupational Therapy, 56*(5), 538-546.

Bricker, D., & Squires, J. (1989). The effectiveness of parental screening of at-risk infants: The monitoring questionnaires. *Topics in Early Childhood Special Education, 9*(3), 67-85.

Davidson, J., & Henderson, V. (2010). Travel in parallel with us for a while: sensory geographies of autism. *The Canadian Geographer, 54*(4), 1-14.

Dickman, I. (1985). *One miracle at a time.* New York, NY: Simon and Schuster.

Dunn, W. (1999). *The sensory profile.* San Antonio, TX: Psychological Corporation.

Dunn, W. (2008). *Bringing Evidence into Everyday Practice: Practical Strategies for Healthcare Professionals.* Thorofare, NJ: SLACK Incorporated.

Dunst, C. (2000). Revisiting "Rethinking Early Intervention," *Topics in Early Childhood Special Education, 20*(2), 95-104.

Epstein, J. (1993, April). Make parents your partners. *Instructor, 19,* 119-136.

Featherstone, H. (1980). *A difference in the family: Living with a disabled child.* New York, NY: Basic Books.

Grinker, R. (2007). *Unstrange minds: Remapping the world of autism.* Cambridge: Basic Books.

Guidotti, R. (1998, June). Rick Guidotti opens our eyes to the beauty of albinism. *Life,* 65-69.

Holm, M. B. (2000). Our mandate for the new millennium: Evidence-based practice—The Eleanor Clarke Slagle Lectureship. *American Journal of Occupational Therapy, 54,* 575-585.

Jette, A. (1995). Physical disablement concepts for physical therapy research and practice. *Physical Therapy, 74*, 380-386.

Judge, S. J. (1998). Parental coping strategies and strengths in families of young children with disabilities. *Family Relations, 47*(3), 263-268.

Lloyd-Smith, W. (1997). Evidence-based practice and occupational therapy. *British Journal of Occupation Therapy, 60*, 474-478.

Muhlenhaupt, M. (1991). Components of the program planning process. In W. Dunn (Ed.), *Pediatric occupational therapy: Facilitating effective service provision* (pp. 125-135). Thorofare, NJ: SLACK Incorporated.

Rogers, E. (2003). *Diffusion of innovation* (5th ed). New York: Free Press.

Rosenberg, W., & Donald, A. (1995). Evidence-based medicine: An approach to clinical problem-solving. *British Medical Journal, 310*, 1122-1126.

Sackett, D., Rosenberg, W., Gray, J., Haynes, R., & Richardson, W. (1996). Evidence-based medicine: What it is and what it isn't. *British Medical Journal*, 312, 71-72.

Sackett, D., Haynes, R., Guyatt, G., & Tugwell, P. (1991). *Clinical epidemiology: A basic science for clinical medicine.* London, England: Little, Brown & Co.

Salisbury, C., & Dunst, C. (1997). Homes, school, and community partnerships: Building inclusive teams. In: *Collaborative teams for students with severe disabilities* (pp. 57-82). Baltimore, MD: Paul H. Brookes Publishing Co.

Wennberg, J. (1990). Outcomes research, cost containment, and the feat of health care rationing. *New England Journal of Medicine, 323*, 1202-1204.

Workgroup on Principles and Practices in Natural Environments (2008). *Mission and key principles for providing early intervention services in natural environments.* Retrieved from http://www.nectac.org/topics/families/families.asp.

Zins, J., Graden, J., & Ponti, C. (1988). Pre-referral intervention to improve special services delivery. *Services in the Schools, 4*(3/4), 109-130.

Additional Web Sites

www.wrightslaw.com/

www.who.int/classifications/icf/en/

www.disabilityisnatural.com/free-articles/

http://specialisterne.com/

www.ted.com

www.access-board.gov/enforcement/rehab-act-text/intro.htm

http://ed.gov/about/offices/list/ocr/504faq.html

www.kcdcinfo.com/index.aspx?NID=224

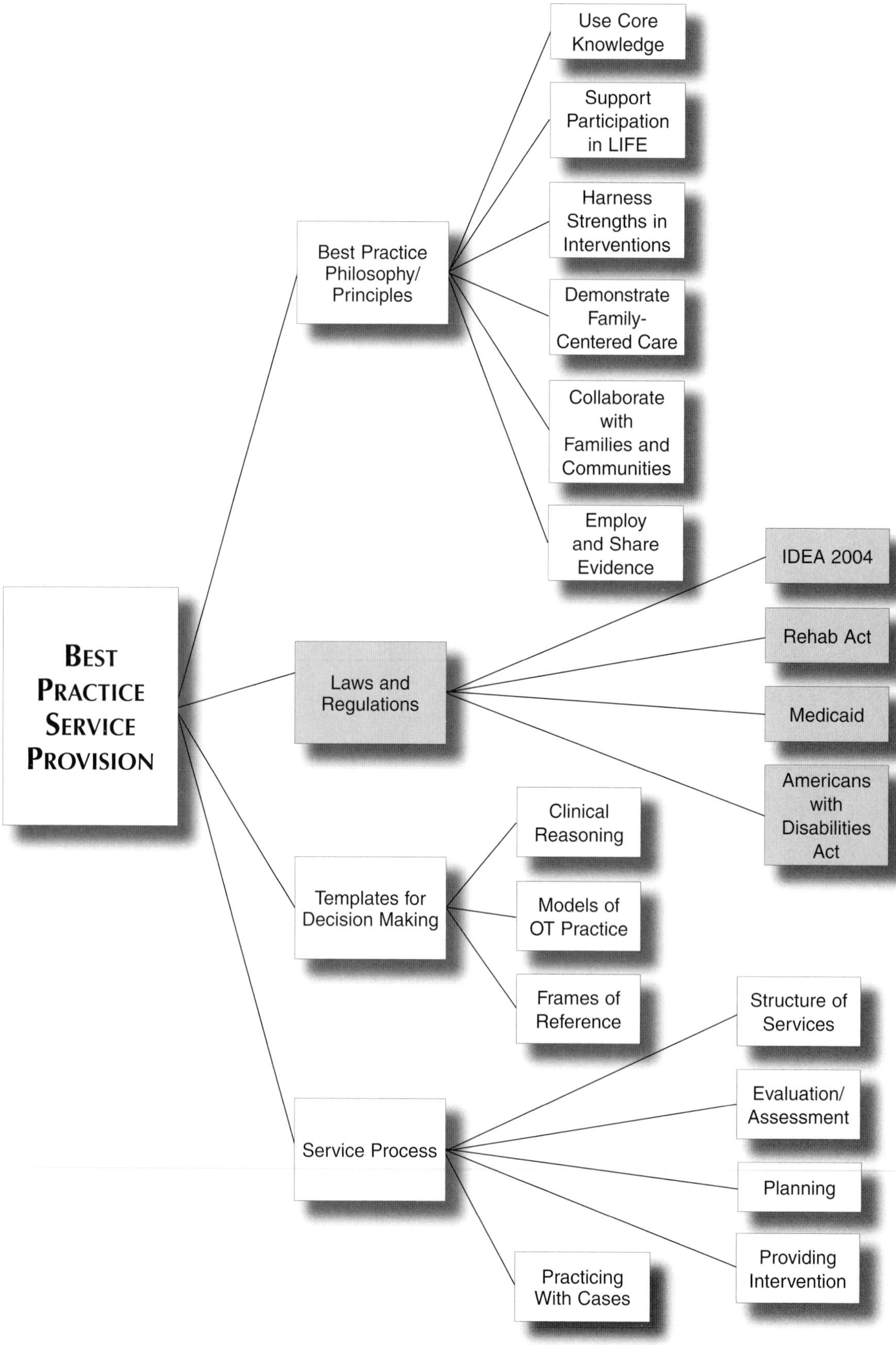
Best Practice Service Provision
Best Practice Philosophy/ Principles
Use Core Knowledge
Support Participation in LIFE
Harness Strengths in Interventions
Demonstrate Family-Centered Care
Collaborate with Families and Communities
Employ and Share Evidence
Laws and Regulations
IDEA 2004
Rehab Act
Medicaid
Americans with Disabilities Act
Templates for Decision Making
Clinical Reasoning
Models of OT Practice
Frames of Reference
Service Process
Structure of Services
Evaluation/ Assessment
Planning
Providing Intervention
Practicing With Cases

CHAPTER 2

Impact of Federal Policy on Services for Children and Families in Early Intervention Programs and Public Schools

Ellen Pope, MEd, OTR

Federal and state laws and regulations guide the practice of occupational therapy with children. These pieces of legislation and regulations provide a map for what we do and how we do our work as occupational therapists within the public systems that administrate these laws. Occupational therapists working with children and families have a responsibility to understand major legislation including IDEA 2004, No Child Left Behind Act (NCLB), Section 504 of the Rehabilitation Act of 1973, the American with Disabilities Act (ADA), and the Developmental Disabilities Assistance and Bill of Rights Act. Therapists working within public school systems or early intervention programs may be directed to administer specific tests, follow specific procedures, and interact with families and children in ways that may or may not be consistent with the laws and regulations. Many times, there are limited laws or regulations that support a particular practice, but instead there are procedures that were developed by a local organization or school system. The practices and procedures that therapists are asked to subscribe to may also not be consistent with best practices (Dunn, 2000). It is up to the therapist to be able to identify and share research, laws, regulations, or guidelines that support best practice philosophy with other team members and administrators. An example of a document published by the National Early Childhood Technical Assistance Center is *Mission and Key Principles for Providing Early Intervention Services in Natural Environments* (2008). This document outlines best practices in Part C Early Intervention Programs and reflects both the law and the most recent research.

IDEA (Individuals with Disabilities Education Act, 2004 Reauthorization, P.L. 108-446) was reauthorized in 2004. Over the years, this particular piece of legislation has had the greatest impact on the practice of occupational therapy with children 21 years of age or younger. The intent of this law has been consistent from the time of its inception in 1975 when it was called the Education for the Handicapped Amendments (E.H.A. P.L. 94-142). The purpose of IDEA for children 3 to 21 years of age is (d)(1)(A) to ensure that all children with disabilities have available to them a free appropriate public education that emphasizes special education and related services designed to meet their unique needs and prepare them for further education, employment, and independent living. This is consistent with Principle 2 of best practice philosophy, "Individuals have the right to participate in daily life activities of their choosing;

Dunn W. *Best Practice Occupational Therapy for Children and Families in Community Settings, Second Edition* (pp. 15-23)
© 2011 SLACK Incorporated.

communities have the responsibility to provide reasonable access to these activities."

When IDEA (P.L. 108-446) was re-authorized in 2004, one of the goals was to better coordinate special education with the NCLB. NCLB focuses on all students, with the general goal of closing gaps in achievement test scores. Application of these two laws for students with special education needs has resulted in more specific recommendations about how students with disabilities are assessed for adequate yearly progress (AYP) and how special education teachers are determined to be highly qualified.

Prior to 1986, the federal law focused primarily on children with disabilities aged 3 to 21 years. In 1986, Congress recognized "an urgent and substantial need" and added Part H (changed to Part C in 1997) to address the needs of infants and toddlers (0 to 3 years) with disabilities and their families. The purpose of this part of the law is stated as follows:

> *To enhance the development of infants and toddlers with disabilities; to reduce educational costs by minimizing the need for special education through early intervention; to minimize the likelihood of institutionalization and maximize independent living; and to enhance the capacity of families to meet their child's needs. In this most recent addition to IDEA, the focus is on the family and building their capacity to meet the needs of their infants and toddlers* (IDEA, 2004).

The implementation of Part H was not the responsibility of any one agency, but of many different agencies; therefore, interagency coordination and collaboration was critical (Shackelford, 2006).

This collaboration reflects best practice philosophy #4.

Table 2-1 shows how this law has evolved over the past 35 years to support children 0 to 21 years of age with disabilities.

In addition to the federal laws and state regulations, some states have written guidelines for occupational therapists working in school-based practice. In Kansas, a document titled "Occupational Therapy and Physical Therapy in the Schools: Frequently Asked Questions" (www.ksde.org/LinkClick.aspx?fileticket=%2FOt9XzqmdPI%3D...mid. This can also be accessed by searching for occupational therapy on the ksde.org Web site.) was developed for OTs and PTs serving children 3 to 21 years of age in the public schools. In Missouri, the Department of Elementary and Secondary Education has also developed a set of guidelines regarding the practice of occupational therapy in school systems.

Locate the provision within IDEA 2004 that addresses changes in transition planning post-high school. What does the law say? What is the role of the occupational therapist in postsecondary transition planning?

The IEP for a student who turns 16 must address newly defined transition services—defined as a coordinated set of results-oriented transition activities for a student with a disability to become an independent adult, e.g., postsecondary education, employment, independent living, and community participation. The 2004 amendments removed the requirement to provide transition services at age 14.

LOOK UP ASSIGNMENT

Find out what guidelines have been developed in your state that guide the practice of occupational therapy serving children under IDEA.

Does your State Department of Education have guidelines for OTs? When were these guidelines developed? Do they reflect current laws and evidence?

A number of resources and Web sites are available to therapists to help them understand and apply the laws and regulations. These include Wrightslaw (www.wrightslaw.com), which is a Web site about special education law and advocacy, National Early Childhood Technical Assistance Center (NECTAC, www.nectac.org), National Dissemination Center for Children with Disabilities (NICHCY, www.nichcy.org), and Office of Special Education Programs OSEP, www.osep.org).

Over time, these laws have defined OT's roles and responsibilities and have guided the occupational therapy practice with children and their families. These laws have also been instrumental in supporting more inclusive practices for all children with disabilities. Education of the Handicapped Act (P.L. 94.142) used the term *least restrictive environment* to describe where services and supports are provided for children with disabilities. In 1986, Education of the Handicapped Act (P.L. No. 99-457) was adopted, which defined the term "*natural environment* for Part H to describe where supports should be provided for infants and toddlers with disabilities and their families. As we have learned more about how children learn and the importance of the context in which they learn, these laws have required that children

Table 2-1.

History of IDEA

Year	Law	Key Features
1975	Education of the Handicapped Act (P.L. No. 94-142)	• Free, Appropriate, Public Education for all children with disabilities (FAPE) • Education must be provided in the Least Restrictive Environment (LRE) • Zero Reject: No child with a disability can be excluded from public education • Nondiscriminatory Evaluation • Individualized Education Plan (IEP) • Procedural Due Process
1986	Education of the Handicapped Amendments of 1986 (P.L. No. 99-457)	• Added Part H Federal Incentive Program for Infants and Toddlers • Amendment of section 619 of EHA, which extended all requirements to 3 to 5 year olds
1997	IDEA Amendments (P.L. No. 105-17)	• Part H for Infants and Toddlers changed to Part C • Having high expectations for children with disabilities and ensuring their access in the general curriculum to the maximum extent possible • Strengthening the role of parents • Coordinating the other local, state, and federal school improvement efforts to ensure that special education is a service for children, rather than a place where they are sent • Providing appropriate special education, related services, aids, and supports in the regular classroom whenever appropriate
2004	IDEA Amendments	• IDEA and NCLB Alignment • Definition of Highly Qualified Teacher • Participation in Assessments: All students with disabilities are required to be included in district-wide and state-wide assessments • Response to intervention • Changes to discipline provisions giving schools more flexibility • Changes to IEP: Defining transition process at age 16, short-term objectives no longer required • Changes to Due Process: Only required to distribute a copy once a year • Modification of Private School Enrollment by Parents • Part C: Establishment of a Seamless System with option for families to continue early intervention services from age 3 through enrollment in kindergarten; required referral to early intervention for all children younger than age 3 who are involved in a substantiated case of child abuse or neglect or are identified as being affected by illegal substance abuse or withdrawal symptoms

(Turnbull, 1986)

with disabilities be included with same-age peers to the greatest extent possible.

The governor of your state has determined the lead agency for Part C. In some states, the Department of Education is lead agency; in other states, the Department of Health is lead agency, and yet other states have lead agencies that pertain to the administration of programs for people with developmental disabilities. For instance, the lead agency for Part C in Missouri is the Department of Elementary and Secondary Education (DESE), while the lead agency for Part C in Kansas is the Department of Health and Environment.

LOOK UP ASSIGNMENT

If you are providing occupational therapy services in Part C, find out what state agency has been appointed the lead agency by the governor.

www.nectac.org/partc/ptclead.asp

Within IDEA 2004, reference will be made to Part C of IDEA and Part B of IDEA. Part C refers to the law as it pertains to infants and toddlers (0 to 3 years of age) with disabilities. Part B refers to the law as it pertains to children 3 to 21 years of age receiving special education. Table 2-2 compares these two parts of IDEA.

Section 504 of the Rehabilitation Act of 1973

Section 504 of the Rehabilitation Act of 1973 forbids discrimination against any person with a disability in programs and activities, public and private, that receive federal funding. Many people consider this act as the first civil rights law for people with disabilities. The purpose of this law was to prevent intentional or unintentional discrimination against people with disabilities. This applies to state and local governments, colleges and universities, schools, child care centers, recreation programs, libraries, and clinics that receive federal financial assistance. This section covers any person who has a physical or mental impairment that substantially limits one or more major life activities, has a record of such impairment, or is regarded as having such an impairment. A major life activity refers to self-care, walking, seeing, hearing, speaking, breathing, learning, and working.

The regulations for both Section 504 and EHA became effective in 1977, but Section 504 is much less known and implemented and has often not been applied by school districts. This was due in part to no funding being attached to this law, making implementation difficult.

Section 504 is extremely broad. It covers individuals with wide-ranging conditions, such as asthma, alcohol and drug addiction, cancer, and HIV. Students who are receiving treatment for chemical dependency may qualify for protection under Section 504, and knowledge that a student is receiving treatment should initiate a referral to discuss a student's eligibility and needs.

The implementation of this law is the responsibility of regular education agencies. An occupational therapist may become involved in providing services for a student under Section 504 regulations. Students with disabilities may be eligible for Section 504-related services whether or not they qualify for special education services. Table 2-3 compares components of Section 504, ADA, and IDEA 2004—including referral, evaluation, meetings, and placement.

Table 2-2.

Comparison of Part B and Part C of IDEA

	Part C	Part B
Age	Birth through age 3	Age 3 to 21
Referral	Parent, doctor, neighbor, etc.	Parent, teacher
Timelines	Evaluation and Individual Family Service Plan (IFSP) must be completed in 45 calendar days	Evaluation and Individual Education Plan (IEP) must be developed in 40 school days
Documents	IFSP	IEP
Emphasis	Enhancing the family's ability to meet the needs of their child as well as enhancing the development of the child	Meeting the educational needs of the child
Eligibility	Determined by each state. Under Part C of IDEA, states must provide services to any child "under 3 years of age who needs early intervention services" because the child: 1. Is experiencing developmental delays, as measured by appropriate diagnostic instruments and procedures in one or more of the areas of cognitive development, physical development, communication development, social or emotional development, and adaptive development; or 2. Has a diagnosed physical or mental condition that has a high probability of resulting in developmental delay. A state also may provide services, at its discretion, to at-risk infants and toddlers. Informed clinical opinion is an additional way that infants may qualify for services. Several states' policies specify only informed clinical opinion as the criterion for eligibility without providing quantitative criteria. ***Inclusion of Risk Factors*** Three categories of risk for adverse developmental outcomes that are frequently described by states are conditions of established risk, biological/medical risk, and environmental risk.	Eligibility is determined by each state

(continued)

Table 2-2. (continued)

Comparison of Part B and Part C of IDEA

	Part C	Part B
Services	Assistive technology Audiology Family services coordination Family information and counseling Health services Medical services for evaluation Nursing services Nutrition services Occupational therapy Physical therapy Psychological services Screening Sign language and cued language services Social work services Special instruction Speech-language pathology Transportation Vision	Special education services means specially designed instruction to meet the individual needs of a child. Special education includes modification of regular instructional program, adaptive physical education, vocational education, and community-based instruction. *Related services include the following:* Assistive technology services and instruction Audiology Counseling services Early identification and assessment Medical services for diagnostic purpose Occupational therapy Orientation and mobility Parent counseling and training Physical therapy Psychological services Recreation School health services Social work services Speech/language pathology Special transportation Transition services
Natural environments	Services shall be provided in the natural environment in which the child is found. This includes home and community settings where children without disabilities participate.	To the maximum extent, appropriate services for children with disabilities shall be provided in the "least restrictive environment"
Occupational therapy	Occupational therapy is a primary service.	Occupational therapy is a related service that helps identified students benefit from special education

Table 2-3.

Comparison of Laws

Issues	IDEA	ADA	Section 504
Purpose	To provide federal financial assistance to states to ensure free appropriate public education for students with disabilities	To prohibit discrimination against individuals with disabilities	To prohibit discrimination against individuals with disabilities in programs and activities, public and private, that receive federal funds
Type	Education Act	Civil Rights Law	Civil Rights Law
Responsibility	Special Education	Public and Private Schools	Regular Education
Funding	State, local, and federal	Public and private	State and local (no federal funding)
Administrator	Special Education Director	Requirement for school districts of 50 or more employees (suggest to use 504 coordinator)	Section 504 coordinator
Free Appropriate Public Education (FAPE)	Yes, requires FAPE to students covered under IDEA	Yes, requires FAPE to students covered under 504	Provides additional protection in combination with 504, and IDEA but does not directly provide FAPE
Eligibility	Child with a disability who is determined to be eligible and who is in need of special education	Child with a physical or mental impairment that substantially limits one or more major life activities; has a record of such an impairment	Child with a physical or mental impairment that substantially limits one or more of the major activities of such individual, a record of such an impairment, or being regarded as having such an impairment
Evaluation/ placement	Comprehensive evaluation of child's cognitive, behavioral, physical, and developmental factors is required. Completed by multidisciplinary team that includes parents.	Information must be gathered from a variety of sources in the area of concern, and decisions are made by a group knowledgeable about the student, evaluation data, and placement options. Requires periodic re-evaluations.	Does not specify evaluation and placement procedures; specified provision of reasonable accommodations for eligible students across education activities and settings
Procedural safeguards	Requires written notice to parents in regards to identification, evaluation, and placement and parent right to participate on the team	Requires written notice to parents in regards to identification, evaluation, and placement	Provisions for complaint procedures, public notice, and hearings

The Americans With Disabilities Act

The Americans with Disabilities Act (ADA) was originally passed in 1990 for the purpose of prohibiting discrimination solely on the basis of disability in employment, public services, and accommodations. The ADA Restoration Act was passed in 2008 to reinforce the prohibition of discrimination on the basis of disability. ADA is also considered a civil rights law for people with disabilities. ADA has a broad definition of disability, which includes physiological disorders or conditions, loss affecting one or more of the body systems, or any mental or psychological disorder (i.e., mental retardation, emotional or mental illness, and specific learning disabilities). It covers employment, public services, public accommodations, services operated by private entities (includes day care centers, nursery, elementary, secondary, undergraduate, or post-graduate private school or other places of education), and telecommunications. Any public entity with 50 or more employees must develop a written plan setting forth the necessary steps to undertake structural changes necessary to achieve program accessibility.

Public schools must comply with ADA in their services, programs, or activities, including those that are open to the public. This includes accessibility to parents and other community members for such school events as graduation, parent-teacher organization meetings, plays, and sporting events.

All schools must have a plan on file that describes any barriers to accessibility, as well as the modifications needed to make buildings and facilities accessible.

The Federal Access Board on Titles II and III of ADA released new information in 1998 for accessibility in new construction and alterations of facilities designed for children. This final rule allows exceptions to various ADA Accessibility Guidelines (ADAAG) requirements based solely on adult dimensions. These exceptions are for drinking fountains, rest rooms, and fixed or built-in seats and tables for buildings or portions of buildings that will be used by children ages 12 and younger. Prior to these exceptions, many modifications made in elementary schools were designed for adults and were not appropriately scaled down for younger children.

Occupational therapists may participate when looking at modifications to community and school facilities. Often, individualized modifications must be made to restrooms and playgrounds for children. The occupational therapist, along with other team members, must consider a number of factors when making modifications (including ADA specifications, safety, durability, and ease of use).

Other Children's Initiatives

Medicaid

Title XIX of the Social Security Act included the passage of Medicaid, which is the largest federal program providing funding for services to individuals with developmental disabilities. The federal government provides partial funds to the states, which provides for medical, social, psychological, and health services to families and individuals meeting income eligibility criteria. The Early and Periodic Screening, Diagnosis, and Treatment program (EPSDT) provides for medical, dental, vision, and health intervention. (This includes occupational therapy services in early intervention programs, schools, clinics, and hospitals.)

Many early intervention and school programs access Medicaid funds for related services to help supplement program costs. Occupational therapists in these settings will be required to complete Medicaid forms and submit documentation in order to receive these funds. It is imperative that therapists make decisions about which children require occupational therapy services and what those services will look like based on best practices in the field and the collective wisdom of the team, rather than based on a child's Medicaid eligibility or possibility of additional funds.

Developmental Disabilities Assistance and Bill of Rights Act

This act protects the rights of children and adults with developmental disabilities and includes 4 programs: basic state grants for planning, protection and advocacy, university-affiliated facilities, and special projects. One of the most visible of these is the University Centers for Excellence in Developmental Disabilities (UCEDD). These programs are affiliated with a university or college and provide interdisciplinary training to prepare professionals (including occupational therapists) to work with individuals with developmental disabilities.

Summary

A number of key pieces of legislation have shaped and continue to shape the practice of occupational therapy for children. Occupational therapists should be proactive as legislative and regulatory actions are taken by federal and state governments. It is the responsibility of occupational therapists to become involved in the design, modification, and implementation of laws that both affect the practice of occupational therapists as well as the lives of the children and families that they serve.

An additional responsibility for occupational therapists and other team members is to assist families in accessing and coordinating services that they are entitled to by law. Occupational therapists must continually strive to be informed of ever-changing laws and regulations.

As we write this, the Affordable Health Care Act is being implemented so you will need to stay current. You may follow the impact of this Act on children and their families at www.HealthReform.gov.

References

Dunn, W. (2000). Best practice occupational therapy. In: *Community Service with Children and Families*. Thorofare, NJ: SLACK Incorporated.

Early Intervention (Part C of IDEA) (2009). Retrieved from Wright's Law, www.wrightslaw.com/info/ei.index.htm. Accessed June 2010.

IDEA 2004 Summary. (2009). Retrieved from FAPE; Helping Parents and Advocates Improve Educational Results for Children with Disabilities, www.fape.org/idea/2004/summary.htm. Accessed June 2010.

Individuals with Disabilities Education Improvement Act of 2004 (IDEA) PL 108-446. See http://idea.ed.gov.

NICHCY Web site: www.nichcy.org/babies/overview/Pages/default.aspx. Accessed June 2010.

Public Law 107-110: The No Child Left Behind Act of 2001 [NCLB].

Shackelford, J. (2006). State and jurisdictional eligibility definitions for infants and toddlers with disabilities under IDEA, NECTAC.

Turnbull, R. (1986). *Free appropriate public education: The law and children with disabilities*. Denver, CO: Love Publishing Company.

Workgroup on Principles and Practices in Natural Environments (2008). Mission and key principles for providing early intervention services in natural environments. OSEP Ta Community of Practice – Part C Settings, www.nectac.org/topics/families/families.asp. Accessed June 2010.

Additional Web Sites

www.nectac.org/topics/families/families.asp

www.ksde.org/LinkClick.aspx?fileticket=%2FOt9XzqmdPI%3D...mid

www.wrightslaw.com

www.wrightslaw.com/info/relsvcs.indepth.htm

www.nectac.org

www.osep.org

www.nectac.org/partc/ptclead.asp

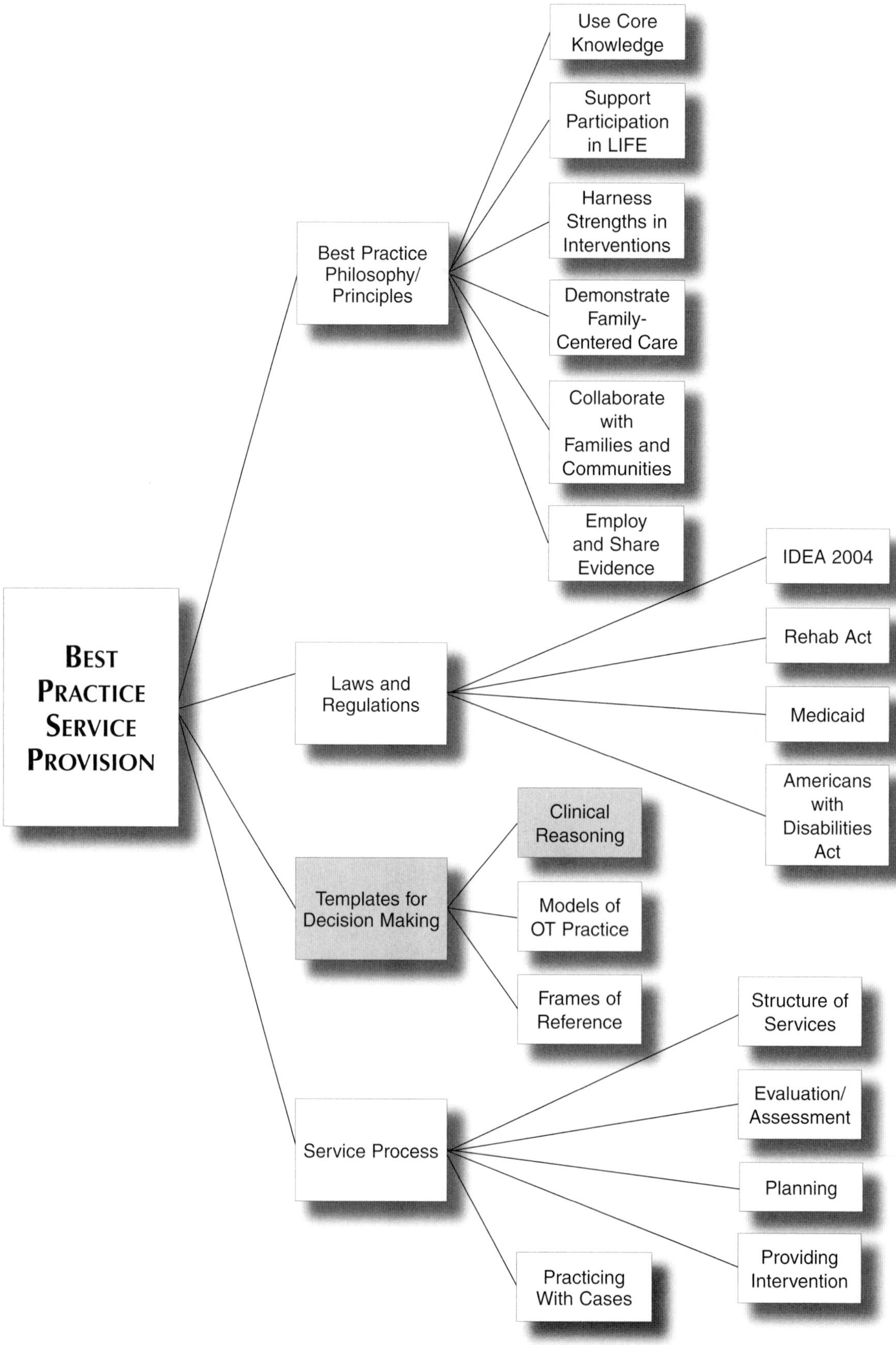

BEST PRACTICE SERVICE PROVISION
Best Practice Philosophy/ Principles
Use Core Knowledge
Support Participation in LIFE
Harness Strengths in Interventions
Demonstrate Family-Centered Care
Collaborate with Families and Communities
Employ and Share Evidence
Laws and Regulations
IDEA 2004
Rehab Act
Medicaid
Americans with Disabilities Act
Templates for Decision Making
Clinical Reasoning
Models of OT Practice
Frames of Reference
Service Process
Structure of Services
Evaluation/ Assessment
Planning
Providing Intervention
Practicing With Cases

3 CHAPTER

Clinical Reasoning for Best Practice Services for Children and Families

Clinical reasoning is a critical skill in artful implementation of practice. Clinical reasoning is a process that professionals use to tap knowledge, organize observations, plan and implement interventions, and reflect on what is happening to revise plans and possibilities for the future. A unique feature of clinical reasoning as a content area is that its focus is on the therapist: what the therapist observes, experiences, understands, and interprets. Most other knowledge and skills a therapist must acquire have a focus on children, their families, other professionals, the environments, and tasks of interest in performance. Therefore, we might characterize clinical reasoning skills development as contributory to the evolution of "therapeutic use of self" because therapists gain insights about themselves as they reflect on their own reasoning processes.

Clinical Reasoning Calls Upon All Facets of Information Processing

Sensorimotor

Schell (1998, 2003) describes clinical reasoning as a "whole body practice," or the process that therapists use to gather information about a situation. While on the surface, it may appear that the therapist is gathering concrete information from records and initial questions; in reality, skilled therapists take in a wealth of information through their own sensory systems. As part of the clinical reasoning process, these initial opportunities to use one's senses to "understand" the situation creates a baseline for gaining insights and making effective plans (Dunn, 1999).

For example, when a therapist meets a mother and toddler, she might engage in initial social interactions, such as greeting the mother and child and inquiring about the mother's concerns. Whole body practice means that the therapist is also "recording" how the mother holds the child, whether they have eye contact with each other, and how the child expresses needs to the mother. The therapist might also touch the child to obtain information about muscle tone and listen to the quality of each of their voices (e.g., is the mother's voice melodic, soft, strained?). The therapist can also smell whether the child needs diapers changed and observe the process of addressing this situation. The purpose in gathering this additional information is not to judge this family, but to use it to aid in decisions about what other information might be needed and what supports this family might require.

Dunn W. *Best Practice Occupational Therapy for Children and Families in Community Settings, Second Edition* (pp. 25-37)
© 2011 SLACK Incorporated.

Cognitive

Clinical reasoning also activates several aspects of the therapist's cognitive processing (Bridge & Twible, 1997). At a very basic level, the therapist must pay attention, remember, organize thoughts, and match new ideas with previously gained knowledge. Additionally, clinical reasoning requires the therapist to use higher cognitive skills, such as problem solving, to reconfigure the current problem in relation to potential solutions.

Experienced therapists also use metacognitive processes to evaluate activities and outcomes (Bridge & Twible, 1997; Schell, 1998, 2003). Metacognition is the ability to analyze how you are thinking about something. When a therapist can think about what he or she has done or planned, the therapist can evaluate the soundness of the action or plan and, hopefully, consider alternatives. Metacognition provides the method for bringing in other information (i.e., checking one's databank [from both experiences and formal learning] and considering its potential impact on the situation). There is also a time feature, in that one can project possible reactions to or outcomes with particular ideas and can change course if deemed necessary to improve outcomes.

In our example with the mother and toddler, the therapist might draw on her knowledge of development to determine what developmental level the toddler has mastered. The therapist might also demonstrate her attending and remembering by reflecting back on what the mother says as she expresses her concerns and needs. At the metacognitive level, having noticed tension in the mother's face and a strained sound in her voice, the therapist might reflect on the meaning of these observations and consider whether she ought to ask the mother if she is anxious and whether she wants to talk about it. During the metacognitive reflection, the therapist will recognize the possibility that a direct question might make the mother stop talking and perhaps end the interaction, but it might also bring relief to the mother to have the opportunity to discuss her concerns further. The therapist would then consider additional information that would assist in making a good decision about how to proceed.

Remember, this metacognitive process is occurring while the therapist, mother, and toddler continue to participate in their "getting to know you" interaction. Metacognition is a transparent filter that supports the therapist to make meaning out of the interaction while still participating with the mother and child.

Aspects of the Clinical Reasoning Process

Many authors have written about the clinical reasoning process (e.g., Bridge & Twible, 1997; Mattingly & Fleming, 1994; Schell, 1998; Schon, 1983, 1987), and each of them organizes the components of clinical reasoning a little differently. I believe that for the novice professional embarking on the journey to become an artful practitioner, Schell's conceptualization is most accessible, and therefore I will use her structure to introduce the aspects of clinical reasoning.

Schell (1998) outlines 4 primary aspects of clinical reasoning: scientific reasoning, narrative reasoning, pragmatic reasoning, and ethical reasoning. Each aspect has a unique contribution to make to the therapist's thinking and planning processes, and they all interact to enable more complex problem-solving. In this section we will discuss the 4 aspects of clinical reasoning and, in the subsequent section, we will consider the power of their interactions for becoming an artful therapist. The tables at the end of the chapter contain a list of questions relevant to each aspect of clinical reasoning.

Scientific Reasoning

Scientific reasoning is a logical process of gathering facts and information and linking this information to "what is known," just as one might do when planning an experiment. Scientific reasoning in practice enables therapists to understand the person's diagnosis or condition, the factors that might be affecting performance, and the possible interventions that are associated with those conditions and factors. Within the scientific reasoning process, therapists must identify and specify the problem (i.e., problem definition) and must decide what interventions are viable for the child and family (i.e., procedural reasoning) (Fleming, 1991; Rogers & Holm, 1991; Schell, 1998).

Problem Definition

Each profession has a particular perspective about the kinds of problems they can consider and address in intervention. For occupational therapists, the focus of the problem must be related to performance in daily life. We review records and referral concerns and solicit information from the family, child, teachers, and other care providers to determine what the child and others need and want the child to do in daily life. For a very young child, the family might wish for the child to play with toys and assist with dressing in the morning. For a school-aged child, the professionals and family may be focused on schoolwork and socialization. An adolescent may want to participate with others in formal clubs or become a driver. In each example, the problem definition stage includes obtaining information about desired and required performance first. It is only then that the occupational therapist investigates contextual, task, or child features that might be contributing to or creating barriers to the primary focus: performance in daily life.

The problem definition process includes a variety of strategies. As discussed previously, the therapist reviews records and other information available about the child. During these reviews, the occupational therapist is considering the concerns from an "occupational therapy" perspective. This means that the therapist is considering all the data through a particular set of filters to see what an occupational therapist would hypothesize about the situation. The occupational therapist is drawing from the "occupational therapy" body of knowledge to consider the possibilities. For example, with a referral about poor seatwork performance, occupational therapists consider *why* the child is having difficulty completing the task (e.g., poor attention, lack of cognitive skills to perform the work, busy environment, spaces too small on worksheet). This is the first step in scientific reasoning because it reflects the domain of concern of occupational therapy and demonstrates that the therapist is beginning to develop hypotheses based on background in the profession (including both experience and literature). This step also informs team members and families about the focus of occupational therapy as part of the interdisciplinary process.

Procedural Reasoning

The second aspect of scientific reasoning is procedural reasoning, which is the process that professionals use to reflect on the information available and consider which intervention possibilities are likely to resolve the performance problems. For this step, the therapist engages in more formal activities (e.g., conduct interviews, skilled observations, or assessments). These procedures are designed to test the original hypotheses with the hope of narrowing the possibilities; when we can focus in on the most precise aspect of the problem, we can improve the effectiveness of the intervention planning process. Chapter 6 provides more detailed information about assessment processes.

Procedural reasoning continues as the therapist initiates intervention. With each activity, the therapist gathers more information, either from the child or from the professional or parent who is carrying out the recommendations. Because of an occupational therapist's perspective, he or she expects to have certain things happen as a result of the suggested activity. During procedural reasoning, the therapist discovers whether the expected outcomes occur, and this provides additional information about how to proceed. Chapter 8 discusses the process of "progress monitoring," which enables the team to determine the effectiveness of strategies.

In the previous example, the child was not completing seatwork. In the records, the therapist saw that the child tended to write bigger than other children, and so hypothesized that the child was having difficulty filling in answers on worksheets with a specified space. Acting on this hypothesis, the therapist suggested to the teacher that she enlarge some worksheets on the copy machine to make the spaces twice as big for the student. The therapist also designed a template with a transparency to make it easy for the teacher to evaluate the child's performance on the new worksheets. When checking back with the teacher, the therapist confirmed the hypothesis about size because the child got more answers completed and therefore got a higher score on several worksheets. The teacher continued to be concerned about the quality of letter and number construction, so they moved to that aspect of the seatwork performance next.

Both aspects of scientific reasoning address the factual aspects of the situation; this is necessary but not sufficient information for an artful occupational therapy practice. Narrative reasoning provides a means for considering the lived experience of people, and not just their technical performance.

Narrative Reasoning

Narrative reasoning is a strategy for understanding the meaning of the experience from the child's, family's, and other care provider's perspectives.

People use the term *narrative* because this form of reasoning occurs in story form (i.e., the parent, teacher, and/or child tell you about their experience) (Mattingly, 1994; Schell, 1998). Factual information from scientific reasoning does not inform us about the meaning of each experience for the people who are living it. When serving children and families in practice, therapists must obtain narrative information from several sources (including the child and the providers), such as teachers and various family members. This is because, in a real sense, all of these people are receiving services from the therapist. Narrative reasoning enables the therapist to discover how everyone is coping with the situation, and this is critical to child and family practice.

For example, although many people have had experiences with the same child who has attention deficit hyperactivity disorder (ADHD) and all would tell you they care for the child, each of them would describe their experiences differently. Grandmother might find the child's high activity level charming, describing it as an "insatiable curiosity," while the teacher might describe the high activity level as "aggravating" during classroom instruction. Both of these people are correct; they are describing the same behavior being manifested (i.e., high activity level—scientific reasoning). Narrative reasoning enables the therapist to consider each perspective when planning recommendations for both the grandmother and the teacher. When using narrative reasoning effectively, therapists make multiple plans so each individual experience can be effective and satisfying for everyone.

Narrative reasoning also provides a method for supporting families to imagine a new life path (Mattingly, 1994). Sometimes, children's disabilities are so unfamiliar to families that they cannot imagine what will happen next, and they have no way of considering a long-term future. In these cases, therapists can provide guidance because we have scientific reasoning to inform us about likely developmental and outcome patterns (from the literature and our experiences with other children with the same disabilities). We do not present our scientific knowledge, but rather use it to guide our narrative process with the family. Therapists first solicit stories from the family about their experience thus far; this often reveals how familiar the family is with the child's current capabilities and limitations. We might also find out if the family has been in touch with other families through church or other support groups, because this is a way for families to gather information for themselves.

Many times, the family's awareness of their child's difficulties becomes clearer with the birth of a sibling who surpasses the first child's capabilities; the complicated feelings associated with this circumstance will affect the family's coping strategies. Through storytelling, the therapist can identify which aspects of the story are consoling (e.g., she has such a great temperament compared to her brother) and which are troubling (e.g., her brother is already walking and we still have to carry her, what will happen when we are too old to care for her). This information guides the therapist's clinical reasoning process by revealing what the family sees as strengths to build on and by suggesting an activity for the therapy process (i.e., life planning so the parents can reduce worrying about the future care needs and enjoy the present with their daughter and son).

Pragmatic Reasoning

Pragmatic reasoning is the form of reasoning that enables therapists to incorporate their knowledge about contexts into their decision-making. Pragmatic reasoning moves the therapists' thinking beyond the child and family to consider the features of the performance environment. In some cases, environmental features can be enhancing to performance, while in other cases they can interfere or prevent performance. In either case, therapists must be aware of features that might affect outcomes in order to design effective interventions.

When therapists serve children and families in their homes, pragmatic reasoning includes consideration of the family's schedule, the arrangement of furniture and toys in the home, and the foods available during visits. For example, if the mother does not cook and therefore does not keep basic food supplies around, the therapist will have to investigate what eating rituals occur in order to support better feeding and eating skills for the toddler she is visiting. Perhaps the mom and therapist will agree on packaged foods to have on hand, or they will visit the nearby fast-food restaurant and conduct their work there. Using pragmatic reasoning in this case means that the therapist recognizes that teaching this mother feeding and eating strategies that one would use when a family sits down to have a meal are not likely to be implemented and, therefore, will not help the child and mother at all. Offering strategies that can actually be part of this family's mealtime experiences is more likely to be repeated and, therefore, impact mealtime.

In public school practice, issues of teacher style and classroom organization become aspects of pragmatic reasoning. Teachers who like to have a clear schedule and expect a very clear set of behaviors from their students need to be dealt with differently than teachers who have a more casual organizational style. The interaction style of the team members affects the way the IEP is constructed and, therefore, how the team will construct the intervention plans. For example, if the therapist recognizes that the team typically focuses on basic skills in reading and math, then the therapist can construct his or her information to make interpretations in relation to reading and math first and then expand to other areas of concern. Pragmatic reasoning provides a means for anticipating the impact of options on the systems within which we work.

Ethical Reasoning

Ethical reasoning is the process that calls upon the therapist to use all the information gathered from the other aspects of clinical reasoning to decide what ought to be done (Schell, 1998). Ethical reasoning requires therapists to stand above the pressures of any particular stakeholder group to determine what is in the person's best interest, considering all factors. Other authors discuss the ethics of clinical reasoning in occupational therapy practice (e.g., Fondiller, Rosage, & Neuhaus, 1990; Neuhaus, 1998), and students are better served to use these references for more details.

When serving children and families, a central ethical reasoning issue is the implementation of family-centered care within various service systems (see Chapter 1). There is much discussion in the literature and in practice settings about the concept of family-centered care, which is a philosophy of intervention in which the family's wishes and perspectives are used to guide practice planning and decisions. However, many professionals were educated during a time when discipline expertise directed the decisions about what would happen with a child and family. This makes it difficult to practice family-centered care because these professionals do not have the background or skill development to implement this philosophy in day-to-day practice. Additionally, service systems have procedures in place that make it "less efficient" to take the time to invite the family to frame the problem. As new practitioners, you will have the opportunity to implement family-centered care as a "best practice," but you will face some barriers. Ethical reasoning directs you to identify the barriers and design solutions to ensure that everyone feels heard and included and that best practices, such as family-centered care, are implemented.

Clinical Reasoning Requires Integration and Flexibility

An artful therapist using a best practice approach considers all four aspects of clinical reasoning throughout the therapy relationship. The insights gained from each type of clinical reasoning have an impact on the other aspects of clinical reasoning as well. In fact, some things cannot be understood without combining information from more than one form of reasoning (Schell, 2003).

For example, scientific reasoning enables the therapist to understand the possible movement restrictions for a child with cerebral palsy. However, the therapist can only understand what this means for the family when he or she learns that the parents are professional dancers. This enables the therapist to understand the meaning of movement as an essential feature of family life; the therapist can use this family feature to build therapeutic movement strategies into their home routines. By taking advantage of the family's unique skills and interests, the family members can feel important to their child's development and can include their child in more activities.

Situations change as children grow older and gain skills, and different possibilities and expectations emerge. Therapists must be able to modify their plans efficiently based on data suggesting that interventions are not working or based on changing circumstances. The clinical reasoning process provides a way to be responsive and to keep the therapy relationship relevant to the child's and family's lives (Schell, 2003).

Clinical Reasoning Develops Over Time

Those entering practice in a profession watch expert practitioners in awe; they cannot imagine how the expert therapist figures out so many things in so little time. What the novice is experiencing is the contrast between beginning the process of learning clinical reasoning and mature, evolved clinical reasoning skills.

Novices are more likely to depend on rules and specific skills to guide practice (Schell, 1998). Because the novice is just trying out new information from theories and initial practice, the novice therapist is less likely to notice contextual cues, reducing the possibility of being quickly adaptable to subtle changes. The novice uses each aspect of clinical reasoning in a more narrow way; for example, conversation (i.e., narrative reasoning) is more likely to be used to establish rapport rather than to gather effective information. The novice focuses on the procedural nature of practice to establish the link between knowledge and intervention.

Within the first year, therapists become comfortable with the procedures necessary to practice, so now they can incorporate more cues from the context (e.g., tone of voice, structure of the physical environment, role of siblings and peers in an interaction). Therapists in this stage of development are beginning to establish a repertoire of experiences from which they can draw to make new interpretations. They also begin to understand the relationship between theoretical concepts and the implementation process.

The therapist's scope broadens in the first 5 years of practice, which also enables the therapist to take in more subtle features of each type of clinical reasoning. In time, therapists gain more and more information about practice from their therapeutic relationships and therefore can be more responsive to subtle changes in the child's and family's needs. After about 10 years, therapists become more intuitive in their ability to process clinical reasoning information, making subtle changes efficiently and effectively.

This process takes a long time; it is not possible to enter the clinical reasoning process anywhere but at the beginning. I advise novices to find a mentor and develop a relationship with an experienced therapist to make this evolution successfully and to participate in work or study groups to provide broader perspectives along the way.

Case Example Illustrating the Integrative and Flexible Process of Clinical Reasoning (With Becky Nicholson, MEd, OTR and Jane A. Cox, MS, OTR/L)

The following tables illustrate one way to apply clinical reasoning principles in practice. This case is about a 4 year old named T.J.; he attends a community preschool program. In this format, the therapist has organized questions under each category as reminders about what to consider. You can design any format that supports you as you think through all aspects of a case. Try out this format, and then design a plan that suits your style of reasoning.

Example of Clinical Reasoning Applied to T.J.: A Preschooler

Note: The structure of these tables (Tables 3-1 through 3-5) illustrates one way to organize material within the "clinical reasoning" structure. There are many ways to do this; the important factor is to have a structure that reminds you what you need to consider with every case.

References

Bridge, C. F., & Twible, R. L. (1997). Clinical reasoning: Informed decision making for practice. In C. Christiansen & C. Baum (Eds.), *Occupational therapy: Enabling function and well-being* (2nd ed.) (pp. 159-177). Thorofare, NJ: SLACK Incorporated.

Dunn, W. (1999). *Sensory profile manual.* San Antonio, TX: The Psychological Corporation.

Fleming, M. H. (1991). The therapist with the three-track mind. *American Journal of Occupational Therapy, 45,* 1007-1015.

Fondiller, E. D., Rosage, L. J., & Neuhaus, B. E. (1990). Values influencing clinical reasoning in occupational therapy: An exploratory study. *Occupational Therapy Journal of Research, 10,* 41-55.

Mattingly, C. (1994). The narrative nature of clinical reasoning. In C. Mattingly & M. H. Fleming (Eds.), *Clinical reasoning: Forms of inquiry in a therapeutic practice* (pp. 239-269). Philadelphia, PA: F. A. Davis.

Mattingly, C., & Fleming, M. H. (1994). *Clinical reasoning: Forms of inquiry in a therapeutic practice.* Philadelphia, PA: F.A. Davis.

Neuhaus, B. E. (1998). Ethical considerations in clinical reasoning: The impact of technology and cost containment. *American Journal of Occupational Therapy, 42,* 288-294.

Table 3-1.

Narrative Reasoning

Personal Information (initials, age, gender, etc.)	T.J. is a male, 4 years and 5 months old
Client History	
Medical history	T.J. received a diagnosis of developmental delay in January 2005. He was born full-term by a C-section due to failure to progress during labor. He was initially hospitalized for 3 days after birth because of feeding problems—he could not latch on to adequately breastfeed. He received ear tubes at 17 months and broke his right arm at the age of 2. T.J.'s current health is good, and he is on no medications.
Social history	T.J. lives with his parents and younger sister. He is usually happy and active. T.J. is easily distracted in large groups of people such as a classroom setting and has difficulty maintaining eye contact.
Educational history	T.J. previously received speech therapy at his home and attended Happy Times preschool and therapy in 2005. He switched from Happy Times to Wonderland Therapeutic Learning Center in July 2006 where he receives speech and occupational therapy. T.J. currently attends St. Agnes preschool 2 days a week. He currently does not receive any special services within his school.
Vocational history	NA
Client's Occupational Profile	
What is the client's occupational history? (life experiences, interests, previous life habits/routines, meaning associated with occupational activities)	T.J. lives with his family in a home in Johnson County. His father works outside the home, and his mother stays at home during the day to care for T.J. and his sister. In addition to preschool and therapy, T.J. also participates in gymnastics. He prefers to lie on the floor at home and play with games or books. For the most part, he does not really interact much with other children. He loves music and likes to dance.
What are current needs, problems, or concerns regarding his/her daily life occupations?	T.J. exhibits some impulsivity and anxiety and has difficulty attending to tasks. He avoids messy activities and dislikes washing his face or hair and getting his hair cut. He does like to wash his hands. T.J. displays difficulty with visual scanning and often does not pay much attention to his environment. He is often clumsy and falls or bumps into things a lot. He will play beside children his age but does not interact with them much. His gross motor skills are below average, and he is aware that the other children can do things that he cannot (catch balls easier, kick and throw, etc.).
What are past/present perceived areas of success and competence regarding his/her daily life occupations?	T.J. has recently begun assisting in brushing his teeth at home. He is fully potty trained and uses appropriate utensils and open cups when eating. He is beginning to assist in basic dressing skills (taking on and off pants, shirts, socks, and Velcro shoes). His verbal skills and ability to follow directions have also greatly improved during the past several months. He also is becoming more aware of his body positioning (not falling as much) and seems less anxious overall.
How has the health/social condition affected his/her ability to continue with his/her life story?	T.J. is aware that some of his skills are below average, and he does not interact with peers as much because of this. He also can become anxious in certain situations, causing him and his family to avoid "high traffic" activities.

(continued)

Table 3-1. (continued)

Narrative Reasoning	
What are the contextual supports and barriers affecting this person's ability to engage in desired occupations?	*Supports:* Involved parents who have good follow through and are willing to incorporate several different activities into his routine, speech and occupational therapy, and a younger sister who allows him to have some peer interaction. *Barriers:* Other children engage in higher level of play (such as playing with the balls together), loud or busy places that cause him to become anxious, "busy" environments that are distracting or keep him from noticing key visual cues.
What are the client's priorities and desired target outcomes/ goals?	T.J.'s mother stated that she would like for T.J. to have the body awareness and tone to function at everyday tasks, would like to see decreased anxiety, and wants to improve his visual scanning so that he can adjust to his environment.
What occupational activities are both meaningful to the person and useful in fulfilling therapy goals?	T.J. likes to play with a specific batman toy. The school does less desirable activities (messy activities, playing with the ball) and then allows T.J. to play with the batman toy.

Rogers, J. C., & Holm, M. B. (1991). Occupational therapy diagnostic reasoning: A component of clinical reasoning. *American Journal of Occupational Therapy, 45,* 1045-1053.

Schell, B. B. (1998). Clinical reasoning: The basis of practice. In *Willard & Spackman's occupational therapy* (9th ed.) (pp. 90-99). Philadelphia, PA: Lippincott.

Schell, B. B. (2003). Clinical reasoning: The basis of practice. In *Willard & Spackman's occupational therapy* (10th ed.) (pp. 131-139). Philadelphia, PA: Lippincott.

Schon, D. A. (1983). *The reflective practitioner: How professionals think in action.* New York, NY: Basic Books.

Schon, D. E. (1987). *Educating the reflective practitioner.* San Francisco, CA: Jossey-Bass.

Table 3-2.

Scientific Reasoning

What is the client's medical, educational, or social condition prompting OT involvement?	T.J. has a diagnosis of developmental delay and displays below-average fine and motor skills, as well as sensory integration issues.
What are the performance skills, body functions, and daily living limitations that typically result from this condition?	**Skills** • Motor—Posture (stabilizes, aligns, positions), coordination • Process—Energy (attends), temporal organization, organizing space and objects, adaptation • Communication—Physicality (gazes, gestures) Information exchange (articulates, engages), relations (conforms, focuses, relates) **Functions** • Mental—Orientation, temperament, attention, sequencing complex movement, emotional • Sensory—Hearing, proprioceptive, touch • Neuromusculoskeletal—Control of voluntary movement function affects the occupations of ADL (dressing), play (participation), and social participation
What contextual factors typically affect performance?	• Physical—Sensory qualities (level of noise, activity, and overall distractions) affect's T.J.'s performance • Social—Expectations of teachers, therapists, family members, and peers • Personal—Participation in different educational opportunities and attempted participation in typical activities that a 4 year old would engage in • Spiritual—Level of motivation (occasionally low, necessary to use specific reinforcing toys) • Temporal—Beginning to attend school, having to separate from Mom for extended periods of time
What theories and research are available to guide my assessment and intervention decisions?	**OA:** Determine through observation and interview the occupational challenges that T.J. faces and help build adaptive responses in order to achieve occupational adaptation. **MOHO:** Look at T.J.'s habits, abilities, and what motivates him to determine his occupations. Engage in specific activities to help shape abilities and increase his level of performance. Focus on habits and educating family to incorporate therapeutic activities into daily routine. **Sensory Processing:** Find out how T.J. reacts to sensory stimuli in his daily environment. Determine areas of difference through parent interview and sensory profile, and look at how this affects his performance. Plan interventions that help T.J. organize the incoming sensory information within daily routines and activities. Interdisciplinary research indicates that imbedding interventions within authentic environments and activities is effective for generalization (e.g., Workgroup on Natural Environments summaries of the literature).
Considering this person's context, resources, and goals, what intervention protocols are applicable to this person's condition?	Identify T.J.'s daily routines. Identify opportunities for imbedding sensory, motor, and cognitive opportunities within these routines. Coach parents and teachers about how to identify and use authentic opportunities in service to T.J.'s development.

Table 3-3.

Pragmatic Reasoning

Who referred this person and why?	T.J. was already receiving services when his mother heard about Wonderland Therapeutic Learning Center by word of mouth. Because the occupational therapist was part of this school, the family had access to services and supports.
Who is paying for these services, and what are their expectations?	The parents are paying for the school as a whole; services are part of the school's structure. They expect verbal updates and a written report every 6 months on T.J.'s progress as well as ongoing goals and home activities. They said they want the preschool to communicate with the school district as well.
What are the family, caregiver, and community resources available to support intervention and follow-up recommendations?	T.J.'s family is actively involved in his schooling and supports. They are ready and willing to try any new activities at home. T.J. receives speech and OT, and will participate in different summer groups in the community as well (e.g., preschool and gymnastics, in which T.J. has the opportunity to engage with other peers).
How much time is there to work with this person?	During his attendance at Wonderland and other times with the family as scheduled. Later, we will work on transitions into public school programs.
What space and equipment is available for therapy/intervention?	The Wonderland School has a lot of equipment available for all the children. There are headphones and CDs for quieter activities, and they have a large room available with scooters, balance beams, a ball pit, trampoline, swings, and a ladder. There are also tables for fine motor activities and hundreds of games/toys/puzzles. There is also an outdoor play area with climbing and moving equipment.
What space and equipment is not available for therapy/intervention?	Because we are in T.J.'s natural environment, we have all the materials, etc., available that other children his age would use.
What disciplines are available and utilized by this client for therapy/interventions?	**OT, Speech, Education** Speech is working mostly on articulation and appropriate responses in social situations. OT also works on improving his social skills (and decreasing anxiety), particularly during movement experiences, because this is an area T.J. needs more experiences with so he can play with peers.
How do these disciplines compare and contrast with OT's role for this client?	The educators are working on sequencing, organizing, and setting structures for T.J. so he can anticipate what is coming next to decrease his anxiety. They are also taking cues from the therapists about how to provide T.J. with additional movement and interaction opportunities.
What are my professional competencies and development needs?	**Competencies:** Ability to identify ways to embellish activities so they incorporate motor skills practice, social interaction, and predictability while remaining fun for T.J. and the other children. **Needs:** Understand the curriculum and school schedule as well as family routines so I can identify all the possible opportunities to support T.J. and give him more chances to practice.

Table 3-4.

	Ethical Reasoning
What were the benefits and risks to the person? Did the benefits warrant the risks?	**Benefits:** Services would promote development and increase independence and interaction with peers. Allow T.J. to engage in a wider variety of activities and increase his safety by increasing his awareness of the environment. **Risks:** Overstimulation caused by too much vestibular input. Increasing anxiety by exposing T.J. to activities he does not like (such as messy activities).
Given the issues of time constraints and limited resources, what were determining factors in prioritizing care for this client?	Looked at parent's goals/wants for child. Also looked at areas of lowest scores on evaluations and what seemed to be affecting his performance the most. Trying to anticipate what T.J. will need when he transitions into public school, so we can provide opportunities to practice those skills as well.
How do you resolve conflicts when there are discrepancies between team members', caregivers', and the client's/family's goals?	We have a weekly team meeting to discuss the children and make plans. At this time, we negotiate the priorities for each child, including T.J. If anyone is concerned about an approach, we identify a way to measure progress and set a short timeline to check on this approach. This keeps us focusing on the evidence from T.J.'s actual performance when we make new decisions.

Table 3-5.

Interactive Reasoning

How did you develop and promote a positive interpersonal relationship with this client and make him/her feel at ease?	Initially, I talked with the parents and teacher about our findings and asked them what their priorities were for T.J. I also spent time in free play near T.J.'s play areas so he could get comfortable with me being around.
How did you answer questions the client had? What if you didn't know the answer?	I answered questions that T.J.'s mother had using jargon-free language to ensure she would understand. I also asked her if she understood my explanation for her question and asked her to let me know if she had any other questions. When questions arose that I did not feel I could supply an adequate answer for, I did my own research for the answer and offered resources as well.
How did you encourage the client to perform at his/her optimal level?	T.J. performs at his optimal level when his sensory needs are met throughout the day. This involves recognizing when he needs soft, dimmer lights, and a less busy atmosphere if he is upset. I coached the teachers about how to recognize when rough play and vestibular activities are becoming overwhelming to him.
What nonverbal strategies were important during the treatment of this client?	It was important to give T.J. positive feedback with smiles, high fives, and hugs when he felt comfortable. The team also discussed the behaviors that served as "precursors" to him feeling overwhelmed so we could redirect him when needed.
How should I interact with this client so that I can support him/her but do not "invade" the person when performing activities?	It was very important to always be aware of my proximity to T.J. to ensure that he felt comfortable with physical prompting and also that I provided adequate physical assistance when he needs additional support. When completing fine motor activities, selection of materials was critical given his dislike for tactile input. Avoiding light touch was very important, and making sure that T.J. had control over the amount of tactile input was critical to his participation.
What cultural factors do I need to consider when treating this person?	T.J.'s parents were highly educated and had specific expectations of therapeutic interventions. The parents were very invested in trying to correct T.J.'s behaviors so he "looked" like the other children. We discussed what exact behaviors they meant when they said this, so the team would understand their meaning.

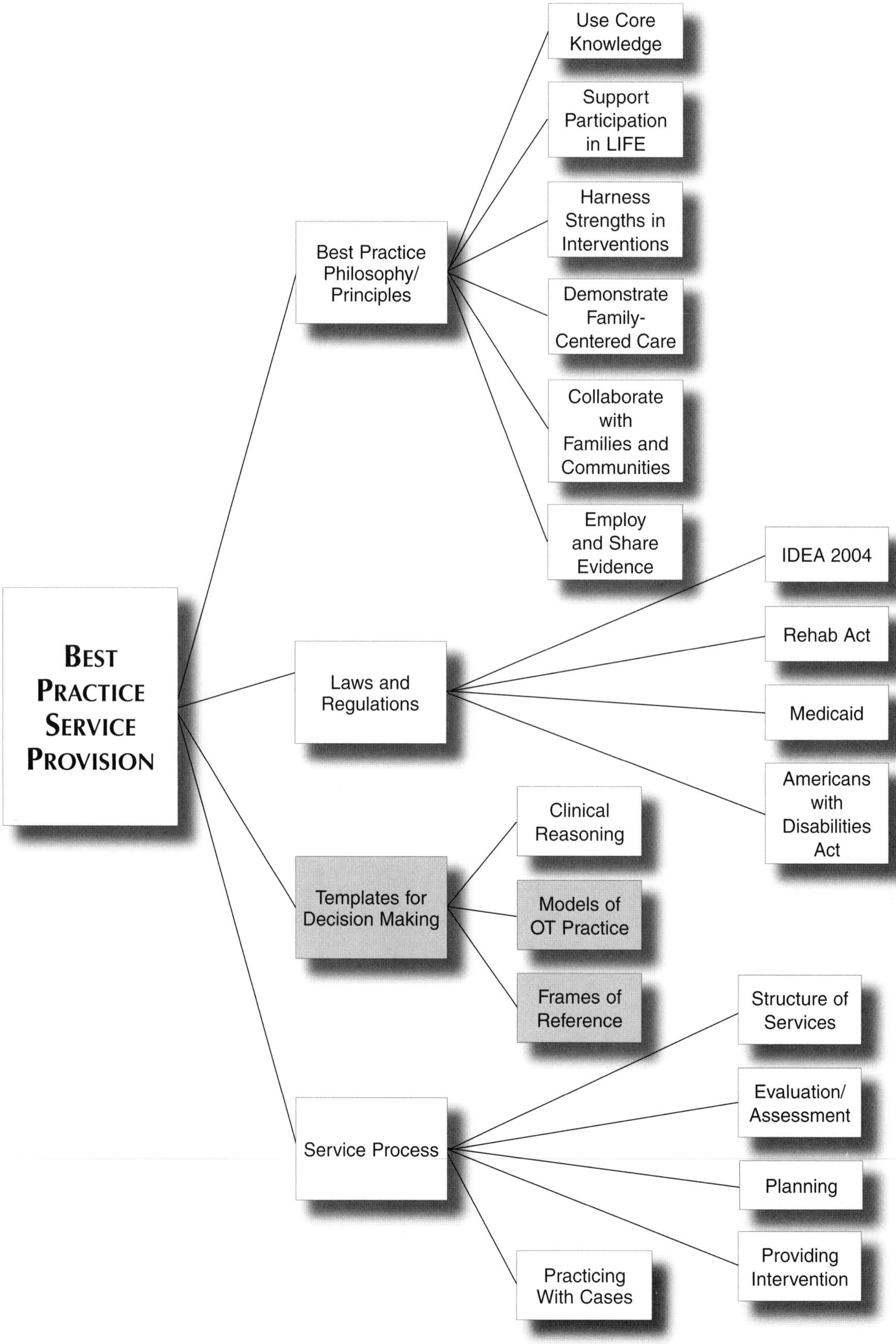
Best Practice Service Provision
Best Practice Philosophy/ Principles
Use Core Knowledge
Support Participation in LIFE
Harness Strengths in Interventions
Demonstrate Family-Centered Care
Collaborate with Families and Communities
Employ and Share Evidence
Laws and Regulations
IDEA 2004
Rehab Act
Medicaid
Americans with Disabilities Act
Templates for Decision Making
Clinical Reasoning
Models of OT Practice
Frames of Reference
Service Process
Structure of Services
Evaluation/ Assessment
Planning
Providing Intervention
Practicing With Cases

CHAPTER 4

Using Frames of Reference and Practice Models to Guide Practice

Practice dictates that professionals base their competent reasoning and decision making on ideas that are consistent with the profession's philosophies. Although much of occupational therapy practice is based on common philosophy, sometimes it is difficult for others to see that consistency in our decision-making. This is illustrated when other professional colleagues and families cannot understand the links between what the occupational therapy professional says, writes about, and does.

For example, if the family expresses concern about the child developing friends, and the occupational therapist administers a gross motor assessment, the family might wonder if the therapist was listening because the family does not easily see the relationship between motor skills and friendship. If a teacher discusses a child's inattention and then sees the therapist spinning the child, the teacher may wonder what "magic therapy" is happening and how spinning relates to attention for schoolwork. Therapists have an obligation to not only be relevant, but to act in ways that demonstrate relevance to others.

That is why the various frames of reference in occupational therapy are so useful. They provide a systematic way to consider participation problems and identify the priorities for intervention to support successful participation. When used properly, frames of reference provide the therapist with the means to link the referral concern to the possible interfering factors and potential solutions. Therapists must study several frames of reference to appreciate the scope and limitations of each one. Frames of reference provide overarching guidance for professional practice, while models of practice provide more specific guidance for assessment and intervention planning.

Overarching Frames of Reference for Occupational Therapy Practice

For this text, we will discuss 3 overarching frames of reference as most consistent with community-based models of practice and most compatible with the philosophy of this book. Each of these conceptual frameworks describes an interactional relationship among people, the tasks they wish to perform (i.e., occupations, activities), and the places in which they must perform (i.e., environment or context). The emphasis on context for performance makes them

Dunn W. *Best Practice Occupational Therapy for Children and Families in Community Settings, Second Edition* (pp. 39-71)
© 2011 SLACK Incorporated.

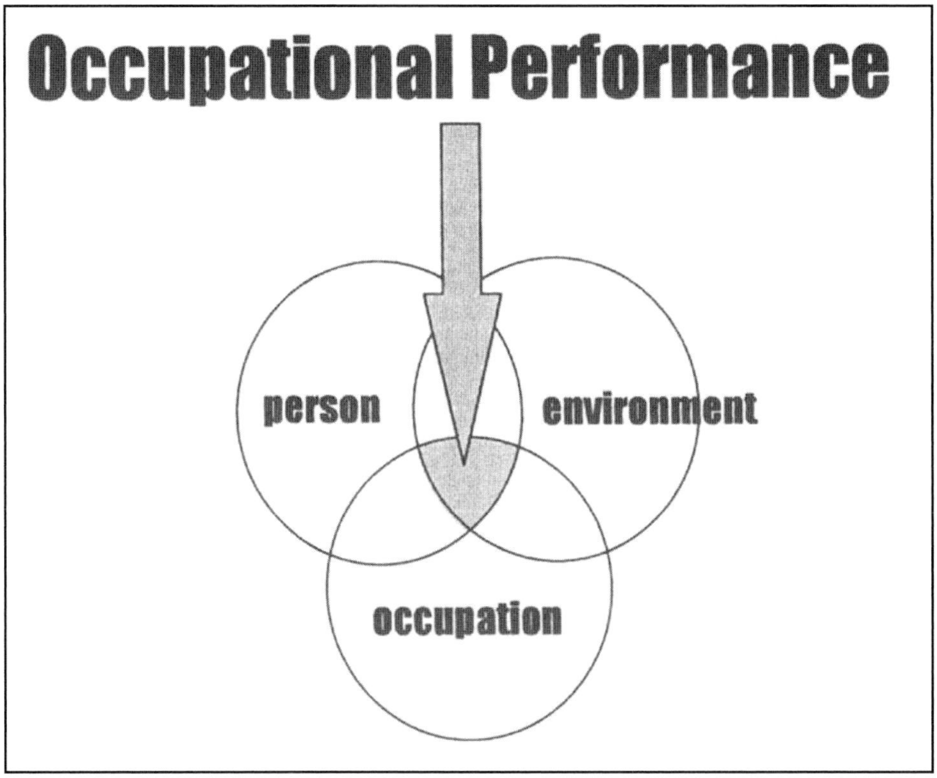

Figure 4-1. Person-environment-occupation relationship. (Adapted from Law, M., Cooper, B., Strong, S., Stewart, D., Rigby, P., & Letts, L. (1996). A person-environment-occupation model: A transactive approach to occupational performance. *Canadian Journal of Occupational Therapy, 63,* 9-23.)

well-suited to community-based practice because daily life settings by their nature have constraints and supports within them. Therefore, by using one of these overarching frames of reference, occupational therapists ensure that they will consider the participation challenge in a manner consistent with both core occupational therapy principles and community-based practice. Dunbar (2007) edited a text that applies various occupational therapy models to service with children and families; it provides much more detail with examples than can be provided in this overview.

Person-Environment-Occupation Conceptual Framework

The Person-Environment-Occupation (PEO) model illustrates a transactive approach to understanding the person's occupational performance (Law, Cooper, Strong, Steward, Rigby, & Letts, 1996; Law & Dunbar, 2007). These authors consider the relationships among the person, the environment, and the occupation as dynamic, such that changes in one aspect can affect the others and in turn can affect overall occupational performance. Readers are encouraged to read the original work for more in-depth study of this conceptual framework and the more recent work by Law and Dunbar (2007) for an application to children and families. Figure 4-1 illustrates the proposed relationships among these factors.

In the PEO model, people are individuals with unique physical, emotional, and spiritual characteristics who engage in various life roles such as student, friend, and family member. In this model, a person's values and beliefs affect the life-roles a person might select or feel satisfied with; values, beliefs, and skills might also contribute to group membership and participation as another way to manifest roles, skills, and interests.

The environment includes physical, social, political, economic, institutional, cultural, and situational contexts within which individuals act (Law, Cooper, Stewart, Letts, Rigby, & Strong, 1994). Each of these environments has inherent features that can enable or disable an individual's performance (Law, 1991). The environment can provide reminders about what to do or what is expected, and then the person interacts with these environmental cues to act in these environments. For example, when a child sees the personal hygiene products on the sink area, they remind the child about what to do (e.g., brush teeth, wash face) and can support the child to be successful in the personal hygiene rituals.

The feature of "occupation" refers to the activities and tasks that people do to conduct their daily lives. Some occupations fulfill needs to be met, while others reflect the person's interests and desires. These authors characterize occupations as sets of tasks that are grouped in some meaningful way so that the person can carry out life roles. For example, the role of parenting might consist of many tasks, such as feeding, diapering, playing, and nurturing the child.

These scholars characterize "occupational performance" as the transaction between the person, the environment, and the occupation. They state that the parts are inseparable if occupational therapists are to be successful in discovering the nature of the person's performance challenges and setting an effective course of action to improve occupational performance. Their model provides a way for occupational therapists to see that intervening with any of the features (i.e., the person, the environment, the occupation) can affect changes in the overall goal: improved occupational performance.

Ecology of Human Performance Conceptual Framework

The Ecology of Human Performance (EHP) is based on very similar constructs as the PEO frame of reference. The EHP outlines "person," "task," and "context" variables and states that the interaction among these variables determines one's performance range (Dunn, Brown, & McGuigan, 1994). Table 4-1 contains a listing of the definitions for the EHP framework. Dunn, Brown, and Youngstrom (2003) and Dunn (2007) provide updated discussions with case studies applying EHP in practice and research programs.

In the EHP framework, the "person" variable is a product of the genetic endowment and the experiences that result in particular sensorimotor, cognitive, and psychosocial abilities and limitations. The "context" variable incorporates the physical (e.g., terrain, furniture), social (e.g., one's friends and family), cultural (e.g., expectations of certain groups), and temporal (e.g., demands related to age or stage of disability) aspects of the environment.

For these authors, "tasks" are objective sets of behaviors, which are generically available to anyone. Individuals select tasks based on their interests, skills, and available contexts; the tasks that fall within the individual's interests and skills and that are supported within a particular context are called the "performance range." Other tasks are available, but outside the performance range (Figure 4-2). When individuals have either limited personal skills or a restricted context, the performance range is narrowed. When occupational therapists provide intervention, they are working to expand the performance range to include more tasks. This can include a number of intervention strategies.

A unique feature of the EHP framework writings is that the authors offer specific therapeutic interventions to meet performance needs (Dunn, Brown, McClain, & Westman, 1994; Dunn et al., 2003). These are listed in Table 4-1 with definitions, and we will discuss them in relation to designing services in a later chapter. The five interventions are establish/restore (addressing person variable needs for performance), adapt/modify (addressing task and context changes that support performance), alter (finding new contexts for performance), prevent (anticipating performance difficulties and intervening to keep them from interfering with performance), and create (using therapeutic knowledge in the best interests of a community). The *Occupational Therapy Practice Framework* from AOTA employs these intervention categories to illustrate the range of options available in occupational therapy practice (2008).

Occupational Adaptation Conceptual Framework

The Occupational Adaptation (OA) framework is based on concepts of normal development, with a process-oriented depiction of how people use occupation and adapt across their lives (Schkade & Schultz, 1992). This conceptual framework provides explicit explanations about the generic constructs that undergird occupational therapy. DeGrace (2007) provides an updated application of this model for children and families that is helpful for your work in community practice.

These scholars discuss the person, the occupational environment, and the interaction among

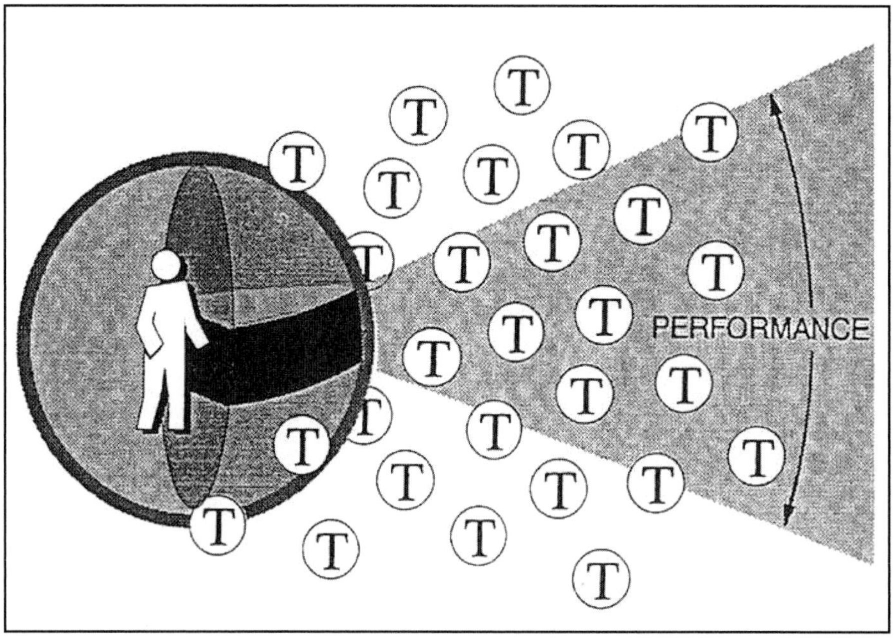

Figure 4-2. Schema of a typical person within the Ecology of Human Performance framework. People use their skills and abilities to "look through" the context at the tasks they need or want to do. People derive meaning from this process. Performance range is the configuration of tasks that people execute. (Reprinted with permission from Dunn, W., Brown, C., & McGuigan, A. (1994). The ecology of human performance: A framework for considering the effect of context. *American Journal of Occupational Therapy, 48,* 600.)

them as the elements of their model. The person has sensorimotor, cognitive, and psychosocial systems to support performance. Additionally, issues related to motivation and adaptation are included as a way to link the person's skills with occupational performance.

Occupational environments are the contexts in which people engage in occupations. Unlike the PEO and EHP frameworks, they organize the environmental variables by the actual places in which persons perform; the other frames of reference discuss more general characteristics of environments, such as "physical" and "social" features. These authors also identify a "demand or press for mastery" feature in the occupational environment, which creates the link to the motivation or "desire for mastery" from the person.

They have also described "occupations" more explicitly. As with the other frames of reference included in this discussion, they describe work, play, leisure, and self-maintenance as the performance areas of interest. However, they go on to discuss three properties of occupations: active participation, meaning, and a product (Law, Cooper, Strong, Stewart, Rigby, & Letts, 1997). It is helpful that they included these properties because their inclusion points out the importance of individuals as the "directors" of their own lives and therefore a critical source of information when making practice decisions.

An intriguing concept that the OA framework emphasizes is the process of occupational adaptation. When people are faced with "occupational challenges," which can be generated from their own desires to perform or from cues in the environment, they must either demonstrate competence in participating or identifying adaptive strategies to enable performance. Individuals are considered "competent" when they are able to generate adaptations to support their occupational performance, evaluate the effectiveness of the adaptation, and, when successful, integrate the adaptation into their performance schemas for the future.

These ideas about OA form the basis for constructing the interventions. Individuals who require occupational therapy are experiencing occupational performance challenges; the focus of intervention is to improve the internal adaptation process. Therapists can manipulate environmental variables and the person's skills, with the emphasis on satisfying active participation.

For example, if working with an adolescent who had difficulty with time management, the therapist would first identify the meaningful parts of the student's schedule and how those parts of the schedule are managed in comparison to the troublesome parts of the schedule. This would provide information about the current adaptive strategies that are successful and those that are ineffective. Within this information, the therapist might also identify person and environmental factors that are contributing to the occupational challenge. The therapist can then interpret the information in light of the student's adaptive

Table 4-1.

Ecology of Human Performance: Definitions

Person: An individual with a unique configuration of abilities, experiences, and sensorimotor, cognitive, and psychosocial skills.
A. Persons are unique and complex and therefore precise predictability about their performance is impossible.
B. The meaning a person attaches to task and contextual variables strongly influences performance.

Task: An objective set of behaviors necessary to accomplish a goal.
A. An infinite variety of tasks exists around every person.
B. Constellations of tasks form a person's roles.

Performance: Performance is both the process and the result of the person interacting with context to engage in tasks.
A. The performance range is determined by the interaction between the person and the context.
B. Performance in natural contexts is different than performance in contrived contexts (ecological validity).

Context: The AOTA Uniform Terminology (3rd ed.) definition for context is as follows:
Temporal Aspects (Note: Although temporal aspects are determined by the person, they become contextual due to the social and cultural meaning attached to the temporal features):

1. Chronological: Individual's age.
2. Developmental: Stage or phase of maturation.
3. Life cycle: Place in important life phases, such as career cycle, parenting cycle, educational process.
4. Health status: Place in continuum of disability, such as acuteness of injury, chronicity of disability, or terminal nature of illness.

Environment:

1. Physical: Nonhuman aspects of context (includes the natural terrain, buildings, furniture, objects, tools, and devices).
2. Social: Availability and expectations of significant individuals, such as spouses, friends, and caregivers (also includes larger social groups which are influential in establishing norms, role expectations, and social routines).
3. Cultural: Customs, beliefs, activity patterns, behavior standards, and expectations accepted by the society of which the individual is a member (i.e., political aspects or laws that shape access to resources and affirm personal rights; opportunities for education, employment, and economic support).

Therapeutic Intervention: Therapeutic intervention is a collaboration between the person/family and the occupational therapist, directed at meeting performance needs.
Therapeutic interventions in occupational therapy are multifaceted and can be designed to accomplish any or all of the following:

Establish/Restore a person's ability to perform in context.
Therapeutic intervention can **establish** or **restore** a person's abilities to perform in context. This emphasis is on identifying the person's skills and barriers to performance and designing interventions that improve the person's skills or experiences.

Adapt contextual features and task demands so they support performance in context.
Therapeutic interventions can **adapt** contextual features and task demands so they are more supportive of the person's performance. In this intervention, the therapist changes aspects of context and/or tasks so performance is more possible. This includes enhancing features to provide cues, or reducing other features to reduce distractibility.

Alter the actual context in which people perform.
Therapeutic intervention can **alter** the context within which the person performs. This intervention emphasizes selecting a context that enables the person to perform with current skills and abilities. This can include placing the person in a different setting that more closely matches current skills and abilities, rather than changing the present setting to accommodate needs.

Prevent the occurrence or evolution of maladaptive performance in context.
Therapeutic interventions can **prevent** the occurrence or evolution of barriers to performance in context. Sometimes, therapists can predict that certain negative outcomes are likely without interventions to change the course of events. Therapists can create interventions to change the course of events. Therapists can create interventions that address person, context, and task variables to change the course, thus enabling functional performance to emerge.

Create circumstances that promote more adaptable/complex performance in context.
Therapeutic interventions can **create** circumstances that promote more adaptable performance in context. This therapeutic intervention does not assume a disability is present or has the potential to interfere with performance. This therapeutic choice focuses on providing enriched contextual and task experiences that will enhance performance.

Reprinted with permission from Dunn, W., Brown, C., & McGuigan, A. (1994). The ecology of human performance: A framework for considering the effect of context. *American Journal of Occupational Therapy, 48,* 600.

and maladaptive strategies and can design interventions to enhance person and environmental elements that support more adaptive performance overall. Perhaps the student uses a list-making strategy that he learned in a business class, but has difficulty prioritizing the lists. The therapist and student might have a weekly planning session for several weeks in which they add deadlines, anticipated length of task, and level of interest to the list, and then together prioritize based on this additional information. Then, the student can evaluate the effectiveness of the extra information and begin to integrate useful parts into future plans.

The Model of Human Occupation

The Model of Human Occupation (MOHO) grew out of the early work of Kielhofner and Burke (1980). MOHO includes an emphasis on "occupational adaptation" through "motivation," "routines and patterns," "nature of skills and performance," and the influence of context on occupations (Kielhofner, Forsyth, & Barrett, 2003). As with the other models, MOHO provides a structure for understanding a person's circumstances and how person factors might impact occupational performance.

MOHO is built on two primary assumptions: (1) behavior is dynamic and depends on context and (2) occupation is a key component of one's ability to be organized. When people do things in their everyday lives, the experiences inform them about their own capacities, interests, and decisions. The therapeutic process supports people to engage in occupations so they can maintain, restore, or reorganize their lives (Kielhofner, Forsyth, & Barrett, 2003).

The core concepts of MOHO enable us to see its unique contribution to occupational therapy knowledge. "Volition" refers to the person's motivation to do things. "Habituation" references the way people organize their actions so they have routines they can access in their daily lives. "Performance capacity" refers to our health status (physical and emotional) and the experiences that have shaped them. Other models infer these aspects of participation, but MOHO explains these aspects in great detail, and this emphasis has been important to our global ability to understand occupations and participation as a discipline.

There are suggested questions to reveal how these concepts are manifesting in a person's life (e.g., see Kielhofner, Forsyth, & Barrett, 2003). For example, to find out about interests, one might ask, "What occupations does this person enjoy doing?" or "What aspects of these occupations does the person enjoy the most?" To find out about habits, one might ask, "What kind of routines does the person have and how effective are they for everyday life needs?" You can see from questions such as these that we want to know not just the factual information (e.g., what are your interests?), but additionally we want to know the person's experience with them (e.g., what parts do you like?). By knowing the person's lived experiences, the therapist applying MOHO concepts can take advantage of these very individual responses to design interventions that will be equally salient for the person.

Some researchers have designed measures to systematically characterize the processing and skills needed for a task. The Assessment of Motor and Process Skills (AMPS) (Fisher, 1998) and the Assessment of Communication/Interaction Skills (ACIS) (Forsyth, Salamy, Simon, & Kielhofner, 1998) provide taxonomies that characterize the person's capacity and skill performance. When combined with information about context and routines, the data from these assessments further illuminates a person's situation so intervention planning can be precise and yield satisfying outcomes. Kielhofner, Forsyth, and Barrett (2003) provide a table of assessments that support MOHO; please review these options as part of model-based comprehensive assessment.

When applying MOHO within a child and family context, Kramer and Bowyer (2007) discuss how children make choices as part of the "volitional process." They describe how children imagine what an experience might be like based on past experiences, interests, and sense of mastery of skills needed to participate. After making choices, children are influenced by their perceptions of the experience, and this in turn contributes the sense of efficacy when the next choice is available. They state that this process contributes to the children's developing sense of "personal causation" and informs their interests, values, and capacities as they mature. Kramer and Bowyer (2007) provide several informative case studies illustrating the application of MOHO in pediatric community practice; please refer to their work for additional examples.

Summary

There are a number of frames of reference to guide occupational therapy practice, and we have reviewed 4 contemporary frameworks here. As you can see, these 4 have many things in common: they all discuss the importance of the person, the environment, and occupational performance. They all have some way to characterize the interaction among these key variables as a means to understand performance and difficulties with performance. Each framework has some unique features as well, primarily in the way that the authors create an emphasis for intervention planning.

So what is a budding occupational therapy professional to do with all of this information? It can certainly be confusing to have many authors go on and on about what seems to be the same issues. First, by studying all of these frames of reference, you might derive the core concepts of the profession (e.g., that a person's performance in context is important to occupational therapy practice). Part of how any profession explicates its discipline's contribution is through "trying out" ways to characterize the ideas and the practice.

Second, by studying these frameworks, you are participating in the evolution of thought in the discipline. Just as different groups of authors have spent time discussing core concepts for the profession and have presented them with their scholarly writings, you must also think about core concepts of the profession and formulate an infrastructure for your own thinking. These authors are reflecting for you the various ways that we might all think about the core concepts of occupational therapy. You and your classmates think a little differently from each other, and scholars do the same. As your mentors, we recognize that one of the frameworks will be easier for each of you to understand and is organized more consistently with your thinking style. It will be important to have a conceptual framework imbedded in your thinking as a way to ensure that your decisions are "occupational therapy" decisions and not good ideas that are outside the practice domain of occupational therapy.

Additionally, from this treasure chest of ways to characterize the core concepts of the discipline of occupational therapy come insights for all of us. Because each framework emphasizes one area a bit differently, or even raises an issue that the others do not, we all have the opportunity to think about that concept. If we only had one perspective, some salient issue would not be raised at all. These points of similarity and difference then must be tested in scholarly work and in practice, so that the ideas can evolve even more.

Models of Practice to Support the Intervention Process

While the overarching frames of reference provide a mechanism for transmitting the general philosophy of occupational therapy, they cannot provide specific guidance for intervention planning. There are other conceptual models that focus the therapist's thinking on what might be supporting or interfering with performance. For example, using an EHP framework, the therapist might determine that contextual features are interfering with seatwork completion. But without additional ways to understand the performance difficulty, the therapist would be offering a litany of suggestions without focus or specificity. The more focused conceptual models provide the means to specify aspects of the context that are interfering, thus narrowing the potentially successful intervention options.

In this section, we will introduce the basic concepts of the most frequently used conceptual models in child and family practice. There are many other sources for more detailed information about these models (see the references at the end of this chapter). The purpose of this section is to summarize salient features of these models of practice for use in community practice settings.

Models of practice provide a perspective about how to think about a problem. Although there is some literature in our profession that suggests that certain models of practice apply to certain diagnoses, I believe that this is an incorrect application of this knowledge. Occupational therapists develop knowledge and learn about diagnoses so we can understand the person's condition and possible risks associated with the condition. Occupational therapists focus on performance in daily life, and at this level the diagnosis or condition is information for scientific reasoning and is less relevant to intervention planning. What takes on more importance for occupational therapy is the impact of the condition on this person and his or her family. We do not provide intervention to change the disease or disorder itself (e.g., children will continue to have cerebral palsy during and after occupational therapy intervention); occupational therapy provides intervention to make life more satisfying. Satisfaction can occur with increased skill, increased ease of access, ability to abandon useless tasks, etc.

Therefore, my perspective here reflects my desire to mentor you to engage in perspective-taking through these models of practice. What options do you have to offer if you use one practice model or another? What might you be missing if you neglect to consider one of the models of practice? What practice model(s) might provide insights to broaden your thinking in solving a particular problem? The models of practice have increased utility when used for perspective-taking.

One reason why people tend to limit the use of models of practice is related to the evidence available to guide practice. For some of the models of practice, research indicating usefulness is limited to certain groups; we cannot always generalize findings from one group to another. This cautiousness is necessary for ensuring appropriate use of knowledge. It does not mean that professionals must not use evolving knowledge to guide practice; it only points out the critical need for professionals to record their decisions and the results of their choices more carefully so that data on effectiveness can accumulate (see Chapter 8).

One more word of caution is necessary. It is very seductive in practice to say, "I use an eclectic approach to practice." This has been a traditional way that therapists have explained their use of more than one model of practice in their thinking. The difficulty with the idea of using an eclectic approach is that it can interfere with evidence-based practice. Researchers do not typically test an "eclectic" approach; they test methods related to theory, frames of reference, and models of practice in the interest of expanding knowledge. It is important for therapists to develop the kind of thinking that enables them to say, "Using the __________ model of practice, I would use these specific assessment strategies and suggest these particular interventions."

This does not mean that therapists must limit their thinking to one model of practice with each child; it is always informative to consider a child's performance needs from multiple models of practice (i.e., multiple perspectives). When professionals require themselves to link each of their thoughts and hypotheses to particular "perspectives," then assessment and intervention options become clearer for the professionals and others. This way, professionals are following each line of thinking consistently with a model of practice, and this reveals both logical hypotheses for action and evidence for future practice decisions.

The Developmental Practice Model

The developmental perspective has a pervasive influence on occupational therapy practice with children and families. This practice model provides professionals with background and guidance about what typically evolves in the course of growing up. In many ways, developmental models have formed the gold standard for children's performance. There are many textbooks and assessment tools that provide detailed information about development, and so I will not review this material here.

One of the most valuable aspects of the developmental model is its universality. Every discipline that serves children and families studies the developmental model, and so it provides information that all team members share. With a common set of concepts and language for discussing the child, the team members can communicate their perspectives on shared ground.

I do have a word of caution about the application of the developmental model when serving children who have various disabilities. An incorrect assumption that has grown out of using the developmental perspective as the gold standard for performance is that our goal with children who have disabilities is to facilitate their development to reach these milestones. Many children who have disabilities will never demonstrate the evolution of movement skill that is represented on a developmental continuum. Furthermore, children who have disabilities are likely to have alternate strategies for task accomplishment that are useful for them. We must not interfere with increasing levels of functional performance because the child's patterns "do not look good" or are not like others. For example, children who have cerebral palsy learn to grasp toys and eating and writing utensils, but their grasping patterns are dominated by spasticity (i.e., they will have a hyperflexed or hyperextended wrist, use a more primitive grasping pattern, and will hold the objects more tightly, providing less opportunity for adjustments). Most of these children will never use a tripod grasp, and it would be inappropriate to interfere with their writing, playing, or eating skill development until they have "better grasp." The developmental model provides a rich backdrop for our considerations of children's performance and, as such, is available for perspective-taking and guidance, but not as a way to limit a child's exploration and discovery of unique and successful ways to do things.

Sensory Processing Practice Model

Sensory-based models of practice are a critical area of knowledge and skill for occupational therapists. They have grown out of occupational therapy literature, and other disciplines and families have come to rely on occupational therapists to contribute this expertise. Other disciplines use this knowledge within their research and practice programs, but they use occupational therapy resources to incorporate this perspective into their work. Additionally, these models have been generated with children, so they are particularly relevant to this text. It is important that we commit time to understanding sensory models thoroughly. This section provides an overview; please use contemporary references to learn more.

Situating Contemporary Sensory Models in a Historical Context

The sensory processing practice model evolved from the work of Dr. A. Jean Ayres, who examined how to apply neuroscience knowledge within her practice with children who had "minimal brain dysfunction" (Ayres, 1972). She used the term *sensory integration* to represent her hypotheses and research. Sometimes, the term *sensory integration* is confusing when discussing these ideas with colleagues from other disciplines because sensory integration is also a term used in neuroscience to describe the generic principle of the brain organizing sensory input. Neuroscientists describe sensory integration as a neurological process of organizing sensory information from the body and environment (Kandel, Schwartz, & Jessell, 2000). Dr. Ayres went on to hypothesize about how children use that information to respond appropriately to environmental demands (i.e., the "adaptive response") using "inner drive" (how a child demonstrates motivation) and termed this application of knowledge *sensory integration* also.

Authors in occupational therapy describe 3 basic concepts upon which sensory integration knowledge has been built (Ayres, 1972; Clark, Mailloux, & Parham, 1985; Fisher, Murray, & Bundy, 1991; Kimball, 1999). First, a person's ability to interact with the environment is related to that person's ability to receive and organize sensory input. Second, this organization of sensory input (i.e., sensory integration) provides the foundation for cognitive development and emotional regulation. Third, the sensory experiences that are part of one's daily routines create meaningful links between the input and the adaptive response; this link advances sensory integration and supports cognitive and emotional development.

Sensory integration was built upon sound neuroscience knowledge. This is important to remember; the foundations for sensory integration are based on well-established features of how the nervous system operates (see Kandel, Schwartz, & Jessell, 2000). Dr. Ayres did not create these features; she built applied science hypotheses on them. Factor analytic studies revealed patterns of performance that are indicative of specific performance difficulties (Ayres, 1972; Ayres & Marr, 1991; Fisher et al., 1991; Kimball, 1999).

In recent years, scholars have conducted summary reviews of the intervention studies that employed sensorimotor and classic sensory integration principles (Baranek, 2002; Pollock, 2009). They report that although anecdotal evidence is positive, outcomes of studies suggest that interventions directed at changing "client factors" and "performance skills" do not produce participation outcomes. They state that the core principles are based on a sound foundation and that employing strategies that address participation directly are more likely to foster both participation and generalization. As Dr. Ayres herself said in her Eleanor Clarke Slagle lecture, "There is a long gap between these basic research data and the assurance that a treatment procedure is effective. We need many studies to test, scientifically, the hypotheses suggested by the theories" (Ayres, 1963; p. 225). We honor her legacy by continuing to examine evidence-based ways to apply her concepts in contemporary practice.

The strong conceptual foundation from Dr. Ayres made it possible to consider the broader application of sensory concepts to the general population in addition to people with disabilities as our culture broadened its ways of serving children (e.g., with legislation, see Chapter 2). Sensory processing concepts are also based on factor analyses of large samples of people without disabilities and comparison studies with people who have various disabilities. This broader view has illuminated some new concepts that can be applied in daily life, thereby honoring her legacy and situating occupational therapy practice in the current milieu of the community and everyday life.

Overview of the Model: Core Principles

The core principles of sensory processing are captured in Dunn's model of sensory processing (Dunn, 1997) (Figure 4-3). There are two underlying constructs that anchor the sensory processing patterns. The first construct is "neurological thresholds," which refers to the way the nervous system operates. The entire nervous system reacts based on an accumulation of excitatory and inhibitory inputs; when there are more excitatory than inhibitory messages to a neuron or brain region, activation occurs (which then transmits a message) (Kandel, Schwartz, & Jessell, 2000). Based on a combination of genetics and experiences, each person has specific set points or thresholds that indicate a particular level of responsiveness. Some people respond very quickly to sensory stimuli, while others have slower or delayed responses to the same stimuli. When responses are quick and frequent, we say that the person has "low thresholds" (i.e., it does not take very much input to activate the system); when responses are slow, we say the person has "high thresholds" (i.e., it takes a lot of input to activate the system).

The second underlying construct is "self-regulation," which refers to the way a person handles incoming sensory input. People tend to manage their own states by engaging in behaviors to maintain a comfortable feeling about their current situation. On one end of this continuum, people tend to let things happen around them and react (a passive approach to self-regulation), while at the other end of this continuum, people tend to engage in behaviors to control the input they receive (an active approach to self-regulation).

When we intersect these 2 constructs, 4 patterns emerge (see Figure 4-3). As you can see from the figure, seeking is the pattern that includes high thresholds and an active self-regulation strategy. Avoiding includes low thresholds and an active self-regulation strategy. Sensitivity represents low thresholds and a passive self-regulation strategy. Registration combines high thresholds and a passive self-regulation strategy. Each pattern illustrates a unique way of responding to sensory experiences in everyday life.

Neurological Thresholds	Self-Regulation	
	Passive	Active
High	Registration	Seeking
Low	Sensitivity	Avoiding

Figure 4-3. Dunn's Model of Sensory Processing. (Reprinted with permission from Dunn, W. (1997). The impact of sensory processing abilities on the daily lives of young children and families: A conceptual model. *Infants and Young Children, 9*(4), 23-35.)

"Seekers" enjoy sensory input and find ways to get more. Their high thresholds mean they need a lot of input to activate, and so they use active strategies to get enough input to meet their threshold needs. Seekers might enjoy spicy foods, want to wear layered clothing, need music or background noise to study (e.g., using an mp3 player, studying with the TV), have cluttered-looking desks, hum while working, or touch others when speaking to them.

"Avoiders" want as little sensory input as possible. They have very low thresholds, so it does not take much to feel overwhelmed. Avoiders find ways to minimize sensory input as their management strategy. They might hold their ears in class, want to wear the same thing every day, have only a few preferred foods, play alone, or prefer computer communication to face-to-face encounters.

"Sensors" are very particular about their experiences. They notice many things that other people do not notice, which makes them precise, but can also be overwhelming. They are likely to talk about the textures or elastic in their clothing being uncomfortable, prefer only certain pens or pencils, work better with structure, tolerate only certain taste, texture, or temperature of foods, and have a specific idea about where everything goes.

People with "registration" characteristics are called "bystanders" because they fail to detect things that others are noticing. With high thresholds, many stimuli occur without their notice; this makes bystanders very easy going, but they might also forget their house key, leave homework on the counter, miss their names being called, or be unaware of tone of voice.

Although the sensory processing literature explains these four patterns as if they are distinct categories, every person actually has some aspects of each pattern in their repertoire. A person might be a seeker for sounds, but an avoider for touch experiences. Knowing the person's patterns is the key to effective use of this model in practice (Dunn, 1999, 2001).

Evidence About the Model

Dunn's model of sensory processing is based on research about how people respond to sensory experiences in their everyday lives (Ben-Sasson et al., 2007; Brown, Tollefson, Dunn, Cromwell, & Filion, 2002; Brown & Dunn, 2002; Dunn, 1999, 2002, 2006a, 2006b; Dunn & Bennett, 2002; Dunn & Brown, 1997; Dunn, Myles, & Orr, 2002; Dunn & Westman, 1997; Ermer & Dunn, 1998; Kientz & Dunn, 1997; Myles et al., 2004; Pohl, Dunn, & Brown, 2001; Rogers, Hepburn, & Wehner, 2003; Tomchek & Dunn, 2007; Watling, Dietz, & White, 2001). Using the Sensory Profile assessments (Brown & Dunn, 2002; Dunn, 1999, 2002, 2006) as the measure of a person's responsiveness to sensory experiences in everyday life, researchers reported about both patterns in the general population and in groups of people with disabilities.

The first studies involved school-aged children without disabilities. With a national sample of more than 1,000 children, Dunn (1999) reported that children's responses were not only characterized by sensory systems (e.g., visual, touch, sound), but could also be characterized by a pattern of responses. From this initial work, hypotheses were developed that evolved into Dunn's model of sensory processing. This model was tested in subsequent studies of infants and toddlers (Dunn, 2002), adolescents, adults, and older adults (Brown & Dunn, 2002). The 4 patterns of sensory processing continued to emerge from factor analyses of these new populations, thus providing supporting evidence about these concepts.

Other researchers have provided evidence about the concepts in Dunn's model by comparing findings with physiological responses (Corbett, Schupp, Levine, & Mendoza, 2009; McIntosh, Miller, Shyu, & Hagerman, 1999; Schaaf, Miller, Seawell, & O'Keefe, 2003). They report that there is a complex relationship between sensory processing patterns and other responses, including stress, vagal tone, skin conductance, and cortisol levels. Findings such as these suggest that we can ask about daily experiences and obtain information that reflects the status of other physiological mechanisms.

Our interest in sensory processing has grown out of our profession's work with children who have particular disabilities. Researchers have also compared children with autism, Asperger disorder, attention deficit hyperactivity disorder (ADHD), and Fragile X syndrome to each other and peers without disabilities (Dove & Dunn, 2009; Ermer & Dunn, 1998; Kientz & Dunn, 1997; Rogers, Hepburn, & Wehner, 2003; Tomchek & Dunn, 2007; Watling, Dietz, & White, 2001). They report that children with these disabilities have more intense reactions to sensory experiences than their peers. Additionally, the groups of children with disabilities have different patterns from each other, suggesting that there are unique sensory patterns across these groups as well.

Model's Relationship to Participation

The sensory processing model addresses children's responses to sensory experiences in everyday life. Articles that discuss the use of the sensory processing concepts in practice emphasize the interface between the child, the demands of the activities, and the context (Dunn, 1997, 2010; Dunn, Myles, & Orr, 2002; Dunn, Saiter, & Rinner, 2002; Myles et al., 2004). The 4 patterns of sensory processing are not a description of the child's capacity, but rather a description of the child within particular situations. Therefore, from a sensory processing point of view, participation challenges suggest that there is not a fit between the child, the activity, and the context. Therapists support participation by finding ways to make a better fit so the child can participate successfully (Dunn, 2009). The very act of participation in meaningful occupations provides feedback about adaptive strategies and broadens the children's repertoire for future engagement.

Intervention Approach Using This Model

When looking at the domain of concern for occupational therapy (AOTA, 2008), the sensory processing model would emphasize "context and environment" and "activity demands" and employ the "modify" intervention approach to support

Table 4-2.

Emphasis Areas for Sensory Approaches (OT Practice Framework, 2008)

Occupational Therapy Practice Framework (AOTA, 2008): Scope of practice	Emphasis in Sensory Processing	Emphasis in Sensory Integration
Activity Demands	*	
Context and Environment	*	
Performance Patterns		
Areas of Occupation		
Client Factors		*
Performance Skills		*

Table 4-3.

Emphasis Areas for Sensory Approaches (OT Practice Framework, 2008)

Occupational Therapy Practice Framework (AOTA, 2008): Intervention Options	Emphasis in Sensory Processing	Emphasis in Sensory Integration
Create/Promote		
Establish/Restore		*
Maintain		
Modify	*	
Prevent		

participation (Dunn, 2009). This means that professionals use the insights they gain from understanding a child's sensory processing patterns and needs to make adjustments so activities and environments are more "friendly" for that child. This approach suggests that the participation challenge is about finding the best fit for the child in particular contexts and activities. In a traditional sensory integration approach, the emphasis is on "client factors" and "performance skills," employing the "establish/restore" intervention approach. Plans would focus on improving the child's sensory, perceptual, and motor capacity and skills so they could participate more effectively. Tables 4-2 and 4-3 illustrate the emphasis areas of these 2 approaches.

By emphasizing the fit among the child, context, and activities, interdisciplinary evidence becomes available to support best practice decisions. For example, the Workgroup on Principles and Practices in Natural Environments (OSEP TA Community of Practice, 2008) outlined 7 key principles to guide practices. These key principles are aligned with the philosophy of this book (see Chapter 1) and are supported by interdisciplinary evidence. Please refer to their Web site for additional information: www.nectac.org/topics/families/families.asp.

There is also a continuing education CD available from AOTA that provides more detail about the links between interdisciplinary evidence and sensory processing approaches (see "Sensory Processing in Everyday Life" CD). Another source for your reference is Dunn (2010), which summarizes the literature for an interdisciplinary audience.

Motor-Based Practice Models

Motor-based models are rooted in rehabilitation with children and adults who have specific disorders. They evolved from the problem solving of practitioners who were serving these individuals and were trying to improve their ability to function. Some efforts led to very detailed methods of looking at muscles, joints, or movements, and, in some cases, these detailed views became the emphasis, and actual participation in everyday life became a secondary consideration. Contemporary researchers and practitioners are using the core principles of the motor models to link back to participation, with promising results.

The Biomechanical Practice Model

Overview of the Model: Core Principles

The biomechanical model has been part of occupational therapy and rehabilitation in general for many decades (Kielhofner, 2009). The biomechanical practice model is based on the application of physics principles to the human body. In applying physical science principles to the human experience as in the study of kinesiology, we make two assumptions. First, motor responses (i.e., the action of the physical object—the body) are based on sensory input that has created maps of the body. Second, there is a predictable pattern of development of the automatic responses that the person will use to move with and against gravity (i.e., postural control) (Colangelo, 1999). Biomechanical perspectives are like physics, in that the movements related to weight, gravity, mass, etc., are going to be similar to the movements of inanimate objects. When using the biomechanical perspective, we must also consider the cognitive and emotional aspects of the human organism as the object of interest because the person has drives to interact with the world. Predictions about movement outcomes have to be mediated from a purely physics point of view. Just as physics will be different on an object that is imperfect (e.g., a sphere with a flat spot on it), variations in the human organism change the way that the biomechanical properties can manifest themselves.

Gravity is a major focus in the biomechanical practice model. Gravity is a constant force on the human body, and the individual's ability to move about in relation to gravity plays a large part in determining effectiveness. Therefore, there are primary areas of focus when using the biomechanical practice model for perspective-taking (Colangelo, 1999). First, we want to reduce the impact of gravity on the individual's ability to move. We can do this by getting the body aligned in relation to gravity. When the body is aligned, there is an equal pull on all the parts radiating from the center of the body's weight. Alternatively, we can reduce the impact of gravity by enhancing postural reactions; when individuals have better control over posture and position due to better muscle actions, they can reduce the power of gravity to pull them over. Second, we want to improve functional performance and skilled limb, hand, and foot use. We do this by finding ways to reduce the impact of gravity and associated postural reactions so that individuals can concentrate their efforts on skilled performance.

The biomechanical practice model also relies on knowledge from development literature. Colangelo (1999) provides an excellent discussion of the reflexive and motor development issues from the biomechanical perspective; I encourage you to obtain this reference for your files. In normal development, infants move reflexively at first and then gain control over those movements, enabling them to explore the environment in increasingly complex ways. The early reflexes provide predictable experiences for the infant, in which certain sensory stimuli (e.g., head movement and touch on a body surface) yield a consistent motor response (e.g., arm extension and grasping, respectively). As the child acquires these sensorimotor experiences, the relationship between the sensory and motor maps in the brain begin to form, and the child can gain more control over movements. We also know from developmental literature that reflexes and other automatic responses to movement and gravity evolve in a predictable manner, increasingly supporting the child to move into upright postures against gravity.

Once the child gains control over these basic movements, the child begins a process of developing stability in one body area to support mobility in another body area. For example, when the child is propping the head up with the forearms in prone position, the forearms, trunk, and legs are providing stability so that eventually the child can shift weight to one side and reach with the "free" arm. At each stage of being more upright (e.g., sitting, kneeling, standing), this pattern of creating a stable base for movement occurs. These milestones of movement and control are related to the effects of gravity on the child as an object in the environment. Therefore, using a biomechanical perspective, we must be aware of children's abilities to control their mass in relation to the force of gravity in order to support their development.

Evidence About the Model

Most of the literature related to the biomechanical practice model is interdisciplinary and has addressed the issues of people with severe and multiple disabilities. These people are the most challenged by gravity, and their ability to engage in daily life is interfered with or prohibited by this lack of ability to master gravitational influences on movement and stability. Studies have shown that we can increase a person's engagement by adding purpose to repetitive movements (Riccio, Nelson, & Bush, 1990). Sharpe (1992) applied the biomechanical practice model to fabricate orthotic devices and showed that they were effective at reducing stereotypic behaviors and increasing toy contact in children who had Rett's syndrome. Children with severe disabilities perform better when the biomechanical practice model is used to design assistive technology support that provides multimodal stimuli (Daniels, Sparling, Reilly, & Humphry, 1995). Hainsworth, Harrison, Sheldon, and Roussounis (1997) showed that children with cerebral palsy have better gait and range when they used their lower extremity orthoses.

Studies are typically done with small numbers of participants and tend to use research designs that are more individualized (e.g., that chart the specific performance goals of the study subjects). This is appropriate for documenting changes in those people, but sometimes it becomes hard to generalize from these small samples to the population at large as one can in a study with many subjects. Be careful to look for similarities and differences between individuals reported in the literature and the individuals you are serving when using this evidence to make practice decisions. You must also have a clear data collection plan to document the effectiveness or ineffectiveness of the intervention.

Model's Relationship to Participation

The musculoskeletal system is the most common target for the biomechanical practice model. We tend to focus on children who have complex physical disabilities in relation to their disorders, such as cerebral palsy and muscular dystrophy. However, it is important to remember that many children do not have control over their postural mechanisms even though they do not have a frank disability, and the biomechanical practice model offers a useful perspective for these children as well because a biomechanical approach can be used to create supports for participation.

The key issue that triggers therapists to take a biomechanical perspective is the child's difficulty with stability and mobility, which is needed for engagement in daily life. Modulation between stability and mobility for successful performance is critical from the biomechanical perspective. Whenever modulation is the issue, we can conclude that children might have difficulty related to too much, too little, or high variability in their responses. For the biomechanical practice model, this translates into considerations of muscle tone (the building block of postural control and movement) and skeletal alignment.

Muscle tone is the ability of the muscle to contract when needed. Normal muscle tone reflects a balance of excitation and inhibition from the nervous system acting on the muscle. Excitation comes from the reflex arc (i.e., the sensory neuron, interneuron, and motor neuron—see your neuroscience text), and inhibition comes from the descending motor neurons that serve that limb or muscle. When children have central nervous system disorders, such as cerebral palsy, muscle tone can be disrupted, resulting in high muscle tone (i.e., excess tension) or low muscle tone (i.e., lack of activation). This occurs because the balance of power in the system is upset; whenever the balance of power is disrupted, we can see either extreme as a result. In the case of high muscle tone (i.e., spasticity), the reflex arc is "released" from inhibitory control due to disruptions in the brain areas that send the descending motor messages. Without the inhibitory control, the reflex arc continues to generate activity in the muscle, so it contracts more and more often, makes the muscle very tense, and interferes with fluid movement. When tone is very low, we believe that the "release" phenomenon is related to lack of activation of the reflex arc, leading to a very unresponsive muscle. In this case, the inactive muscle makes the limb and joints very mobile and therefore unable to support either stability or active movement for function. It is the lack of control over the musculoskeletal movements that interferes with performance.

When children have more subtle difficulties with body control, we can still see the interference of poor postural stability and mobility in their daily life. These children may hang on furniture and other people for support, may lay on their desks during seatwork, and may tire more easily than children the same age. They may have difficulty learning skills even when motivated, such as riding a bike or climbing on the play equipment at school. The biomechanical practice model can be useful for these children as well, because it offers options for supporting these children's performance.

Intervention Approach Using the Model

Kielhofner (2009) summarizes the biomechanical intervention approach by discussing the intersection of movement and performance. In his summary of the model, he states that addressing one's capacity for movement is at the heart of this model's intervention approach. When we consider movement during occupations, the emphasis for intervention is on establishing a useful relationship with gravity through positioning to support and facilitate functional movements. Therapists can establish useful relationships with gravity in two ways. First, we can engage the child in activities that will facilitate the child to have better postural control. Second, we can supply adaptive equipment and devices that provide external support for parts of the body, thereby reducing the load on the child to meet the constant challenge of gravity. Once the child has a stable relationship with the forces of gravity, it is possible to introduce skilled movements and interactions with the environment, including manipulation with hands, looking at toys and friends, reaching and grasping, and moving about in space.

It is important to gauge the therapeutic emphasis when using a biomechanical perspective. There are times when it is appropriate to emphasize increased postural control by requiring the child to exert personal effort to improve muscle control to hold the body up against gravity. At other times, this type of exertion may yield very little progress overall and exhaust the child, making the child unavailable for other interactions. In these cases, it is more useful to introduce adaptive devices that provide the postural support; the device "erases" the impact of gravity on the child without the child's effort and thereby reserves the child's personal resources for skilled movements that stimulate cognitive and emotional development.

Therapists must consider the cost-benefit analysis of each choice. It is inappropriate to set up situations in which the child has to "earn" the right to participate by improving postural control before participation is made available. Whenever a participation opportunity is available, best practice dictates that occupational therapists provide adaptations to make participation possible; these are not the times for the child to work on postural control. We ask ourselves, "What would I have to introduce here to erase the effects of gravity on this child's body so this child can participate with the others?" For example, we would supply a child who has a severe disability with a wedge when in prone position, so the child can see friends playing on the floor instead of making the child develop head control to see friends. This is one of the best features of the biomechanical practice model; it provides you with explicit information for giving the child access to living. The disability can become "transparent" for a bit of time so the child can learn the enjoyment of engaging in daily life activities.

Think about yourself. If you want to watch a movie with your friends, and your shoulders and neck are sore from a previous workout, you are likely to create a supported sitting spot with pillows, rather than make yourself "work on" those sore muscles while you watch the movie. You do not need to miss your time with your friends when there are ways to make it easy to participate in spite of your current difficulty.

The biomechanical practice model also informs us about how to use gravity to the child's benefit. When we position a child properly in relation to gravity, we can make it easier to generate active movement. For example, when a child is placed in a sidelying position, the child can move the arms along the lines of gravity, making the weight of the arms less troublesome. The ground can support one arm as the child reaches, and the child does not have to support the weight of the head to look at the hands as the child makes contact with toys in proximal space. In a prone support, the child's arms can move toward gravity to touch and manipulate objects. When children become more active with objects, they can develop the cognitive and perceptual skills they need for more complex activities.

These principles are also applicable to children with more subtle disabilities. Children who have poor trunk control may be squirmy in their desk chairs or may fall out of them during class. Changing to a chair with arms and making sure the child's feet are firmly placed on the floor can be enough to support the child in the chair for seatwork. Sometimes, turning a chair backwards so the child can lean on the backrest while working is enough support for successful school performance. To apply the biomechanical practice model during daily life, always think, "if I changed this child's relationship to gravity or reduced the power of gravity by supporting body parts, would performance improve?"

Situating Contemporary Motor Models in a Historical Context

The Neurodevelopmental Practice Model

Some characterize several treatment models as "neurodevelopmental," referring to those approaches that look at the developmental aspects of the nervous system (Kielhofner, 2009; Trombly & Radomski, 2002). When serving children, professionals typically consider the Bobath approach the neurodevelopmental treatment model (NDT). NDT has evolved from work of medicine, physical therapy, human development, and brain injury literature. The original work evolved out of Karel and Berta Bobath's service to individuals who had brain injury, similar to Dr. Ayres' early work. NDT is a sensorimotor approach that serves to enhance the child's motor and postural capacities so that the child can participate more actively in tasks. This model incorporates attention to the developmental sequence that enables a child to gain mastery over primitive reflexes for purposeful movement and knowledge about how the sensorimotor system receives and interprets input for motor responses (Schoen & Anderson, 1993). There must be a good working knowledge of normal development to apply this practice model, because concepts of abnormal movement are judged in relation to "normal developmental milestones."

Normal development contains core principles related to sensory motor feedback patterns, movement components, and motor sequences (Bly, 1991; Schoen & Anderson, 1993). The principles of normal development include the ideas that movement control occurs from head to foot, from the center of the body to the limbs and hands or feet, and from large to small movements. Sensory motor principles address the fact that most movements, even reflexive ones, originate based on a sensory stimulus or sensory input. For example, in the rooting reflex, the child turns toward a touch stimulus on the cheek; in the grasping response, the child clutches an object touching the palm. Eventually, the child internalizes this information about the body and movement and can gain control over the movement, but the sensory input paired with the movement is part of the memory of that movement pattern.

The child develops components of movement as building blocks for more complex movements later. The primary principle that guides development of movement components is the interaction between the need for stability and the desire for mobility. NDT and the biomechanical practice model share this concept and emphasis. Stability occurs when complementary muscle groups can contract in synchrony, thereby holding a body area or joints in place. We need stability to "ground" us and to mediate the effects of gravity on our control of body in space. It creates a base of support for movements required for interaction. Mobility occurs as the child attempts to explore and engage in the environment. Mobility requires stability, the ability to shift one's body mass, and the ability to separate movements of the trunk and limbs from the point of stability. For example, a child might establish stability in the shoulders by co-contracting the front and back chest muscles and pulling the clavicle and scapula down so that the child stays upright when reaching out for a cup.

Finally, the child must develop patterns of movement that support more complex interactions. There are movement patterns in each stage of motor development from lying on the ground, to sitting, kneeling, and standing. A key feature of the patterns of movement is the child's ability to engage in many combinations of movement and to demonstrate fluidity, i.e., an ability to move into and out of movement patterns easily. NDT has an assumption that these normal movement patterns are essential to all children's development, even children with movement disorders (i.e., cerebral palsy). From this perspective, competence is compromised when the child develops a reliance on compensatory patterns of movement to accomplish tasks in daily life (Schoen & Anderson, 1993); because normal movement patterns are most efficient, they must be preferred.

Model's Relationship to Participation

Because this practice model was developed out of work with people who had brain injury, it is essential for a therapist to understand abnormal motor development associated with brain injury in order to employ this practice model. Some believe the abnormal movements are the result of poor inhibitory control in the nervous system, while others characterize the difficulty as obstructions in particular sections of the trunk and postural control areas or persistence of primitive reflexes (e.g., Bly, 1980; Bobath, 1971).

From an NDT perspective, children do not have control over their own movements. Children can lack control in several ways. A child with very low muscle tone will have poor control because the effects of gravity are so powerful that the child does not have the power to move the body away from gravity. These children have a hard time being upright without supports from equipment or people, and movements can lead to the child falling over (i.e., towards gravity) because there is no stability to support the movement. Children with very high muscle tone (e.g., spasticity) also do not have control over their own movements, but their bodies tend to look "locked up." Any movement attempts move the whole body as a mass (e.g., whole body rolls over when the child was trying to reach for a toy); the child has a great deal of difficulty separating one body part from another for functional movements. Children create compensatory strategies to minimize the effects of these motor impairments. For example, a child with poor head and trunk control may stay curved over in sitting, but push the head and neck out to see others rather than work to obtain co-contraction in the trunk muscles for sitting upright.

The traditional application of NDT does not emphasize participation the way contemporary practice does. As you can see, the emphasis was on posture and alignment. In contemporary practice, we might learn the core principles of NDT because they help us learn about how normal and atypical movement evolve and then consider how these factors might affect participation using other problem-solving and evidence-based strategies.

Evidence About the Model

A number of research teams have investigated the effectiveness of NDT with varying results. In earlier work, researchers compared NDT to "no therapy," early intervention, motor learning, and other traditional therapies, with mixed results. Some findings indicated that there were no differences between NDT and other interventions (e.g., Breslin, 1996; Jonsdottir, Fetter, & Kluzik, 1997; Scherzer, Mike, & Olson, 1976; Wright & Nicholson, 1973), some supporting alternative interventions over NDT (e.g., d'Avignon, 1981; Palmer et al., 1988), and one demonstrating the benefit of NDT (Carlsen, 1975). These studies used heterogeneous samples of children in relation to age and severity of disability.

In more recent work, Lilly and Powell (1990) found no differences in dressing skills after either NDT or play interventions with two children who had cerebral palsy. Law, Cadman, Rosenbaum, Walter, Russell, and Dematteo (1991) investigated the effects of upper extremity inhibitory casting and NDT on motor and performance skills and found that casting and NDT together improved the quality of upper extremity movements and wrist extension in children with cerebral palsy. Additionally, more intensive NDT and NDT alone did not have an effect on these measures; hand function improvements were equivocal. Jonsdottir, Fetter, and Kluzik (1997) compared practice to NDT and found no differences in head or shoulder displacement; there were some indications that postural alignment measures might show differences, with NDT being preferred.

All of the evidence points out the difficulty in deciding the proper focus of measurement in intervention studies. Although we might see changes in motor component movements, we must question the utility of spending the child's and family's resources for this type of intervention if those do not translate into functional outcomes. Work needs to be done to investigate possible links between NDT and daily life.

Intervention Approach Using the Model

The traditional application of the NDT practice model in intervention involves individual interactions between the therapist and the child. In this model, the therapist prepares the child by engaging the child's body in passive movements at first and then increasingly provides sensory input and task demands to engage the child in more active movements. Patterns of engagement encourage co-contraction for stability with controlled movements of selected body parts as the child interacts with others and objects. Eventually, the child takes over more responsibility for stability and mobility with actions such as propping and other weight-bearing tasks; weight-bearing also provides intense sensory support for stability (i.e., proprioception and touch pressure). Therapists also take advantage of supportive devices and equipment to reduce the child's load while learning new skills, as we would when using the biomechanical model. Therapists must have a working knowledge of the sensory inputs that facilitate and inhibit muscle activity, a clear picture of developmentally appropriate movement sequences, and specialized skill in the NDT techniques to provide this type of intervention.

This traditional form of providing NDT intervention may or may not be effective in particular circumstances (as summarized previously); it is not useful in its traditional form for serving children and families in community settings. At home and in school, the focus is on the child's participation. The principles of NDT intervention are very useful for other service models that are appropriate for community practice. The methods for reducing the negative effects of tone can be applied to caregiving routines. For example, when a child has high muscle tone, the legs are frequently pushed together in adduction, making it difficult to remove and insert diapers. We can teach parents and other care providers how to increase hip flexion and release this tightness, which enables them to complete diaper changing efficiently. We can also teach some of the handling strategies for carrying the children as care providers transport them throughout the day.

We must be cautious in applying the traditional NDT model of practice; the current evidence does not support its broad use. As best practice therapists, we must convey the equivocal nature of the evidence when discussing options with families. For example, we might say, "researchers have found some changes in the trunk when we activate the muscles evenly (i.e., postural activation study of Jonsdottir, Fetter, & Kluzik, 1997), but findings are not consistent, so we will need to collect data on your child to see if it is working with her." We would also need to be prepared with other options if the family does not select this more equivocal option.

Motor Control and Motor Learning: Contemporary Motor Models

Overview of the Models: Core Concepts

The motor control and motor learning literature contains more contemporary views of movement acquisition. They account for the variability of the use of muscles and joints in a way that traditional motor models did not (Kielhofner, 2009). Shumway-Cook and Woollacott (1995) define motor control as "the study of the nature and cause of movement" (p. 3) and motor learning as "the study of the acquisition and/or modification of movement" (p. 23). We might also view these areas of study as the basic science of movement (i.e., motor control) and the applied science of movement (i.e., motor learning).

There are many theories guiding knowledge development about motor control. While earlier theories of motor control focused on reflexive and hierarchical structures within the central nervous system (Magnus, 1926; Sherrington, 1947; Weisz, 1938), more recent theories have incorporated more complex hypotheses about body position and gravity (e.g., Shumway-Cook & Woollacott, 2007), the central nervous system (e.g., Bernstein, 1967; Forssberg, Grillner, & Rossignol, 1975; van Sant, 1987), models of action separate from the central nervous system in particular (e.g., Kugler & Turvey, 1987; Schmidt, 1988; Thelen, Kelso, & Fogel, 1987), and considerations of task and environmental influences (e.g., Gibson, 1966; Greene, 1972; Woollacott & Shumway-Cook, 1990). As with all emerging theoretical knowledge, each of the scholars have contributed particular information to our understanding of motor control mechanisms. As therapists, the information from the motor control literature provides us with scientific reasoning knowledge for our decision-making; the more we understand the underlying mechanisms that support or create barriers to performance, the better our intervention planning options can be.

Complex concepts require many perspectives. Researchers in motor control are looking at an integrated model that acknowledges the need to understand the CNS, the mechanisms for actions, and the person-task-environment interface (Mathiowetz & Bass-Haugen, 2002; Shumway-Cook & Woollacott, 1995). With this integrated view, it becomes necessary for motor control researchers to consider cognitive, sensorimotor, and ecological factors in their quest to fully understand motor control mechanisms. It is interesting that, although this area of research has evolved from other disciplines, these researchers have also determined that they need to understand person-task-environment interactions to make progress in knowledge development.

The motor learning literature concerns itself with acquisition, practice, generalization, and adaptation of movements for action. There are 4 concepts that underlie the motor learning literature (Schmidt, 1988): learning is a process of acquiring skills, learning emerges from practice and experience, we surmise what learning has occurred from the behaviors we observe, and learning by its nature produces relatively permanent changes.

There are also several theories guiding the motor learning knowledge development. Some of the earlier theories emphasized the sensorimotor feedback loop and motor programs as the core building blocks to support motor learning (e.g., Adams, 1971; Schmidt, 1988); in these models, the motor programs got stronger with practice. Newell (1991) proposes that people must increase the coordinated efforts between perceptual information and one's actions to have motor learning occur. Newell also considers the task and context as factors that have an impact on motor learning. All of the motor learning theories address the hypothesized processes for people to acquire skills; this is in contrast to the motor control theories that concerned themselves with the actual mechanisms that support movement. The motor learning literature is more directly applicable to practice decision-making.

Evidence About the Models

The research in motor learning has informed us about effective (and ineffective) ways to support people to learn. One critical factor to motor learning is feedback, which can be from internal mechanisms (i.e., body sensations) or from external sources (i.e., from the environment, including from other people). Bilodeau, Bilodeau, and Schumsky (1959) showed that it is important to know the effectiveness of movement in order to learn. However, it is still unclear what parameters we must place on this feedback about the results of performance. For example, experimenters have been unable to identify the optimal time to wait between practice trials, or how long to wait (or not wait) to give the feedback about performance (also called "knowledge of results") (Schmidt, 1988). People also seem to profit most from a summary of their performance, rather than feedback after each trial; Schmidt (1988) hypothesizes that giving feedback after each trial may be too encumbering and leads the person to rely on external feedback too much. Children and adults profit from feedback that is consistent with their information levels; adults may profit from more precision and detail because they understand the material (e.g., providing information about inches, pounds).

Motor learning researchers have also studied the aspects of practice that make learning more effective. Although people fatigue with repeated practice on a task and get worse when they get tired, this type of practice enables generalization of routine tasks (Schmidt, 1988). People also perform better when they have been able to practice variations of the task (Catalano & Kleiner, 1984), when they practice the whole task rather than isolated parts that are not explicitly part of the functional performance (see Kaplan & Bedell, 1999, for a discussion related to children), and when the practice and performance contexts are similar (Schmidt & Young, 1987). Rawlings, Rawlings, Chen, and Yilk (1972) showed that when individuals practice mentally, they perform almost as well as those who practice physically. Other studies have suggested (see Schmidt, 1988; Singer, 1980) that we must be careful in our use of guidance for learning; it seems that individuals profit from initial guidance for learning (i.e., physically supporting the movement or verbally directing the movement), but not as a long-term strategy.

More recently, occupational therapy researchers have been interpreting the motor control literature from our discipline's point of view (e.g., Giuffrida, 2003). For example, Mathiowetz and Bass-Haugen

(2002) describe the need for individuals to find the best solution for movement for the situational demands. This is a great place to keep current on reading for future developments.

Model's Relationship to Participation

Within the motor learning literature, some authors focus on the skills the person cannot perform successfully (Kaplan & Bedell, 1999), while other authors consider the aspects of learning that seem to be supporting or interfering with function (Shumway-Cook & Woollacott, 1995). Those who consider a more global view will also look at task and environmental variables to see what might be interfering with the person's ability to function; this information is very helpful for intervention planning (e.g., Held, 1987; Mathiowetz & Bass-Haugen, 2002). For example, age is an important variable in recovery of task performance; there is a complex interaction between central nervous system areas and age, with some being vulnerable or invulnerable at different ages from infancy to adulthood (Shumway-Cook & Woollacott, 1995, 2007). The environmental variable of training conditions interacts with the state of the system (i.e., the CNS) to affect recovery. People who receive training that is more immediate to the injury and when there are forced-use conditions (i.e., we make the person use the more involved limbs to function) seem to have better functional outcomes (Held, 1987).

Intervention Approach Using the Model

In the motor control and motor learning literature, researchers discuss the process of recovery of function. From a strict perspective, recovery means that the person returns to his or her abilities prior to the injury without any changes in the pattern of performance (Almli & Finger, 1988). Bach-y-Rita and Balliet (1987) discuss the "forced recovery" process in which we specifically design interventions to require movements that we believe are having an impact on reorganizing the neural mechanisms that support motor movements. These perspectives reflect the idea of "fixing" the person; more contemporary views acknowledge the person's interactions with the environment as an additional factor in function and recovery (Christiansen & Baum, 1997; Law et al., 1997). With a broader view, it is possible to consider both restorative strategies and compensatory strategies to support motor learning and recovery of function.

The motor learning literature informs us that knowledge of results of performance and practice is important for positive functional outcomes. Practice must be variable to have the most lasting effects, including changing order and demands (Catalano & Kleiner, 1984). When people can practice in a natural setting, they do better than when we create isolated practice opportunities for them; this also facilitates generalization (Winstein, 1991; Winstein & Schmidt, 1990). People also improve with mental practice of movements, not just physical practice (e.g., Rawlings, Rawlings, Chen, & Yilk, 1972). We must also balance skill acquisition with skill generalization (Singer, 1980) (i.e., when we make tasks more difficult at first, acquisition will be slower, but generalization might be better). We must also avoid the temptation to give feedback about performance continuously; data suggest that people perform better in the long run when they receive summary feedback (Schmidt, 1988).

Psychosocially Based Practice Models

We also have practice models that emphasize the psychosocial aspects of children's development. These models remind us of the importance of interacting with others in an appropriate and satisfying way. These models are likely to be familiar to our colleagues in other disciplines, so they can form a basis for communication among professionals as well.

The Coping Practice Model

Overview of the Model: Core Principles

The coping practice model is based on theoretical constructs from child development and psychology (Compas, 1997; Werner & Smith, 1982). Coping is defined as the "process of making adaptations to meet personal needs and respond to the demands of the environment" (Williamson, Szczepanski, & Zeitlin, 1993, p. 396). There are 2 unique features of this practice model: coping addresses the adaptive features of a child's skills regardless of the child's background or type of disability, and coping is best used along with other models of practice (Williamson & Szczepanski, 1999).

Coping is a feature of the adaptive process. As such, coping can only occur as part of the interaction between the child and the context, which includes the people, objects, and settings for performance. There is a level of stress that accompanies these interactions that stimulates the child to act; children learn coping strategies through these interactions. The stressors can be internal (e.g., anxiety, excitement, interest) or external (e.g., complexity of the physical surroundings, requests or demands for performance, changes in routines) and yet can have the same impact on the effectiveness of the coping strategies. It is through skilled observation and interviews that the therapist can uncover the features of the child, the environment, and the behavioral repertoire that relate to the coping process for the child.

The coping literature contains research about the construct of coping (Lazarus & Folkman, 1984; Zeitlin, Williamson, & Rosenblatt, 1987), but this work was not designed to address the application of these coping constructs to practice. Williamson, Szczepanski, and Zeitlin (1993) designed a model for applying the coping constructs to support better understanding of coping in children and, therefore, make it possible for these ideas to impact practice for children with disabilities. The model proposes 4 steps in the coping process. The first step involves determining the meaning of the event for the child who has internal and external stressors to contend with, some demand for action, and some skills and ideas about how to perform. As we observe these aspects of the event and the child's behavior, we might determine that the event is upsetting, challenging, or thrilling (i.e., the meaning or interpretation) for the child.

The second step is to design an action plan. This step is dependent upon the child's awareness and the actual availability of internal and external resources to support an action. Younger children tend to be more reactive related to immediate needs (e.g., I am very hungry), while older children can use their cognitive skills and life experiences to consider options for responding. The action plan that is developed is framed by the child's consideration of these resources as possible supports to solve the problem.

The third step in the coping process is to implement a coping effort. After developing a plan or options, the child must act. The authors state that the coping effort is focused on one of several intended impacts. The child might select an action that deals with the stressor directly (e.g., asks for help in getting the snack food), manages the emotions created by the stressor event (e.g., moves away from the kitchen to stop the frustration of not getting the snack food), or changes the associated physical tension (e.g., begins to play a tumbling activity to enable the body to "regroup"). Whatever actions the child takes, there will be corresponding internal feedback from the movements and external feedback from the impact of the action on the environment.

Therefore, the fourth step in the coping process is evaluating effectiveness of the coping effort. As stated above, the child receives feedback internally and externally from the coping effort. The child will tend to demonstrate positive behaviors if he or she determines that the intended outcome is reached (e.g., the stressor is reduced) or will demonstrate negative behaviors if the child perceives that the coping effort was unsuccessful (e.g., physical tension remains). When the child interprets the outcome as negative, this triggers another coping cycle. The authors point out that as more coping opportunities occur, the child accumulates information that influences his or her sense of self-efficacy and identity.

It is very important to remember that this model of coping is in relation to the child's perspective about the effectiveness of the coping effort. There are many situations in which the child's and an observing adult's decisions about the effectiveness of the coping effort will be different. A child may be delighted with the exploration of a new activity, while the adult may feel uncomfortable that the child is unable to participate "successfully" (i.e., according to some rule or standard). A child may be overwhelmed by a request deemed to be simple by the adult making the demand.

Model's Relationship to Participation

From a coping frame of reference, the demands of the activity, the setting, and the child's skills/strategies converge to enable successful participation. Therefore, children have difficulty with coping when there is a bad fit between their skills and resources and the demands of a particular situation. This condition is universal in the sense that every type of disorder or disability has the potential to acquire good or poor coping skills. Additionally, even without a disorder, we all have to manage demands with our current resources. Therefore, the behaviors that are associated with the coping model could be present in any child or even with parents or teachers with whom we work.

We would identify a child as having a challenge with coping when the child is unable to meet the demands of daily life. This could manifest itself in many ways. A child could simply not be able to get ready for the day or could demonstrate frustration over the requirements for getting ready (e.g., saying "the toothpaste is too hard to squeeze" or throwing it down). The child could appear active but be ineffectual in the morning routine or could express negativity regarding self or the ability to be successful (e.g., "I can not..."). The child could also demonstrate rigidity in behavior and performance as an indicator of poor coping skills.

Evidence About the Model

Scholars in related disciplines have studied the features of coping. Researchers have found a relationship between self-concept, academic achievement, and coping skills in children with and without disabilities (DiBuono, 1982; Kennedy, 1984). Zeitlin (1985) reported relationships between coping behaviors and a child's sense of personal mastery. Generally, children with disabilities have inferior coping strategies when compared to their peers without disabilities (Lorch, 1981; Yeargan, 1982). Children in poor socioeconomic conditions also demonstrate less success in coping than do their peers with better socioeconomic conditions (Brooks-Gunn & Furstenberg, 1987). In a series of studies conducted by Williamson, Zeitlin, and Szczepanski (1989) and Zeitlin and Williamson (1990), they found consistent differences between infants and toddlers with and without disabilities. They comment that although both groups had wide ranges of performance capabilities, the children with disabilities seemed "...more vulnerable to the stress of daily living" (p. 406). This may be due to having fewer internal resources (e.g., because of the neuromuscular system working less effectively) or the reduced capacity of external resources due to high caregiving demands (Turnbull & Turnbull, 1990).

Other authors have pointed out the critical role that families play in the coping process. Following up with at-risk populations, Zeitlin, Williamson, and Rosenblatt (1987) designed a counseling model to support families with children who had disabilities. They demonstrated success at infusing more adaptable coping strategies into these family constellations.

More recent applications of coping models address contextual factors in participation. For example, studying elementary school-aged children, researchers found that anxiety is related to asking for social support and that anger is associated with externalizing the situation (Vierhaus & Lohaus, 2009). Mayr and Ulich (2009) identified 6 dimensions of well-being that include coping: social contact, self-control, assertiveness, coping, task orientation, and pleasure in exploring. Others have taken the coping literature and created interventions to assist children in gaining insights about what they can learn from challenging situations (Borders, 2009). Woolfson and Brady (2009) examined coping with teachers who had students with learning difficulties and found that teacher experience and professional development did not contribute to attitudes, but self-efficacy was a positive predictor of how a teacher viewed a student, and sympathy was a negative predictor. So you can see that there are many interdisciplinary applications of this model.

Intervention Approach Using the Model

The primary focus for intervention when using a coping practice model is to find the best match between the child's resources and the demands of the environment. When there is a better match, children can be available for learning (just as the biomechanical practice model provides external supports to reduce impact of gravity, enabling the child to interact). There must be a "just right" challenge before the child; when the challenge is too simple, a "stressor" is not created and the child does not have to call upon coping resources. When the challenge is too great, the child becomes overwhelmed and cannot interact or interacts inappropriately, creating more stress.

There are 3 categories of emphasis for intervention using the coping practice model (Williamson, Szczepanski, & Zeitlin, 1993). Other models of practice provide guidance about the many ways that therapists can design changes to support a child's work toward more effective coping.

We can modify the demands placed on the child. The environment has many features that can be adjusted to become more consistent with a particular child's abilities. We can remove extra objects that might be distracting or emotionally upsetting, or we can create and demonstrate more simplified directions. The cognitive practice model offers ways to adjust strategies for children with varying cognitive abilities.

Second, we can improve the child's resources for coping. This can include the child establishing more skills or redesigning the environment to make possibilities more available. The sensory integrative practice model provides guidance about how to enhance a child's sensory processing abilities to be able to notice salient stimuli and screen out other stimuli; both strategies would enhance coping.

Third, we can ensure the child receives and interprets feedback. For coping to improve, the child must be able to derive meaning from the changes in self and environment that occur with coping efforts. First, we must attend to the child recognizing the feedback, then to interpreting it, and, finally, to generalizing the feedback for new events. The behavioral practice model offers insights about how to create more salience in feedback.

We can also consider strategies for addressing the coping skills of the adults who care for the children, primarily the teachers and the parents. As stated earlier, Woolfson and Brady (2009) found that teachers with self-efficacy were more likely to have positive coping related to students with learning challenges; perhaps we can advocate for students to be placed with teachers who have positive coping on their behalf.

The Behavioral Practice Model

Overview of the Model: Core Principles

The behavioral practice model has emerged from social sciences and includes cognitive learning and social interaction theoretical constructs. A core concept in the behavioral perspective is that all behavior is learned; this learning is based on the child's capacities (including developmental level, skill development, cognitive ability), the child's drive to engage or perform, the situation or environment, the demands for learning and performance, and the feedback or support for the behavior or performance (Bruce & Borg, 1987). Like the developmental model, many disciplines study the behavioral model, so this model provides another common ground for understanding children's needs and potential interventions.

The behavioral literature is concerned with learning and what supports learning to occur. From a behavioral point of view, we consider the characteristics of the desired behavior, the stimulus for the desired behavior (sometimes called the "antecedent behavior" or "cue"), and the reinforcement for the desired behavior (sometimes called the "subsequent event"). We want the cue to trigger the desired behavior, and we want to provide a reinforcer just after the desired behavior to encourage this desired behavior to occur more often. We also want to reduce undesirable behaviors or inappropriate uses of the desired behavior; in this case, we ignore the behavior (called "extinguishing") (Bruce & Borg, 1993).

Both reinforcing and extinguishing are ways to provide feedback. For example, if the teacher wishes for children to be quiet when she turns off the lights, she would turn the lights off (cue), watch for some children to be quiet (desired behavior), and say, "I am so proud of Thomas and Marsha for being quiet when I turn the lights off" (reinforcer), while also ignoring children who continue to talk (extinguishing).

We must be aware of the features of the cue or stimulus, and which of these features are salient to the desired behavior. In the above example, the teacher wishes for the lights going off to be the salient cue; however, in order for the lights to go off, she must be standing in a particular location in the room (e.g., by the door where the light switch is located). One arm is probably going to be in an upward bending pattern to reach the switch. If a child focuses in on these features, the child may get quiet every time the teacher goes toward the door or raises her hand to point, thereby missing the cue of interest to the teacher (i.e., the lights off). Another child may be oblivious to the teacher's behavior and may only get quiet when a peer pokes him or her (the peer notices the correct cues). In this case, the child would begin to pair being quiet with the peer behavior; therefore, if the peer is moved or absent, the child's behavior will be inappropriate.

Second, we must understand what is reinforcing to the person whose behavior we wish to change. In our classroom example, the teacher is counting on her positive attention to be desirable to the children (and therefore "reinforcing"). For a child who does not care about the teacher's approval, her praise will have no effect on being quiet. If there is a shy child in the room, the child may not wish to be "singled out" by the teacher and, therefore, may find ways to avoid this attention. We must take the time to find out what is reinforcing to the person we are serving and construct our reinforcement to meet that person's needs and desires if we want a behavioral approach to improve behavior.

Model's Relationship to Participation

The behavioral and coping models of practice both consider the relationship between the person's behavioral repertoire and participation, rather than focusing on the factors associated with diagnoses or conditions. Therefore, anyone can be a candidate for the behavioral practice model if they have behaviors that interfere with successful performance or if they lack needed behaviors to participate. Because of the intimate relationship between behaviors and the context for performance, most applications of the behavioral model will be environmentally specific (i.e., the dysfunctional behavior may only be present in certain environments). Behaviorism is not concerned with the internal or past reasons for a person's dysfunctional behavior, unlike psychoanalytic approaches that might address one's earlier experiences or one's feelings about what is happening. The behavioral practice model considers that dysfunction is in relation to the environment (e.g., poor cues for behavior or lack of reinforcement for the precise behavior of interest).

Evidence About the Model

During the 1970s, there was a period of rapid expansion of behavioral practice model ideas. A corresponding number of authors in occupational therapy reported on the effective application of behavioral principles to improve outcomes in people who have disabilities (Ford, 1975; Jodrell & Sanson-Fisher, 1975; Leibowitz & Holcer, 1974; Lemke & Mitchell, 1972; Ogburn, Fast, & Tiffany, 1972; Weber, 1978; Wehman & Marchant, 1978). These studies investigated the effectiveness of behavioral applications for work outcomes, learning, play, socialization, and skill development. Stein (1982) provides a review of the application of the behavioral strategies within occupational therapy as well. In the 1990s, there was less emphasis on studying the impact of behaviorism within occupational therapy practice, but the application of behaviorism within intervention programming is prevalent (Bruce & Borg, 1993). Behaviorism has grown as a discipline in the past two decades, and much of the current work comes out of behavioral psychology and interdisciplinary research entities. Odom and Karnes (1988) provide an excellent resource for some of the seminal work; if you anticipate working on an interdisciplinary team with a behavioral paradigm, I recommend you become familiar with this and other related works. Ask a colleague who is a behavioral specialist to provide you with the most current material.

Intervention Approach Using the Model

Behaviorism is concerned with getting rid of behaviors that interfere with successful performance and increasing the number and complexity of behaviors that are functional for the child and family in daily life (Bruce & Borg, 1993). The behavior and coping models of practice share an intervention feature also; both are appropriate models of practice to use as complementary models with other perspectives. This is helpful when we work on interdisciplinary teams. Other team members may be familiar with the behavioral model, but not with a more traditional occupational therapy practice model, such as sensory integration. When we can converse in a language that is familiar to our colleagues, we create common ground for more refined intervention planning.

We must recognize ways to build behavioral schemas. Many times, children do not have the behaviors they need in their repertoire, and so we must find ways to reinforce the child along the way to learning the desired skill. One strategy is to "shape" the behavior; this means that we reinforce behaviors that are approximations of the desired behavior and systematically increase the preciseness needed for reinforcement. For example, if we want a child to wash her face, we may initially praise her for getting water on her face, then for rubbing over the whole face, and, finally, for using soap in the routine. Another strategy is called "chaining." In this procedure, we recognize the smaller steps in a complex task and construct reinforcers for each part. For young children, it is often best to begin with the last step so the child can feel the sense of accomplishment and then move to involvement with earlier parts. For example, when learning to tie shoes, children get discouraged by the complexity and give up before their shoes are tied; when parents have to finish the job, the children have no sense of having participated. If, however, the parent does all the early steps and involves the child in pulling the loops at the end, the reinforcement can be paired with "tying your shoes." The parent then slowly involves the child in earlier steps until the child is doing the whole job alone.

We must also recognize ways to sustain desirable behaviors. It is unreasonable to think of constructing a child's life so that the child will receive reinforcement from you each time a task, or portion of a task, is completed. Additionally, with an "every time" reinforcement schedule, the child's behavior can deteriorate very quickly without the reinforcer. Less frequent reinforcement and unpredictable (i.e., "intermittent") reinforcement schedules actually lead to more sustained behavioral patterns. When a child does not know when he will get a sticker for his homework, he will do it more often than if he knows he will get one every time. Intermittent reinforcement provides a mechanism for the child to internalize the behavior and a sense of accomplishment.

The Cognitive Practice Model

Overview of the Model: Core Principles

The cognitive practice model originates from work in psychology, education, medicine, and neuroscience. In all of these fields, professionals have been fascinated with the way the brain is organized and how it receives, interprets, and uses information. There are a number of theories about how the cognitive processes work; they are not so much conflicting with each other as emphasizing different aspects of the evolution and use of cognitive abilities (Bruce & Borg, 1993). From an information processing perspective, the person receives input from sensory channels, processes this information (and stores aspects in memory), and produces a response based on the interpretation. You will notice that this way of describing processing is similar to the way that the sensory processing practice model describes it; this is because both of these models of practice are based in neuroscience. The difference between these models of practice lies in their chosen emphasis of interest, which also leads to different ideas for intervention planning. The information processing perspective leads us toward a consideration of knowledge, memory, problem solving, and methods of processing, while the sensory integration perspective leads us toward a consideration of the receipt and meaning of sensory events for developing responses. Occupational therapy, psychology, and education are the team disciplines most likely to have studied the cognitive model and, therefore, can use this common ground for intervention planning.

Within information processing models, scholars discuss the content of knowledge as declarative (facts, concepts, ideas) and procedural (processes, actions). People use declarative knowledge as content for their procedural knowledge; procedural knowledge advances an interest or cause. When the person faces a problem, the person must call upon the relationships developed among the declarative and procedural information available to organize thinking and identify possible strategies. Each person finds particular strategies more (or less) helpful. For example, some people use post-it notes as a cueing strategy for tasks, while others might find all those "flags" on their work distracting.

As people gain insight about what works for them, their problem-solving ability improves because they do not spend effort considering or trying ineffectual approaches. In the past decade, cognitive psychologists termed this process of gaining insights *metacognition*. Metacognition is the ability to think about what you are or have thought about; it is a process of considering your own perspective and deciding about the wisdom of it. The reflective nature of metacognition facilitates growth and enables people to consider others' points of view. It also enables individuals learning new knowledge and skills to receive explicit guidance about their own learning from a teacher, coach, or therapist.

A complementary perspective on the cognitive practice model is the structural perspective (Bruce & Borg, 1993). You are probably familiar with the work of Jean Piaget; he describes an evolutionary process that supports the development of cognitive skills. He discusses assimilation (i.e., the process of taking new information into the current cognitive structures) and accommodations (i.e., the process of revising and advancing one's cognitive structures due to increasing awareness of differences and complexities that will not fit into the current way of thinking). Throughout the developmental period, individuals use assimilation and accommodation to incorporate information into their cognitive structures. The developmental nature of this perspective enriches the cognitive practice model application options because it points out the discovery aspects of cognitive development. Bruce and Borg (1993) provide a very good summary of cognitive development.

Model's Relationship to Participation

Within the cognitive practice model, participation is related to how the brain processes information for use in daily life demands. In traditional views, cognitive models were related to frank disruption in the brain structures, making cognitive centers of the brain inaccessible or inoperative (as with brain injury) or more subtle brain dysfunction (e.g., learning disability or attention deficit hyperactivity disorder). More contemporary cognitive approaches include consideration of environmental and task demands that may be so great that they surpass the person's ability (Kielhofner, 2009). Occupational therapy researchers have developed cognitive assessments for adults (e.g., Abreu & Toglia, 1987), but it is more common to have formal cognitive assessments for children from interdisciplinary team members (e.g., measures of intelligence and psychoeducational abilities); therapists can derive insights from these findings. However, as occupational therapists, we identify cognitive contributions to participation most frequently as we observe and interact with children in daily life activities. This is vital information for the team because it represents the "operationalizing" of cognitive abilities. Sometimes children can demonstrate isolated cognitive skills, but cannot use those skills when needed. This must be part of the team's information for planning.

For example, the therapist observes an adolescent in home economics class and sees that the student can clean up after cooking but places objects in the wrong places (e.g., puts the cups in the refrigerator, bowls with ingredients with the clean dishes). The therapist might also report that the student can follow single directions, but cannot put them in the right order (e.g., puts the cheese on the griddle and then butters the bread). These observations can shed light on the student's ability to use cognitive abilities in a daily routine. These are applied cognition errors in performance that indicate the adolescent's difficulty with perceptual skills, organization, and sequencing—all cognitive processes.

Evidence About the Model

Studies in occupational therapy intervention indicate that there is a relationship between cognitive capacity and self-care performance in adults who have had a stroke (Bernspang, Viitanen, & Ericksson, 1989; Carter, Oliveira, Duponte, & Lynch, 1988). However, we do not know whether a self-care performance approach or a cognitive approach would be most effective in intervention.

For those of us who work with children and families, the literature has provided us with data validating the relationship between cognitive and perceptual difficulties and various disabilities (Goodgold-Edwards & Cermak, 1990; Menken, Cermak, & Fisher, 1987; O'Brien, Cermak, & Murray, 1988); but there also is a paucity of occupational therapy literature on effectiveness of cognitive interventions with children. Cognitive effectiveness literature is more commonly found in the education and psychology arenas. Educators are particularly likely to use cognitive models of practice in their styles of teaching along with other models of practice (e.g., behavioral, developmental). For example, Spence (1994) reported that younger children benefit less from cognitive approaches than older children, perhaps due to evolving cognitive ability. A confounding variable in these studies is that cognitive and behavioral strategies are used together, making it difficult to identify the effects of each model on the outcomes (Spence, 1994). Prout and Prout (1998) conducted a meta-analysis of cognitive approaches used in counseling in public schools and found that these interventions were more effective in groups. When combined with behavioral strategies, the best effects were found on the children's reporting of their improved internal state.

Intervention Approach Using the Model

The cognitive approach to intervention in occupational therapy is multifaceted and based on the premises that the brain is plastic, engagement in occupational performance can enhance brain organization, and adaptations can minimize the effects of cognitive impairments (Kielhofner, 1992). Authors also discuss the need to consider perception, attention, memory, problem solving, and generalization (Abreu & Toglia, 1987; Todd, 1993). Many of the scholars in occupational therapy who investigate cognition are concerned with adult populations (Abreu & Peloquin, 2005; Allen, 1992; Giles, 2005; Toglia, 2005). Polatajko and Mandich (2005) apply cognitive knowledge to the needs of children with Developmental Coordination Disorder (DCD) with an approach called Cognitive Orientation to Occupational Performance (CO-OP). Kielhofner (2009) provides a summary table of the cognitive interventions used in the occupational therapy literature. Katz (2005) is an excellent resource for the application of cognitive models in occupational therapy across the lifespan.

The CO-OP intervention is a problem-solving approach that enables children to select their goals and to plan systematically to meet these goals. The therapist guides the child through the process of discovery to figure out what works and what does not work as they strive together to accomplish what the goals reflect. The sequence is called "goal-plan-do-check" to reflect the process we guide the student through to determine effective strategies to improve participation. In studies, researchers have shown that CO-OP is effective at improving participation (Missiuna, 2001).

Another application of the cognitive model is cognitive behavioral therapy (CBT), which is based on the cognitive theories. CBT is based on the idea that a person's perspective about a situation determines the reactions rather than the actual situation. The basic assumptions of CBT include (1) how we think about a situation affects how we act; (2) we can be aware of how we think; and (3) when we think differently, we can behave differently (Dobson & Dozois, 2010; Taylor, 2006). CBT has been extensively studied, primarily with adults who have the capacity to reflect on their own thoughts, behaviors, and experiences. Concepts of CBT are applied within family systems and school-based therapy programs by anchoring behaviors of concern to the ways that families, teachers, and children think about the situations in which the behaviors occur. It is not common in community-based practice with children to follow the precise regimen of CBT. Let's look at a simple example.

Tom believes that the teacher does not like him. A CBT perspective would say that this perception can affect the child's behavior. Perhaps this particular teacher expects certain behaviors that are challenging for the child (staying in the seat and working). The teacher may only be reminding the child about the expectation ("Remember Tom, you need to stay in your seat during work time"), while the child sees this reminder as a reminder that the teacher does not like him. If Tom acts based on his belief, he might blow up in class at a simple reminder, rather than simply adjusting his behavior based on the reminder. CBT intervenes to change the pattern of perception that leads to negative behaviors, so that situations can be evaluated more realistically. The teacher might talk to Tom and discuss what other things happen in the school day that indicate she likes him, or she might make a more explicit list of her expectations of all students so Tom can observe that she corrects everyone on these particular behaviors to support him to see more aspects of the situation.

Because the occupational therapist's unique contribution to the team is an awareness of performance in daily life, intervention to change the impact of cognitive difficulties on performance is critical (Kielhofner, 1992). The occupational therapist can design adaptations to minimize the effects of cognitive limitations (e.g., placing cues around the bedroom about the morning routine to minimize the effects of memory loss on efficiency), design restorative interventions to improve cognitive abilities (e.g., working on alternating attention in the kitchen by making the person prepare lunch and fold the laundry), or find activities or environments with demands that are more congruent with the person's current cognitive abilities (e.g., working with the teacher to select a better-matched reading group). It is our expertise at translating cognitive data about a person into the impact on his or her life that is extremely valuable to families and educators.

Summary

Occupational therapists serving children and families in community practice engage in several processes so others can have confidence in their work. First, we employ a systematic thinking process, called clinical reasoning, which ensures that we consider all relevant areas of the person's life. We also work within occupational therapy theories that contain the core constructs of occupational therapy practice. Then, as we think about the participation challenges, we use contemporary conceptual models of practice, which provide a structure for planning evidence-based interventions. Each practice model emphasizes different aspects of person, context, and participation and so support different needs. Knowing about these theories and models provides a mechanism to link decision-making to evidence-based practices.

References

Abreu, B., & Peloquin, S. (2005). The quadraphonic approach: A holistic rehabilitation model for brain injury. In N. Katz (Ed.), *Cognition and occupation across the life span: models for intervention in occupational therapy* (2nd ed.) (p. 73-112). Bethesda, MD: American Occupational Therapy Association Press.

Abreu, B., & Toglia, J. (1987). Cognitive rehabilitation: A model for occupational therapy. *American Journal of Occupational Therapy, 41*, 439.

Adams, J. (1971). A closed loop theory of motor learning. *Journal of Motor Behavior, 3*, 110-150.

Allen, C. (1992). Cognitive disabilities. In N. Katz (Ed.), *Cognitive rehabilitation: Models for intervention in occupational therapy* (p. 1-21). Boston, MA: Andover Medical.

Almli, R., & Finger, S. (1988). Toward a definition of recovery of function. In T. LeVere, R. Almli, & D. Stein (Eds.), *Brain injury and recovery: Theoretical and controversial issues* (pp. 1-4). New York, NY: Plenum Press.

American Occupational Therapy Association. (1994). Uniform terminology for occupational therapy—Third edition. *American Journal of Occupational Therapy, 48*, 1047–1054.

American Occupational Therapy Association. (2008). Occupational therapy practice framework: Domain and process (2nd ed.). *American Journal of Occupational Therapy, 62*, 625-683.

Ayres, J. (1963). The development of perceptual motor abilities: A theoretical basis for treatment of dysfunction. *American Journal of Occupational Therapy, 17*, 221-225.

Ayres, A. (1972). *Sensory integration and learning disorders*. Los Angeles, CA: Western Psychological Services.

Ayres, A., & Marr, D. (1991). Sensory integration and praxis tests. In A. Fisher, E. Murray, & A. Bundy (Eds.), *Sensory integration: Theory and practice* (p. 203). Philadelphia, PA: F. A. Davis.

Bach-y-Rita, P., & Balliet, R. (1987). Recovery from stroke. In P. Duncan & M. Badke (Eds.), *Stroke rehabilitation: The recovery of motor control* (pp. 79-107). Chicago, IL: Yearbook Medical Publishers.

Baranek, G. T. (2002). Efficacy of sensory and motor interventions for children with autism. *Journal of Autism and Developmental Disorders, 32*(5), 397-422.

Ben-Sasson, A., Cermak, S., Orsmond, G., Tager-Flusberg, H., Carter, A., Kadlec, M., & Dunn, W. (2007). Extreme sensory modulation behaviors in toddlers with autism spectrum disorders. *American Journal of Occupational Therapy, 61*(5), 584-592.

Bernspang, B., Viitanen, M., & Ericksson, S. (1989). Impairments of perceptual and motor functions: Their influence on self-care ability 4 to 6 years after stroke. *Occupational Therapy Journal of Research, 9*, 27.

Bernstein, N. (1967). *The coordination and regulation of movement*. London, England: Pergamon Press.

Bilodeau, E., Bilodeau, I., & Schumsky, D. (1959). Some effects of introducing and withdrawing knowledge of results early and late in practice. *Journal of Experimental Psychology*, 142-144.

Bly, L. (1980). Abnormal motor development. In D. Slaton (Ed.), *Development of movement in infancy*. Chapel Hill, NC: University of North Carolina at Chapel Hill.

Bly, L. (1991). A historical and current view of the basis of NDT Pediatric. *Physical Therapy, 3*, 131-135.

Bobath, B. (1971). Motor development, its effect on general development and application to the treatment of cerebral palsy. *Physiotherapy, 57*, 526-532.

Borders, M. (2009). Project hero: A goal setting and healthy decision making program. *Journal of School Health, 79*(5), 239-243.

Breslin, D. (1996). Motor learning theory and the neurodevelopmental treatment approach: A comparative analysis. *Occupational Therapy in Health Care, 10*(1), 25-40.

Brooks-Gunn, J., & Furstenberg, F. (1987). Continuity and change in the context of poverty: Adolescent mothers and their children. In J. Gallagher & C. Ramsey (Eds.), *The malleability of children* (pp. 171-188). Baltimore, MD: Paul H. Brookes Publishing.

Brown, C , Tollefson, N , Dunn, W., Cromwell, R., & Filion, D. (2002). Sensory processing in schizophrenia: Missing and avoiding information. *Schizophrenia Research, 55*(1-2), 187-195.

Brown, C., & Dunn, W. (2002). *The adult sensory profile*. San Antonio, TX: Psychological Corporation.

Bruce, M., & Borg, B. (1987). *Frames of reference in psychosocial occupational therapy*. Thorofare, NJ: SLACK Incorporated.

Bruce, M., & Borg, B. (1993). *Psychosocial occupational therapy: Frames of reference for intervention* (2nd ed.). Thorofare, NJ: SLACK Incorporated.

Carlsen, P. N. (1975).Comparison of two occupational therapy approaches for treating the young cerebral-palsied child. *Am J Occup Ther, 29*, 268-272.

Carter, L., Oliveira, D. O., Duponte, J., & Lynch, S. U. (1988). The relationship of cognitive skills performance to activities of daily living in stroke patients. *American Journal of Occupational Therapy, 42*, 449.

Catalano, J., & Kleiner, B. (1984). Distant transfer and practice variability. *Perceptual and Motor Skills, 58*, 851-856.

Christiansen, C., & Baum, C. (1997). *Occupational therapy: Enabling function and well-being* (2nd ed.). Thorofare, NJ: SLACK Incorporated.

Clark, F., Mailloux, Z., & Parham, D. (1985). Sensory integration and children with learning disabilities. In P. Clark & A. Allen (Eds.), *Occupational therapy for children* (p. 384). St. Louis, MO: C.V. Mosby.

Colangelo, C. (1999). The biomechanical frame of reference. In P. Kramer & J. Hinojosa (Eds.), *Frames of reference for pediatric occupational therapy* (2nd ed.) (pp. 257-322). Baltimore, MD: Williams & Wilkins, Inc.

Compas, B. (1997). Coping with stress during childhood and adolescence. *Psychological Bulletin, 101*, 393-403.

Corbett, B., Schupp, C., Levine, S., & Mendoza, S. (2009). Comparing cortisol, stress & sensory sensitivity in children with autism. *Autism Research, 2*(1), 39-49.

Daniels, L., Sparling, J., Reilly, M., & Humphry, R. (1995). Use of assistive technology with young children with severe and profound disabilities. *Infant Toddler Intervention, 5*(1), 91-112.

d'Avignon, M. (1981). Early physiotherapy ad modum Vojta or Bobath in infants with suspected neuromotor disturbance. *Neuropediatrics, 12*(3), 232-241.

DeGrace, B. (2007). The occupational adaptation model: application to child and family interventions. In: Dunbar, S. (Ed.), *Occupational therapy models for intervention with children and families*. Thorofare, NJ: SLACK Incorporated.

DiBuono, E. (1982). *A comparison of the self-concept and coping skills of learning disabled and non-handicapped pupils in self-contained classes, resource rooms and regular classes* [Dissertation]. West Covina, CA: Walden University.

Dobson, K., & Dozois, D. (2010). Historical and philosophical bases of the cognitive-behavioral therapies. In K. Dobson (Ed.), *Handbook of cognitive behavioural therapies* (3rd ed.). New York, NY: The Guilford Press.

Dove, S., & Dunn, W. (2009). Sensory processing patterns in learning disabilities. *Occupational Therapy in Early Intervention, Preschool and Schools, 2*(1), 1-11.

Dunbar, S. (2007). *Occupational therapy models for intervention with children and families*. Thorofare, NJ: SLACK Incorporated.

Dunn, W. (1997). The impact of sensory processing abilities on the daily lives of young children and families: A conceptual model. *Infants and Young Children, 9*(4), 23-35.

Dunn, W. (1999). *Sensory profile manual*. San Antonio, TX: The Psychological Corporation.

Dunn, W. (2001). The sensations of everyday life: theoretical, conceptual and pragmatic considerations. *American Journal of Occupational Therapy, 55*(6), 608-620.

Dunn, W. (2002). *The infant toddler sensory profile*. San Antonio, TX: Psychological Corporation.

Dunn, W. (2006a). *School companion sensory profile manual*. San Antonio, TX: The Psychological Corporation.

Dunn, W. (2006b). *Sensory profile supplement*. San Antonio, TX: The Psychological Corporation.

Dunn, W. (2007). Ecology of human performance model. In Dunbar, S. (Ed.), *Occupational therapy models for intervention with children and families*. Thorofare, NJ: SLACK Incorporated.

Dunn, W. (2009). *Sensory processing concepts and applications to practice* [CD]. Rockville, MD: American Occupational Therapy Association.

Dunn, W. (2010). Sensory processing: Tools for supporting young children in everyday life. In S. Maude (Ed.), *Proven Strategies and Instructional Practices in EI/ECSC* (Vol. 2). Santa Barbara, CA: Praeger.

Dunn, W., & Bennett, D. (2002). Patterns of sensory processing in children with attention deficit hyperactivity disorder. *Occupational Therapy Journal of Research, 22*(1), 4-15.

Dunn, W., & Brown, C. (1997). Factor analysis on the Sensory Profile from a national sample of children without disabilities. *American Journal of Occupational Therapy, 51*(7), 490-495.

Dunn, W., Brown, C., McClain, L., & Westman, K. (1994). Ecology of human performance: A framework for thought and action. In C. B. Royeen (Ed.), *ATOT self study series on occupation*. Bethesda, MD: American Occupational Therapy Association.

Dunn, W., Brown, C., & McGuigan, A. (1994). The ecology of human performance: A framework for thought and action. *American Journal of Occupational Therapy, 48*(7), 595-607.

Dunn, W., Brown, C., & Youngstrom, M. (2003). Ecological model of occupation. In P. Kramer, J. Hinojosa, & C. Royeen (Eds.), *Perspectives in human occupation: Participation in life*. Baltimore, MD: Lippincott, Williams & Wilkins.

Dunn, W., Myles, B., & Orr, S. (2002). Sensory processing issues associated with Asperger Syndrome: A preliminary investigation. *American Journal of Occupational Therapy, 56*(1), 97-102.

Dunn, W., Saiter, J., & Rinner, L. (2002). Asperger Syndrome and Sensory Processing: A conceptual model and guidance for intervention planning. *Focus on Autism and other Developmental Disabilities, 17*(3), 172-185.

Dunn, W., & Westman, K. (1997). The sensory profile: The performance of a national sample of children without disabilities. *American Journal of Occupational Therapy, 51*(1), 25-34.

Ermer, J., & Dunn, W. (1998). The Sensory Profile: A discriminant analysis of children with and without disabilities. *American Journal of Occupational Therapy, 52*(4), 283-290.

Fisher, A. (1998). Uniting practice and theory in an occupational framework. *American Journal of Occupational Therapy, 52*, 509-520.

Fisher, A., Murray, E., & Bundy, A. (1991). *Sensory integration theory and practice*. Philadelphia, PA: F. A. Davis Company.

Ford, A. (1975). Teaching dressing skills to a severely retarded child. *American Journal of Occupational Therapy, 29*(2), 87-92.

Forssberg, H., Grillner, S., & Rossignol, S. (1975). Phase dependent reflex reversal during walking in chronic spinal cats. *Brain Research, 85*, 103-107.

Forsyth, K., Salamy, M., Simon, S., & Kielhofner, G. (1998). *A user's guide to the assessment of communication and interaction skills (ACIS)*. Bethesda, MD: American Occupational Therapy Association.

Gibson, J. (1966). *The senses considered as perceptual systems*. Boston, MA: Houghton Mifflin.

Giles, G. (2005). A neurofunctional approach to rehabilitation following severe brain injury. In N. Katz (Ed.), *Cognition and occupation across the life span: Models for intervention in occupational therapy* (2nd ed.) (pp. 139-165). Bethesda, MD: American Occupational Therapy Association Press.

Giuffrida, C. (2003). Motor control theories and models guiding occupational performance intervention: Principles and assumptions. In E. Crepeau, E. Cohn, & B. Schell (Eds.), *Willard and Spackman's occupational therapy* (10th ed.) (pp. 587-594). Philadelphia, PA: Lippincott Williams & Wilkins.

Goodgold-Edwards, S., & Cermak, S. (1990). Integrating motor control and motor learning concepts with neuropsychological perspectives on apraxia and developmental dyspraxia. *American Journal of Occupational Therapy, 44*, 431.

Greene, P. (1972). Problems of organization of motor systems. In R. Rosen & F. Snell (Eds.), *Progress in theoretical biology* (pp. 304-338). San Diego, CA: Academic Press.

Hainsworth, F., Harrison, M., Sheldon, T., & Roussounis, S. (1997). A preliminary evaluation of ankle orthoses in the management of children with cerebral palsy. *Developmental Medicine and Child Neurology, 39*(4), 243-247.

Held, J. (1987). Recovery of function after brain damage: Theoretical implications for therapeutic intervention. In J. Carr, R. Shepherd (Eds.), *Movement sciences: Foundations for physical therapy in rehabilitation* (pp. 155-177). Rockville, MD: Aspen Systems.

Jodrell, R., & Sanson-Fisher, R. (1975). Basic concepts of behavior therapy: An experiment involving disturbed adolescent girls. *American Journal of Occupational Therapy, 29*(10), 620-624.

Jonsdottir, J., Fetter, L., & Kluzik, J. (1997). Effects of physical therapy on postural control in children with cerebral palsy. *Pediatric Physical Therapy, 9*(2), 68-75.

Kandel, E., Schwartz, J., & Jessell, T. (2000). *Principles of neural science* (3rd ed.). New York, NY: Elsevier.

Kaplan, M., & Bedell, G. (1999). Motor skill acquisition frame of reference. In P. Kramer & J. Hinojosa (Eds.), *Frames of reference for pediatric occupational therapy* (2nd ed.) (pp. 401-430). Baltimore, MD: Williams & Wilkins, Inc.

Katz, N. (Ed.) (2005). *Cognition and occupation across the life span: models for intervention in occupational therapy* (2nd ed.). Bethesda, MD: American Occupational Therapy Association Press.

Kennedy, B. (1984). *The relationship of coping behaviors and attribution of success to effort and school achievement of elementary school children* [Dissertation]. Albany, NY: State University of New York.

Kielhofner, G. (1992). *Conceptual foundations of occupational therapy*. Philadelphia, PA: F. A. Davis Company.

Kielhofner, G. (2009). *Conceptual foundations of occupational therapy practice*. Philadelphia, PA: F. A. Davis Company.

Kielhofner, G., & Burke, J. (1980). A model of human occupation, part one. Conceptual framework and content. *American Journal of Occupational Therapy, 34*, 572-581.

Kielhofner, G., Forsyth, K., & Barrett, L. (2003). The model of human occupation. In E. Crepeau, E. Cohn, & B. Schell (Eds.), *Willard & Spackman's occupational therapy* (pp. 212-219). Philadelphia, PA: Lippincott Williams & Wilkins.

Kientz, M. A., & Dunn, W. (1997). Comparison of the performance of children with and without autism on the Sensory Profile. *American Journal of Occupational Therapy, 51*(7), 530-537.

Kimball, J. (1999). Sensory integrative frame of reference. In P. Kramer & J. Hinojosa (Eds.), *Frames of reference for pediatric occupational therapy* (2nd ed.) (pp. 169-204). Baltimore, MD: Williams & Wilkins, Inc.

Kramer, J., & Bowyer, P. (2007). Application of the model of human occupation to children and family interventions. In S. Dunbar (Ed.), *Occupational therapy models for intervention with children and families*. Thorofare, NJ: SLACK Incorporated.

Kugler, P., & Turvey, M. (1987). *Information, natural law, and self-assembly of rhythmic movement*. Hillsdale, NJ: Erlbaum.

Law, M. (1991). The environment: A focus for occupational therapy. *Canadian Journal of Occupational Therapy, 58*, 171-179.

Law, M., Cadman, D., Rosenbaum, P., Walter, S., Russell, D., & Dematteo, C. (1991). Neurodevelopmental therapy and upper extremity inhibitive casing for children with cerebral palsy. *Developmental Medicine and Child Neurology, 33*, 379-387.

Law, M., Cooper, B., Stewart, D., Letts, L., Rigby, P., & Strong, S. (1994). Person-environment relations. *Work, 4*, 228-238.

Law, M., Cooper, B., Strong, S., Steward, D., Rigby, R., & Letts, L. (1996). The person-environment-occupational model: A transactive approach to occupational performance. *Canadian Journal of Occupational Therapy, 63*(1), 9-23.

Law, M., Cooper, B., Strong, S., Stewart, D., Rigby, P., & Letts, L. (1997). Theoretical contexts for the practice of occupational therapy. In C. Christiansen & C. Baum (Eds.), *Occupational therapy: Enabling function and well-being* (2nd ed.) (pp. 73-101). Thorofare, NJ: SLACK Incorporated.

Law, M., & Dunbar, S. (2007). Person environment occupation model. In S. Dunbar (Ed.), *Occupational therapy models for intervention with children and families* (pp. 27-50). Thorofare, NJ: SLACK Incorporated.

Lazarus, R., & Folkman, S. (1984). *Stress, appraisal, and coping*. New York, NY: Springer Publishing.

Leibowitz, J., & Holcer, P. (1974). Building and maintaining self-feeding skills in a retarded child. *American Journal of Occupational Therapy, 28*(9), 545-548.

Lemke, H., & Mitchell, R. (1972). A self-feeding program: Controlling the behavior of a profoundly retarded child. *American Journal of Occupational Therapy, 26*(5), 261-264.

Lilly, A., & Powell, N. (1990). Measuring the effects of neurodevelopmental treatment on the daily living skills of two children with cerebral palsy. *American Journal of Occupational Therapy, 44*(2), 139-145.

Lorch, N. (1981). *Coping behavior in preschool children with cerebral palsy* [Dissertation]. Hempstead, NY: Hofstra University.

Magnus, R. (1926). Some results of studies in the physiology of posture. *Lancet, 2*, 531-585.

Mathiowetz, V., & Bass-Haugen, J. (2002). Assessing abilities and capacities: Motor behavior. In C. A. Trombly & M. V. Radomski (Eds.), *Occupational therapy for physical dysfunction* (5th ed.) (pp. 137-159). Philadelphia, PA: Lippincott Williams & Wilkins.

Mayr, T., & Ulich, M. (2009). Social emotional well being and resilience of children in early childhood settings—PERIK: An empirically based observation scale for practitioners. *Early Years: An international Journal of Research and Development, 29*(1), 45-57.

McIntosh, D., Miller, L., Shyu,. V., & Hagerman, R. (1999). Sensory modulation disruption, electrodermal responses and functional behaviors. *Developmental Medicine and Child Neurology, 41*(9), 608-615.

Menken, C., Cermak, S., & Fisher, A. (1987). Evaluating the visual-perceptual skills of children with cerebral palsy. *American Journal of Occupational Therapy, 41*, 646.

Missiuna, C. (2001). *Children with developmental coordination disorder: Strategies for success*. Binghamton, NY: Haworth Press.

Myles, B. S., Hagiwara, T., Dunn, W., Rinner, L., Reese, M., Huggins, A., & Becker, S. (2004). Sensory issues in children with Asperger syndrome and autism. *Education and Training in Developmental Disabilities, 3*(4), 283-290.

Newell, K. (1991). Motorskill acquisition. *Annual Review of Psychology, 42*, 213-237.

O'Brien, V., Cermak, S., & Murray, E. (1988). The relationship between visual-perceptual motor abilities and clumsiness in children with and without learning disabilities. *American Journal of Occupational Therapy, 42*, 359.

Odom, S., & Karnes, M. (1988). *Early intervention for infants & children with handicap*. Baltimore, MD: Paul H. Brookes Publishing Co.

Ogburn, K., Fast, D., & Tiffany, D. (1972). The effects of reinforcing working behavior. *American Journal of Occupational Therapy, 26*(1), 32-35.

Palmer, F., Shapiro, B., Wachtel, R., Allen, M., Hiller, J., Harryman, S., Mosher, B., Meinert, C., & Capute, A. (1988). The effects of physical therapy on cerebral palsy: A controlled trial in infants with spastic diplegia. *New England Journal of Medicine, 318*, 803-808.

Pohl, P., Dunn, W., & Brown, C. (2001). The role of sensory processing in the everyday lives of older adults. *Occupational Therapy Journal of Research, 23*(3), 99-106.

Polatajko, H., & Mandich, A. (2005). Cognitive orientation to daily occupational performance with children with developmental coordination disorder. In N. Katz (Ed.), *Cognition and occupation across the life span: models for intervention in occupational therapy* (2nd ed.) (pp. 237-259). Bethesda, MD: American Occupational Therapy Association Press.

Pollock, N. (2009). Sensory integration: A review of the current state of the evidence. *OT Now, 11*(4), 6-10.

Prout, S., & Prout, H. (1998). A meta-analysis of school-based studies of counseling and psychotherapy: An update. *Journal of School Psychology, 36*(2), 121-126.

Rawlings, E., Rawlings, I., Chen, C., & Yilk, M. (1972). The facilitating effects of mental rehearsal in the acquisition of rotary pursuit tracking. *Psychonomic Science, 26*, 71-73.

Riccio, C., Nelson, D., & Bush, M. (1990). Adding purpose to the repetitive exercise of elderly women. *American Journal of Occupational Therapy, 44*, 714.

Rogers, S., Hepburn, S., & Wehner, E. (2003). Parent report of sensory symptoms in toddlers with autism and those with other developmental disorders. *Journal of Autism and Developmental Disorders, 33*(6), 631-642.

Schaaf, R., Miller, L., Seawell, D., O'Keefe, S. (2003). Children with disturbances in sensory processing: a pilot study examining the role of the parasympathetic nervous system. *American Journal of Occupational Therapy, 57*(4), 442-449.

Scherzer, A., Mike, V., & Olson, J. (1976). Physical therapy as a determinant of changes in the cerebral palsied infant. *Pediatrics, 58*, 47-51.

Schkade, J., & Schultz, S. (1992). Occupational adaptation: Toward a holistic approach for contemporary practice, part 1. *American Journal of Occupational Therapy, 46*, 829-837.

Schmidt, R. (1988). *Motor control and learning* (2nd ed.). Champaign, IL: Human Kinetics.

Schmidt, R., & Young, D. (1987). Augmented kinematic information feedback for skill learning: A new research paradigm. *Journal of Motor Behavior, 24*(3), 261-273.

Schoen, S., & Anderson, J. (1993). Neurodevelopmental treatment frame of reference. In P. Kramer & J. Hinojosa (Eds.), *Frames of reference for pediatric occupational therapy* (2nd ed.) (pp. 83-118). Baltimore, MD: Williams & Wilkins, Inc.

Sharpe, K. (1992). Comparative effects of bilateral hand splints and an elbow orthosis on stereotypic hand movements and toy play in two children with Rett's syndrome. *American Journal of Occupational Therapy, 46*(2), 134-140.

Sherrington, C. (1947). *The integrative action of the nervous system* (2nd ed.). New Haven, CT: Yale University Press.

Shumway-Cook, A., & Woollacott, M. (1995). *Motor control: Theory and practical applications*. Baltimore MD: Williams & Wilkins.

Shumway-Cook, A., & Woollacott, M. (2007). *Motor control: translating research into clinical practice* (3rd ed.). Philadelphia, PA: Lippincott Williams & Wilkins.

Singer, R. (1980). *Motor learning and human performance* (3rd ed.). New York, NY: Macmillan.

Spence, S. (1994). Practitioner review: Cognitive therapy with children and adolescents: From theory to practice. *Journal of Child Psychology and Psychiatry and Allied Disciplines, 35*(7), 1191-1228.

Stein, F. (1982). A current review of the behavioral frame of reference and its application to occupational therapy. *Occupational Therapy Mental Health, 2*(4), 35-62.

Taylor, S. (2006). The interface between cognitive behavior therapy and religion: Comment on Andersson & Asmundson. *Cognitive Behavior Therapy, 35*, 125-127.

Thelen, E., Kelso, J., & Fogel, A. (1987). Self-organizing systems and infant motor development. *Developmental Review, 7*, 39-65.

Todd, V. (1993). Visual perceptual frame of reference: an information processing approach. In P. Kramer & J. Hinojosa (Eds.), *Frames of reference for pediatric occupational therapy* (pp. 177-232). Baltimore, MD: Williams & Wilkins.

Toglia, J. (2005). A dynamic interactional approach to cognitive rehabilitation. In N. Katz (Ed.), *Cognition and occupation across the life span: models for intervention in occupational therapy* (2nd ed.) (pp. 29-72). Bethesda, MD: American Occupational Therapy Association Press.

Tomchek, S., & Dunn, W. (2007). Sensory processing in children with and without autism: A comparative study utilizing the short sensory profile. *American Journal of Occupational Therapy, 61*(2), 190-200.

Trombly, C., & Radomski, M. (Eds.) (2002). *Occupational therapy for physical dysfunction* (5th ed.). Philadelphia, PA: Lippincott Williams & Wilkins.

Turnbull, A., & Turnbull, H. (1990). *Families, professionals, and exceptionality: A special partnership* (2nd ed.). Columbus, OH: Merrill Publishing.

van Sant, A. (1987). Concepts of neural organization and movement. In B. Connolly & P. Montgomery (Eds.), *Therapeutic exercise in developmental disabilities* (pp. 1-8). Chattanooga, TN: Chattanooga Corporation.

Vierhaus, M., & Lohaus, A. (2009). Children's perception of relations between anger or anxiety and coping: Continuity and discontinuity of relational structures. *Social Development, 18*(3), 747-763.

Watling, R., Dietz, J., & White, O. (2001). Comparison of Sensory Profile scores of young children with and without autism spectrum disorders. *American Journal of Occupational Therapy, 55*(4), 416-423.

Weber, N. (1978). Chaining strategies for teaching sequenced motor tasks to mentally retarded adults. *American Journal of Occupational Therapy, 32*(6), 385-389.

Wehman, P., & Marchant, J. (1978). Improving free play skills of severely retarded children. *American Journal of Occupational Therapy, 32*(2), 100-104.

Weisz, S. (1938). Studies in equilibrium reaction. *Journal of Nervous Mental Disorders, 88*, 150-162.

Werner, E., & Smith, R. (1982). *Vulnerable but invincible: A study of resilient children*. New York, NY: McGraw-Hill.

Williamson, G., & Szczepanski, M. (1999). Coping frame of reference. In P. Kramer & J. Hinojosa (Eds.), *Frames of reference for pediatric occupational therapy* (2nd ed.) (pp. 431-468). Baltimore, MD: Williams & Wilkins.

Williamson, G., Szczepanski, M., & Zeitlin, S. (1993). Coping frame of reference. In P. Kramer & J. Hinojosa (Eds.), *Frames of reference for pediatric occupational therapy* (pp. 395-436). Baltimore, MD: Williams & Wilkins.

Williamson, G., Zeitlin, S., & Szczepanski, M. (1989). Coping behavior: Implications for disabled infants and toddlers. *Infant Mental Health Journal, 10*, 3-13.

Winstein, C. (1991). Knowledge of results and motor learning-implications for physical therapy. *Physical Therapy, 71*, 140-149.

Winstein, C., & Schmidt, R. (1990). Reduced frequency of knowledge of results enhances motor skill learning. *Journal of Experimental Psychology (Learning, Memory, and Cognition), 16*, 677-691.

Woolfson, L., & Brady, K. (2009). An investigation of factors impacting on mainstream teachers' beliefs about teaching students with learning difficulties. *Educational Psychology, 29*(2), 221-238.

Woollacott, M., & Shumway-Cook, A. (1990). Changes in posture control across the life span—A systems approach. *Physical Therapy, 70*, 799-807.

Wright, T., & Nicholson, J. (1973). Physiotherapy for the spastic child: An evaluation. *Developmental Medicine and Child Neurology, 15*, 146-163.

Yeargan, D. (1982). *A factor-analytic study of adaptive behavior and intellectual functioning in learning disabled children* [Dissertation]. Denton, TX: North Texas State University.

Zeitlin, S. (1985). *Coping inventory*. Bensenville, IL: Scholastic Testing Service.

Zeitlin, S., & Williamson, G. (1990). Coping characteristics of disabled and nondisabled young children. *American Journal of Orthopsychiatry, 60*, 404-411.

Zeitlin, S., Williamson, G., & Rosenblatt, W. (1987). The coping with stress model: A counseling approach for families with a handicapped child. *Journal of Counseling and Development, 65*, 443-446.

Workgroup on Principles and Practices in Natural Environments. (2008). Retrieved from: www.nectac.org/topics/families/families.asp

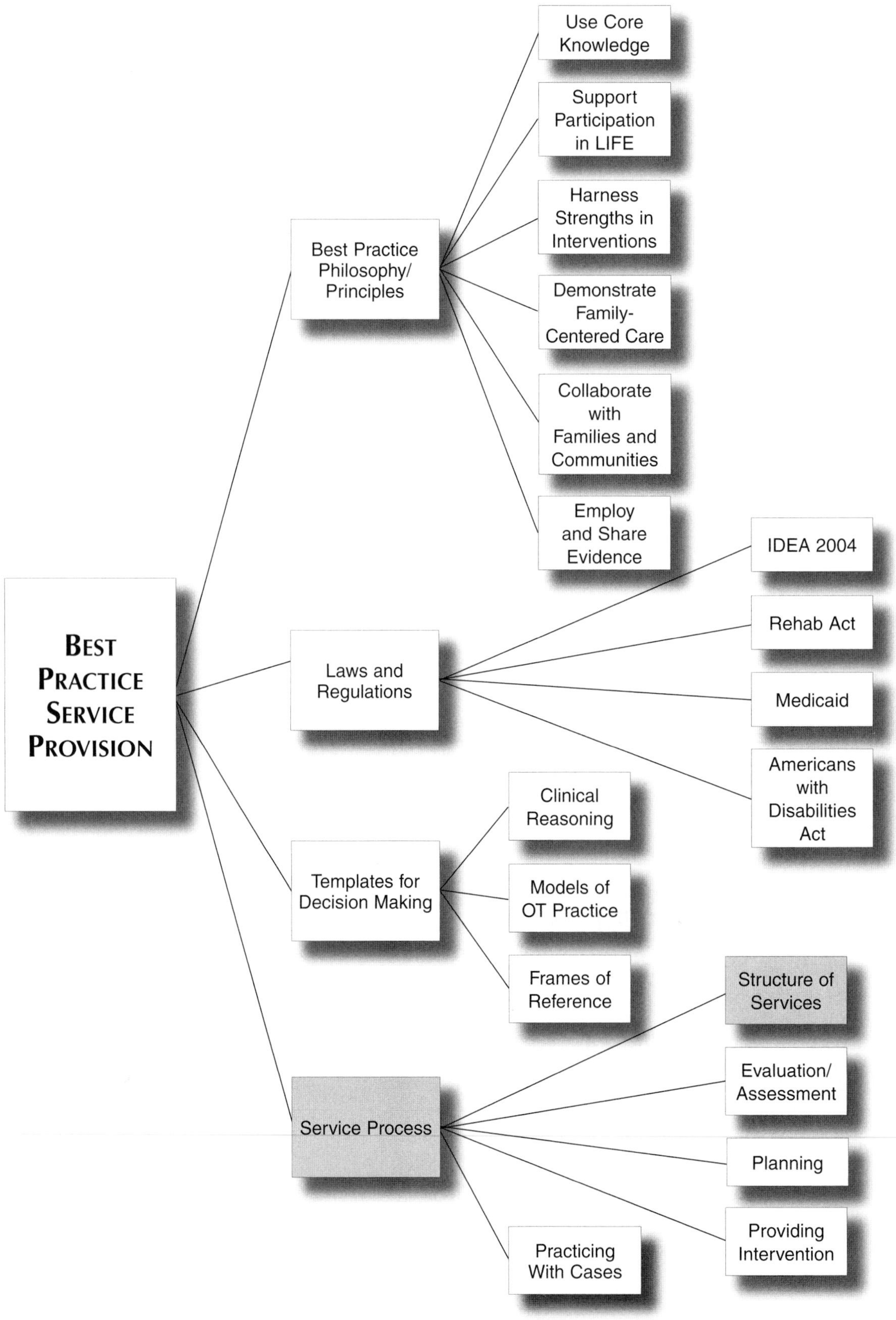

Best Practice Service Provision
Best Practice Philosophy/ Principles
Use Core Knowledge
Support Participation in LIFE
Harness Strengths in Interventions
Demonstrate Family-Centered Care
Collaborate with Families and Communities
Employ and Share Evidence
Laws and Regulations
IDEA 2004
Rehab Act
Medicaid
Americans with Disabilities Act
Templates for Decision Making
Clinical Reasoning
Models of OT Practice
Frames of Reference
Service Process
Structure of Services
Evaluation/ Assessment
Planning
Providing Intervention
Practicing With Cases

5 CHAPTER

Structure of Best Practice Programs

We can have all the laws, regulations, theories, practice models, and problem-solving processes in the world, but they all must still be situated in a structure that enables us to practice efficiently and affords families a way of understanding how to participate on their children's behalf. In this chapter, we will describe the structures for teams, occupational therapy services, and recommended communication methods to support effective community-based services.

Recognizing the Nature of Services and Professional Activities

Community-based agencies have different purposes when providing services. The purpose of early intervention is to provide services designed to meet the developmental needs of children and to build capacity of families. Public education programs are structured to provide education and related services necessary for children to benefit from education. Hospitals and other community agencies have as their missions to provide services for special purposes, such as medically related health, financial assistance, work preparation and training, or mental health programs.

Occupational therapists may be employed in any number of settings and by a wide variety of agencies. Occupational therapy services provided under that agency's administration and financing must be aligned with the purpose of the agency. For example, services provided in public education settings enable children to benefit from educational opportunities. Therefore, in the school setting, it is only appropriate to address the concerns that negatively impact the child's participation in education. Areas of concern that do not influence a child's educational performance are addressed by other community agencies or resources.

Each occupational therapist has professional goals, with professional knowledge and skills underlying these desired outcomes. It is important for therapists to define professional goals clearly for themselves so they choose professional activities that enhance goal attainment. Employment choices play a major role in either enhancing or blocking professional goal attainment, with the best outcomes occurring when the mission of the employing agency and one's professional goals are aligned.

Dunn W. *Best Practice Occupational Therapy for Children and Families in Community Settings, Second Edition* (pp. 73-89)
© 2011 SLACK Incorporated.

Agencies often require professionals to play a variety of roles and to engage in a wide range of responsibilities. For example, a role that occupational therapists may be required to play in early intervention programs is that of a case manager or service coordinator for families. Similarly, many therapists employed in school settings may be responsible for coordinating children's therapy services with those being provided by other community agencies or medical facilities. Traditional roles of occupational therapists are expanding as current practices with infants and children change to better reflect current public policy and legislation.

The laws and regulations outlined in Chapter 2 provide the overarching guidance for many of the places occupational therapists will be employed. You will also have responsibility for learning about any specific missions that your employer has made a commitment to address. These additional commitments might be due to a passionate board member's cause, funding that became available, or because there was a gap in services that needed to be filled. Find out about these things so you can align your professional career goals with agencies that are synchronous with you.

TEAMS PROVIDE A STRUCTURE FOR YOUR PRACTICE

All group members contribute to a team's operation (Lacoursiere, 1980). Their personal values, commitment, sense of professional identity, and comfort within the particular system influence the roles each member adopts and the dynamics used within the group. The laws and regulations specify which professionals need to be considered as agencies provide services; the professionals themselves determine how these teams operate.

There are several approaches to designing a team structure. Each approach focuses on developing programs to meet the child's need to participate in living. Systems select a particular team planning approach based on legal requirements, program philosophies, traditions, experience, or preference of staff members. Only collaborative structures are compatible with a best practice philosophy and approach.

Historically, professionals from various disciplines might gather together periodically to discuss their individual recommendations or summarize their findings. People have referred to these models as multidisciplinary teams to reflect the gathering of disciplines (Bailey, 1984); some have described the process as "co-existing" (Sparling, 1980). This parallel team structure has fallen out of favor for community-based services because it is cumbersome, costly, and violates family-centered care principles and because effectiveness of services in this format has been called into question.

It is much more common to see interdisciplinary and transdisciplinary team structures in community-based practice. An interdisciplinary team is also comprised of professionals from several disciplines. However, the team members of an interdisciplinary team collaborate with each other to interpret their findings and design intervention programs. Sometimes, these professionals conduct evaluations together, as in a play-based assessment. They may also conduct separate evaluations. When designing the intervention program, it is typical for more than one discipline to be responsible for goals. For example, the speech pathologist, occupational therapist, and mother may work together to design and implement a feeding and eating program for a toddler. Team members negotiate about what the priorities are, and the intervention plan reflects the consensus of the group.

In a public school, the educators or school psychologists are frequently the coordinators for the interdisciplinary activities. The regular and special education teachers might plan classroom goals that reflect the combined knowledge gained from the psychological, social work, educational, occupational, and speech therapy evaluations. The teacher's assistant reinforces the student's learning, using strategies developed by the occupational therapist and special education teacher. Teachers and related service personnel (such as occupational therapists) can incorporate language goals into all daily and weekly routines. The music and art teachers might collaborate with the occupational therapist to incorporate postural control activities into their class sessions (e.g., movement activities, standing to work on projects).

Coaching team members work together throughout assessment, diagnostic, planning, and implementation phases. The unique feature of the coaching approach (sometimes people use the term "transdisciplinary" when using a key contact person) is that the team members decide who is the logical person to implement services with the child and family, and that person acts on behalf of the team, representing all disciplines (Conner, Williamson, & Siep, 1978; Sparling, 1980). Each discipline contributes information to the team assessment and goal setting process. Then, one person implements the program and becomes the child's primary provider or "coach" (Rush, Shelden, & Hanft, 2003). The primary service provider reports progress to the team, which meets to review and revise the program plan as appropriate. The other professionals on the team "coach" their primary provider colleague when issues arise that require a particular discipline's expertise (Orelove and Sobsey, 1987; Rush, Shelden, & Hanft, 2003). The model facilitates building rapport between parent, child, and service providers, and it is easier to implement consistent programming.

Classroom teachers serving children with physical disabilities frequently serve as the primary provider for the child on a coaching team. The school's occupational and physical therapists in these situations provide the teaching staff with ongoing training related to handling and positioning children with cerebral palsy during various school activities. They collaborate with each other and with the teachers, developing classroom interventions to facilitate performance during daily classroom activities. Specific interventions might include training in toilet transfer techniques and the use of adaptive equipment for snack and lunch periods. This is an excellent team model for classrooms because the teachers are there every day and the related service personnel are not. The children's achievement of specific goals is reinforced through consistency and ample opportunities for practice within the routines of the day.

The coaching approach requires administrative support; parent and staff training, which depends upon agency and program philosophies; parent and staff commitment; time; and financial resources. Professionals working within a coaching team have the opportunity to learn more about the child and about different approaches through the cross-disciplinary sharing that is essential in the model. However, the resulting role blurring (Conner et al., 1978) can be confusing to the new practitioner who is developing a professional role identity.

Another aspect of team structure revolves around specialty teams. States and communities sometimes gather together a group of professionals because they have expertise that requires advanced training or experience. For example, states have Assistive Technology Centers that house equipment and resources for those who might need applications that are not routinely available. Perhaps a small community has a child who needs a communication device that is costly and that the child may not find useful. The Assistive Technology Center might have this device and be able to lend it to the school, so purchasing is not necessary until they know if the device is appropriate. Larger school districts have Assistive Technology Teams whose members keep up on the latest innovations. It is common for occupational therapists to serve on these teams because we are concerned with the interfaces between a person and his or her context. Assistive technology bridges the gap, affording participation.

States also have family-based teams, such as Families Together. Families Together provides resources to support families as they navigate service systems. Their expertise revolves around knowing what families are likely to need; understanding the resources, service systems, structures, and access points within the state; and keeping in contact with professionals in the state to link everyone together in service to children's needs. This is also a team structure that operates across agencies.

Managing Effective Services

Supervision and Use of Others to Implement Services

Traditionally, we think of supervision as the relationship between a worker and a boss. In practice with children and families, other patterns of supervision are more common. Occupational therapists who serve children and families engage in supervision when they oversee or guide activities that others implement with children for a therapeutic benefit. This can include the therapist supervising parents who are carrying out a feeding program, a teachers' assistant facilitating a toileting routine, a teacher supporting a cognitive development routine, or a job coach providing social supports for a young adult to stock shelves with co-workers. In these relationships, the occupational therapist is responsible for designing the programs (which includes collaborating with others), training the service provider, checking the service provider's skill to carry out the program, providing guidance about precautions, creating a documentation process, and constructing ongoing contact and feedback mechanisms. Occupational therapists maintain overall accountability for these programs and their outcomes.

When occupational therapists supervise others to carry out programs, we extend our impact on the child's participation in daily life. It is inappropriate for occupational therapists to spend the amount of time with the children that would be needed to provide enough practice; our time needs to be spent designing programs that fit into the everyday life routines, coaching those within the everyday life routines, and evaluating progress. We are providing best practice when we imbed our therapeutic expertise into the daily routines.

More formal supervisory relationships can occur with paraprofessionals, COTAs, and less senior occupational therapists who are employed as part of occupational therapy services. The AOTA (2009) defines supervision as a "cooperative process in which 2 or more people participate in a joint effort to establish, maintain and or elevate a level of competence and performance" (p. 797). This document outlines the parameters that must be considered for supervision of these relationships. For example, we need to consider a COTA's experience, the level of complexity of the child's needs, regulatory requirements, and the agency's requirements when identifying the exact supervision requirements of a COTA. Table 5-1 provides an example of a role delineation and supervision planning document that we are using in an early intervention program in Kansas.

Entry-level occupational therapists will be in close and routine supervision relationships, moving toward general supervision as the therapist gains experience. In systems that serve children and families, occupational therapists are likely to have supervisors from other disciplines. Supervisors from other disciplines can provide mentoring and guidance related to collaborative practice and system level knowledge and functions. Entry-level therapists in these situations may design a strategy for obtaining occupational therapy mentoring during their initial years of practice to enhance their professional identification and development. Therapists can do this in a variety of ways:

- They can contract through their agency for time and resources to engage with a more experienced therapist.
- They can participate in study groups in the community.
- They can take graduate courses to provide a forum for formal learning and dialogue.
- They can participate in data collection for research.

Planning Caseload to Reflect Best Practices

A critical aspect of best practice service provision is the determination of an appropriate caseload. When there are too many children on a therapist's caseload, it interferes with effective services because there is not sufficient time to give proper attention to individual needs. Therapists establish caseloads that acknowledge the variety of tasks that are required within the service provision process and provide a mechanism for interacting with significant individuals such as family members, other team members, referral sources, and administrators.

There are many ways to conceptualize how a professional spends time. For this discussion, we will consider 2 overall task categories when determining caseload. The first category includes the function tasks, such as travel, lunch, and supervisory responsibilities. Novices need to include some time for mentoring/supervision for themselves to learn the system expectations and obtain guidance for the work. You can calculate the function category by adding the actual time spent in each of these tasks. For example, a therapist might spend an average of 4 hours per week traveling and receive 1 hour per week of supervision. Additionally, 30 minutes per day for lunch becomes 2.5 hours per week. These 7.5 hours are not available for other duties. Early intervention providers are likely to have more travel time because they see families in their homes and neighborhoods; time is related to our work settings and agencies.

The second category is composed of service tasks, which include team meetings about the children, assessments, documentation, planning, and providing interventions (which include seeing children and meeting with teachers or families to guide them about how to make everyday life activities therapeutic for the children). Best practice services involve more collaboration and team planning, so we need to conceptualize our caseloads with the understanding that team meetings about children and meetings to coach everyday providers (e.g., teachers, parents) are critical aspects of service provision.

Table 5-1.

Plan of Supervision for Occupational Therapist/ Certified Occupational Therapy Assistants

Based on the Kansas State Board of Healing Arts licensing regulations (www.ksbha.org; choose "Licensure Booklets" and then find the occupational therapy booklet), AOTA's position paper on delineation of roles of OTR and COTA and Kansas para-educator supervision guidelines (www.ksde.org; in the search box, put "para educator supervision").

Determining the Frequency of Supervision by OT

Twelve visits per quarter to family (approximately one time weekly)	Supervision provided by OT One home visit monthly
Six visits per quarter to family (approximately every other week)	Supervision provided by OT Two home visits quarterly
Four visits per quarter to family (approximately monthly)	Supervision provided by OT One home visit quarterly

- Supervision visit does not have to be entire home visit
- OT supervisor will attend team meeting with COTA
- OT/COTA will develop a plan to meet on a regular basis for general supervision (weekly to begin with)

Delineating Roles/Tasks Between OT and COTA

OT	COTA
Designate tasks to COTA only for which they have been specifically trained and are qualified to perform (established service competency).	Carry out only the activities that have been delegated.
Complete the initial evaluation to determine eligibility.	COTA cannot complete evaluation or interpret child's performance on evaluations.
Develop IFSP (plan of care) with family and team including frequency and duration of services.	Attend IFSP meetings at discretion of OT. COTA cannot make recommendations regarding the need for OT services or frequency and duration.
Attend and participate in team meetings.	Attend and participate in team meetings.
Implement IFSP with family and team.	Implement IFSP with family and team.
Make changes to outcomes on IFSP.	COTA cannot make changes to the IFSP outcomes.
Timely review of COTA documentation and countersigning official documents including home visit notes and billing. Work with COTA to develop method of data collection to measure progress.	Complete home visit notes, billing, and quarterly reports as agreed upon by supervising OT. Have all official documentation countersigned by OT.
Request joint visit by other team.	COTA cannot request joint visit from other team member; however, a family member can request this at any time.
Participate in transition/discharge planning, completing all documentation.	COTA may help prepare transition/discharge documentation with OT supervision.
Attend final home visit prior to discharge.	

Additionally, your services are not complete until you have documented them. Documentation provides a written record of the actions taken and decisions made on behalf of the individual. Chapters 6 through 9 provide information and examples about effective documentation strategies. It is sometimes difficult for therapists to maintain documentation and preparation time in the schedule. We want to make ourselves available to as many children as possible, so it is easy to put off documentation. Professionals must consider this situation very carefully. There is a point at which one's caseload is so big that the children are not actually receiving quality occupational therapy services because the therapist is simply too busy to be effective. Taking too large a caseload can lead administrators and others to conclude that occupational therapy is not necessary because they see no impact from it, which is an undesirable outcome.

An exact amount of time for these tasks is difficult to determine, due to variance from week to week or by time of year (e.g., more assessments at the beginning or end of the school year for school-based therapists). Estimate an average amount of time spent per week across the whole year. For example, if you spend an average of 2.5 hours per week in assessments and planning, adding this to the 7.5 hours of function tasks above means 10 hours of your weekly time is accounted for already. In a 40-hour work week, this leaves 30 hours for all the tasks involved in applying your expertise to support the children, their families, teachers, and/or community settings.

When there are more children requiring services than the current therapists can handle, then we must join with administrators to solve the problem. The solution is *not* to take more and more children onto the caseload, because the effectiveness of services will diminish. First, all the therapists in a system must examine their service patterns to make sure that they are providing the correct models and approaches for each child. For example, a school practice caseload that involves the therapist pulling students out of classrooms is inappropriate for most public school settings. Vulnerable students need to spend the most time in their educational settings so they can profit from instruction; occupational therapists support the student and teacher so that learning can take place. We identify those students who cannot profit from their education without our support; these are the only students on our caseloads.

Therefore, we continuously re-evaluate children's participation and make changes in services as needed. For example, when children present delays based on a specific assessment, a novice therapist may feel they must continue to serve these children until they reach the typical range. Many of the children we serve have developmental delays and differences throughout their lifetime; that does not mean that they will need occupational therapy services indefinitely to remediate all deficit areas. Our job is to identify ways for them to participate in their everyday lives (including home, school, and community) regardless of inherent delays. The standard we set is based on successful and satisfying participation.

We can also partner with administrators to examine whether other duties can be changed to enable a higher concentration of service provision time. For example, an early intervention program may shift to a primary coaching model, which assigns one service provider to each family for visits, and the whole team supports the family through team meetings and joint visits. This reduces the amount of travel time expended by team members and creates more time for team collaboration and family visits. We might also consider a few weeks of frequent visits, sometimes called front-loading, to get the family started and then have contact by phone with less frequent visits after a family feels like they have the capacity to implement and practice the plan.

Finally, we can assist in finding additional therapists when there are still children needing services and there is no time available in current therapists' schedules. Because we have ongoing shortages in Kansas despite having programs nearby, we have created partnerships among agencies to provide supports to unserved and underserved areas. For example, we identify experienced therapists who want professional development opportunities and use communication technology so they can consult with teams who need occupational therapy expertise but who do not have an occupational therapist. We also use technology to conduct live skilled observations in schools and homes so we can coach teachers and families about how to adjust contexts and activities to support the children's participation.

Let's consider some of the factors that affect caseload in practice.

Managing Caseloads in School Practice

With Becky Nicholson, MEd, OTR

When therapists take positions in school-based practice, it is common to inherit a caseload from a previous therapist who used an older structure for organizing services. Sometimes, changing old patterns is not easy. As an incoming therapist, you have to envision what you would like your service provision structure to look like so you can look beyond the obstacles and think about changes that can improve service to children and families.

Analyze the Current Situation

The first step in making a change in service patterns is to do a careful analysis of the caseload as it exists. When you carefully analyze the services being provided, you can then prioritize how and where it might be possible to alter service patterns. Evidence indicates that services are most effective when they are imbedded in the routines of the student's day (Bayona, McDougall, Tucker, Nichols, & Mandich, 2006; Dunn, 1988, 1990; Kemmis & Dunn, 1996), so this is a way to suggest changes rather than continuing with patterns that have been passed along by previous therapists.

At the same time you are analyzing the services currently in place, you need to also learn who the key players are in your setting and determine where you might have the most success in making changes. It is essential that you secure administrative support in the initial stages. When you have your administrators on board and fully informed of your process, they will provide support when you encounter barriers. Change is very difficult for people, and it is our responsibility to make sure that educators, parents, and support staff recognize the reasons behind the decision to practice in a new way. In this informing process, we provide information in user-friendly formats that illustrate how these changes are beneficial to students.

To examine an existing caseload, analyze each student's service pattern, considering the following information carefully: amount and type of services provided, the goals on the IEP, the length of time the student has been receiving services, and other service providers supporting the student. All this information enables you to critically evaluate whether services have been effective for the student and if there are opportunities for providing services in a different way.

For example, if there has been little progress, this provides an opportunity to make adjustments in the goals, which in turn will affect the service patterns. If a former therapist has developed deficit-based goals and objectives, shifting to goals that are strengths-based and focused on participation in the educational setting can trigger the need for changes in service patterns also. A core philosophy of best practice suggests we focus on children's strengths and the impact of services on participation. When we focus on participation, we employ different service options. Best practice intervention methods involve putting supports in place so that the students can be successful learners.

Taking a strengths-based approach, we identify opportunities to impact the student's ability to participate in education. Although we understand the impact of underlying person factors that may interfere with participation, our focus remains on strategies to support participation, rather than on fixing the underlying deficit. For example, a student has difficulty remembering directions given orally, but he sticks with tasks once he starts them. In a deficit approach, the team might work on his auditory processing skills. In a strengths-based approach, the teacher and therapist would provide support for remembering directions (e.g., a cue card, a buddy to ask for help) so that the student's great persistence can support getting more work completed. Over time, the therapist would coach the student to identify other strategies to reduce the impact of his forgetting (e.g., text self with a message, audiotape directions).

Collaborate With Teachers and Other Team Members to Design New Services

We must be in a partnership with the teachers to provide best practice services. Many teachers have become accustomed to traditional "pull-out" services (i.e., the therapist takes the student out of the classroom to provide individualized therapy activities in another location) from experiences with prior therapists. They may not have had the opportunity to collaborate with a therapist to design activities that are integrated into the classroom and school routines. As you get to know your teachers, the structure of their classrooms, and the student's needs, you may begin to identify opportunities to provide services throughout the school day to address the student's needs while supporting the teacher to be successful with the student. To illustrate this point, let's take a look at Heidi.

Heidi is a 5-year-old girl who attends the neighborhood kindergarten program. The prior occupational therapist had been providing direct "pull-out" services to Heidi to increase fine motor skills. During an initial meeting with the new occupational therapist, the teacher and parents indicated they want Heidi to play with peers on the playground. They also want her to be successful with classroom work.

The therapist observed Heidi on the playground. Although she can physically access the playground equipment, she tended to stay in close proximity to the supervising adults during recess. Because Heidi has moderate spastic quadriplegic cerebral palsy (she has high muscle tone, reduced range of motion, difficulty with balance, contributing to delays in motor skills), her hesitancy to use the equipment seemed understandable. The therapist imagined that, with supports, Heidi could easily be more involved with peers during recess.

Heidi has difficulty with writing and completing seatwork but she loves cutting, which they work on a lot in class. Although writing was difficult for her, she participated in daily seatwork and was progressing well with the support of a paraprofessional.

After discussion with the parents and teacher and observation at recess and in the classroom, the new occupational therapist designed a collaborative team approach based on the needs described by parents and teachers. The occupational therapist spoke with the teacher and paraprofessional and identified students who were attempting to interact with Heidi. The occupational therapist collaborated with the physical therapist to develop a repertoire of playground games/activities that Heidi could do successfully and taught the selected students how to play these games with adaptations.

The occupational therapist collaborated with the speech therapist to develop a social story that involved playing with friends on the playground; they also designed a reward system so Heidi could graph the number of students she played with at recess. Prior to recess, the paraprofessional would read the social story with Heidi. Building on her strength of cutting, Heidi cut out pictures of children and placed them on her graph after every recess.

In addition, the occupational therapist provided an in-service with the school personnel and used Heidi's story as a highly successful example of how a change in services could be in children's best interest.

So, you can see from Heidi's story that the occupational therapist took many steps to investigate the situation at school and included other team members in designing the new services. With the occupational therapy services imbedded within her daily routine, Heidi got many opportunities to practice socialization with her peers, which also provided motor development opportunities, and she got to use her current skills (cutting) to mark her own progress.

Collaborate With Parents to Design Best Practice Activities for Life as Part of Caseload

Parents are part of a student's team, and any plans made must reflect the parents' priorities. When analyzing the caseload, it is essential to make sure you have a clear understanding of what parents want and need for their child. When occupational therapists take the time to make even a brief phone call to talk with parents about their child's program, they communicate the importance of the family in planning and decision making. This conversation also affords the opportunity to find out the family's priorities and may also reveal other daily life needs and opportunities that have been overlooked in IEP meetings. In school-based practice, the team's focus is on the student's ability to profit from education. However, when students have more severe disabilities, the school team emphasizes functional skills; because functional skills intersect between school and home life, it is appropriate in these cases to discuss home routines as part of intervention planning. Let's look at an example of caseload planning when a student has more severe disabilities to illustrate how school and family life are both involved.

Fran is a middle school student who attends her community school. She has been in school with the same students since kindergarten, so everyone knows her. Fran is an electric wheelchair user, has an audio communication board on her lap tray, and wears orthoses to keep her feet positioned properly.

During elementary school, she had a number of service providers, all of whom had their own goals for Fran. She spent a lot of time out of her home classroom getting therapy. Fran was receiving traditional services, with her team taking a developmental approach to intervention; they focus their goals on deficits rather than participation in the school setting.

As Fran transitioned into middle school, her parents decided they wanted a different approach. They saw many of Fran's strengths and were tired of hearing that she was delayed. They knew that she was different from other children and felt that there were ways to prepare her for the life she would have, not a life she would never have. The middle school had a different occupational therapist who shared the family's dreams and hopes for Fran, so they decided to work on a new IEP direction.

During the team meeting, the parents talked about how they wanted the school's help to prepare Fran for life as a young adult who has disabilities. They asked for a functional rather than academic emphasis for her middle school years. They explained that having Fran sit in a social studies classroom without any expectations of Fran was not helping her. The middle school team started to brainstorm what functional skills and expectations could be built into Fran's day. In the transition meeting with the elementary team, everyone indicated that Fran is personable and well-liked. They decided to look for opportunities for her to greet peers, such as at school arrival, during lunch, and during departure. The parents indicated her interest in the kitchen, so they planned for her to take the foods units in the kitchen labs so she could learn how to use adaptive devices for cooking. The school agreed to keep parents informed of devices that worked so they could get them for home as well. They signed her up for the life skills curriculum to learn some personal hygiene skills; Fran was also interested in her hair, so the occupational therapist agreed to help her find ways to fix her hair.

An open discussion of this nature provides the opportunity to bridge the gap between performance at home and performance at school and fosters consistency in all settings. Consistency is important for all children and is especially important for children with severe and complicated disorders. As occupational therapists, we have the opportunity to provide interventions linking performance in the home to performance in the school. When the team has developed a functionally based curriculum, we provide examples of the child's participation in functional activities across settings. A functional approach affects our caseloads as well because we build in time to collaborate with teachers and family members to make sure consistency occurs across all settings.

Recognize the Long-Term Process in Making Changes in Caseload

It is not possible to change a caseload all at once because change requires trust and trust takes time. Sometimes, it is useful to make changes when the IEP renewal dates occur; this gives you time to understand exactly what service pattern a particular student might need to profit from education. At other times, it might seem more urgent to make changes, and at these times, any team member can call an additional meeting to discuss changes in the IEP. Let's look at an example when this strategy is important.

Holly is a third grader who has been receiving individual OT services outside the classroom three times per week to address her handwriting needs (based on her IEP). The new OT meets with the teacher to find out about Holly; the teacher says that Holly is missing some important classroom time, including seatwork time to practice new skills when the teacher is available to answer questions. The OT observes Holly in this class time period and sees several ways that Holly can practice her handwriting while doing her seatwork. The teacher and OT feel that it is in Holly's best interest to be in the classroom more, and they want to find ways to support her during learning activities. Because her IEP renewal is several months away, they call a meeting to update her plan. The OT suggests that she visit Holly in her classroom and give Holly and the teacher strategies for the seatwork time so Holly can practice her handwriting in an activity where handwriting matters and she can be available for teacher support and instruction about the content as well.

The change in Holly's services represents only one student's situation, and occupational therapists have many students on their caseloads. The task of adjusting one's caseload may feel overwhelming, but as you begin to make changes to increase efficiency and consolidate some of your time, you create additional time to make further changes. The key to making a successful transition to best practice services and a corresponding caseload that reflects best practice services is being organized and efficient so that you do not miss opportunities to make changes when the IEPs are due.

As one last illustration, we provide Figure 5-1 (you can view or download a color-coded version of this at www.slackbooks.com/bestpracticeforms if this is helpful to your learning), which illustrates the change in a therapist's schedule before and after working on caseload issues such as those described above. This therapist inherited the "before" schedule and then worked across a school year to consolidate visits to the schools. Although there was still work to do, this example shows the impact of the changes on the therapist's time.

> *The therapist completed an analysis of the inherited caseload. In collaboration with the educational team, the therapist identified schools and classrooms where there were paraprofessional and teacher supports that had not been used to the fullest extent. For instance, the children in yellow (Will, Nick, Josh, Heidi, Walt) were all in a preschool classroom within one school. Each of the classrooms had three to five paraprofessionals to support daily educational activities. In the original schedule, the therapist was implementing a direct pull-out model and was working with the children in isolation with minimal interaction with the paraprofessionals and teachers. The occupational therapist began coaching the educational staff so they could provide opportunities for the students to practice needed skills within the student's daily routine. This change provided time in the schedule for the teachers and paraprofessionals to collaborate with the occupational therapist regularly. The students continued to make gains in the ability to participate in educational activities with occupational therapy services provided once per week. The continuity of services improved as the therapist was available to observe and participate in classroom activities throughout the day. Additionally, the changes made thus far opened up 3 hours of time that could be used for planning, documentation, meetings, or for other students requiring services.*
>
> *The therapist also needs to work on the school reflected in purple (Lisa, Andy, Jacob, David, Phillip, Candy, Haley, Caleb, Drew) to consolidate her time there as well. You can see in the "after" schedule, she has time on Tuesdays when she can be available to the teachers. When a therapist is trapped in a fragmented schedule, there is very little flexibility regarding how time is used. When a therapist can consolidate intervention time, it opens up opportunities for a greater variety of observations and collaborative experiences.*
>
> *For schools that were in remote areas with very few students, the team decided to have the therapist come to the building one time per week but increase the amount of time spent for a single visit using a range of service models. So, for Hunter, Ryan, and Triston, the therapist spent 1 hour per week providing services within the classroom and coaching the teacher about strategies throughout the week. Just this one small change reduced the amount of travel time per week by 1 hour.*

Therapists in school-based settings often ask, "What is an appropriate number of children to have on a caseload? " There is no simple answer. The therapist who tries to accommodate too many schools and too many children will not be able to effectively influence the child's participation in the educational setting. Therapists must learn to *manage* their caseload in order to provide effective services. Ongoing analysis of the caseload and investigating ways to increase effectiveness are critical to the success of an occupational therapy program in school-based settings.

Managing Caseloads in Early Intervention
With Ellen Pope, MEd, OTR

Although the structure of Early Intervention (EI) services is different, therapists face similar issues when managing their caseloads. Best practice in EI programs dictates that children and families be supported within their everyday routines in authentic environments (Workgroup on Principles and Practices in Natural Environments, 2007).

Just as we do in school practice, occupational therapists in EI observe the typical routines, interview the parents, and identify what is supporting and interfering with the child's ability to participate in desired activities. These activities set the ground work for creating best practice services and managing one's caseload accordingly.

There have been 2 forms of traditional services in EI. Some programs schedule families to bring their children to a treatment center or hospital for therapy. Caseload management in this service option is based on the number of slots available for scheduling throughout the day. Therapists do not typically

Schedule Before

	M	T	W	TH	F
8-8:30	Plan	Lisa Andy	Home bound	Lisa Andy	Home bound
8:30-9		Jacob	Travel	Jacob	Office
9-9:30	Will Nick Josh	David Phillip	Will Nick Josh	David Phillip	
9:30-10	Heidi Walt	Candy Haley	Heidi Walt	Candy Haley	
10-10:30	Travel	Caleb Drew	Travel	Caleb Drew	Consult
10:30-11	Dakota	Travel	Dakota	Travel	
11-11:30	Ty Tailor	Kaitlin Melissa	Ty Tailor	Kaitlin Melissa	
11:30-12	Jenny Shawn	Chalee Morgan	Jenny Shawn	Chalee Morgan	
12-12:30	Lunch	Travel/ Lunch	Lunch	Travel/ Lunch	Lunch
12:30-1	Jessi Jane Allison	Walter	Jessi Jane Allison	Walter	
1-1:30	Gilbert Ray	Gregg Kelly	Gilbert Ray	Gregg Kelly	
1:30-2	Travel	Jessica Taylor	Travel	Jessica Taylor	
2-2:30	Ryan	Travel	Ryan	Travel	OT Meeting
2:30-3	Hunter	Triston	Hunter	Triston	

Schedule After

	M	T	W	TH	F
8-8:30	Plan	Lisa Andy		Lisa Andy	Home bound
8:30-9		Josh		Josh	Travel
9-9:30	Will Nick	David Phillip		David Phillip	Home bound
9:30-10	Heidi Walt	Candy Haley		Candy Haley	
10-10:30	Josh	Caleb Drew	Consult	Caleb Drew	
10:30-11	Consult		Consult	Travel	
11-11:30			Kaitlin Melissa	Dakota	
11:30-12			Chalee Morgan	Ty Tailor	
12-12:30	Lunch	Lunch	Lunch	Jenny Shawn	Lunch
12:30-1	Walter		Travel	Lunch	
1-1:30	Gregg Kelly		Ryan	Jessi Jane Allison	
1:30-2	Jessica Taylor	Travel		Gilbert Ray	
2-2:30	Consult	Triston	Hunter		OT Meeting
2:30-3					

Figure 5-1. Before and after schedule for a therapist working on consolidating the caseload.

travel from the center, so they have the maximum amount of time available to see children and families. However, this approach violates the principles of family-centered care and natural learning environments, and it is not convenient for families to meet these schedules.

Other programs visit families and children in their homes, but the therapist provides the individualized therapy to the child as an expert. Similar to the "pull-out" services in a school, the therapist is removing the child from natural routines and environments and creating a "therapy" environment within the home. As the Workgroup documents indicate, when you observe behaviors such as the therapist bringing specialized equipment or toys into the home that come and go with the therapist, best practice services are not occurring. Caseloads with this method can be challenging; there is a lot of traveling when each discipline that is relevant for a child's development visits the family regularly. There is a high risk of fractionated care if the disciplines are not talking and coordinating their work, and families can become overwhelmed and confused about what is happening across all providers.

Best practice EI services take advantage of the interdisciplinary evidence to design the caseloads of all the professionals. For example, one network might employ 3 to 5 different disciplines for their team. When a child and family are referred, 2 team members from different disciplines visit the family to find out their needs and priorities, document the child's eligibility for services, and gather initial information for the team. At the next meeting with the family, the team writes the IFSP with outcomes and services and decides which team member (i.e., which discipline) is the most logical person to be the primary provider with the family.

Each week, the whole team meets, and the primary provider for each family reports in and asks for guidance on any issues that have arisen. With this structure, all disciplines participate in planning and problem-solving, but do not have the time constraint of visiting all the families. Similarly, the families do not have to be available to all those other professionals for visits each week. The team can serve more families because they have less travel time allotted, and because they are the most familiar with their "primary provider" families, they remain current on needs and plans. Let's look at an example.

Donna is a 7 month old who lives with her parents and older brother. Parents are concerned that Donna is not getting the food she needs and that she is small for her age. The EI network in their area completed their eligibility work so Donna can receive EI services. The occupational therapist visits during lunch to see what is going on with Donna's eating and to hear from mom what is concerning her. After this first meeting, they plan to meet three times per week for 2 weeks; the therapist detected a lot of anxiety from mom and wanted to make sure she had some effective strategies really quickly to both allay mom's fears and to get Donna on a positive path to getting her calories and nutrition.

After the first two visits, the therapist met with her team. She described Donna's eating, which included sensitivities to certain aspects of the foods. For example, mom had figured out that Donna wanted food at room temperature and rejected foods with more texture. The occupational therapist noticed that she only ate beige-colored foods. She asked the dietitian on the team to help with a food plan that included other foods that had these characteristics and also contained the necessary nutrients for a child Donna's age.

After these first six visits (2 weeks), they had tried 10 foods, and Donna would eat seven of them. The occupational therapist assured mom about Donna getting the calories and nutrients she needed with these foods and her drinks. They decided to meet once a week for 2 weeks with phone calls as needed, and then they switched to phone calls weekly and a visit each month.

You can see with this scenario that the therapist has a short, intense period to get the family on track and then shifts her time as mom feels more competent. With a flexible schedule, the therapist is available to begin new families frequently, which is a much more pressing need in EI services.

Communication Strategies That Support Best Practices

With Jane Cox, MS, OTR/L

Communicating Among Professionals

Effective team communication facilitates members' understanding of their roles and functions (Losen & Losen, 1985). Formal and informal communications that take place during both group meetings and in casual contacts between members are important influences that generate an atmosphere of understanding and commitment toward program-planning activities. At times, it is difficult for team members with diverse backgrounds to communicate effectively with each other and with parents. Two critical communication strategies are for members to use jargon-free language and to describe behaviors in observable terms; these strategies equalize everyone's understanding and invite all members to participate in the dialogue. Because occupational therapists are trained in group process and communication skills, they can facilitate effective group behavior through their participation.

Jargon-free language is using only words that everyone understands. It is not necessary to use technical terms; they do not help anyone understand what you are trying to communicate. "Johnny has poor vestibular and proprioceptive support for postural control" leaves the reader wondering what that means and why it matters. Instead, we can say, "Johnny is not getting enough sensory feedback from his body to stay in his desk during math"; this invites everyone to understand or ask questions. If a therapist believes that a technical word will be needed, the therapist explains the situation in regular words and then includes the technical word in parentheses.

We also describe what we observe in behavioral terms. This means we write what we see, not our interpretation of what we see. When we write what we see, we leave the door open to multiple interpretations as we get others' observations. We also have the opportunity to measure the behavior to chart progress. Let's look at the example in the shaded box on this page.

As you can see, there are many interpretations of the same situation. Using the facts to record what happens keeps the possibilities open for team discussion.

Some teams function with rotating roles and responsibilities. A teacher, therapist, social worker, or other staff member may lead the team in planning meetings and take responsibility for coordinating the necessary procedures required for the team to develop and implement the program. This approach allows members to experience different responsibilities in planning the child's program, broadening their understanding of various team member roles in the program-planning process.

When a team experiences challenges working together to plan a child's program, they must assess the source of the problem and make a plan to resolve it. Team function can be impeded by problems with the team's evolution as a group, composition, or group process used (Bailey, 1984). In discussing factors that influence team function, Bennett (1982) has raised the issue of territoriality and "protection of turf" in relation to the increasing specialization in childhood services. This territoriality can occur within a team, across teams, and across agencies in interagency work. It is important for team members to avoid competition and respect varied backgrounds; this diversity provides the resources for developing the child's service plan. When professionals tap expertise from diverse backgrounds, they can enhance the resulting plan, and members share an ownership toward the common programs they have developed together (Maher & Bennett, 1984). Sometimes, professional development as a team can be useful for developing group process skills, which are essential to effective team planning.

One area of professional communication that needs direct attention is the relationship between clinic-based professionals and community-based professionals (e.g., school therapists). These agencies have different purposes, and so there is ample possibility for either conflict or fractionation of services, leaving the families to find their way between them. Just as it would be inappropriate for a school therapist to dictate what a clinic-based therapist does with a family, it is inappropriate for clinic-based services to dictate school practices. Certainly, anyone can participate in the school team, but the

OBSERVATIONS

Margo completes half of her math worksheet.

Margo completes the problems down the left side of the page.

Margo holds her head tilted 45 degrees while writing.

Margo looks up 12 times while doing her math sheet.

Margo stays in her seat during the work period.

INTERPRETATION POSSIBILITIES

Margo is distracted and cannot finish her math sheet.

Margo has a visual perception problem.

Margo is bored with the math sheet.

Margo has neglect of the right side.

school team as a unit is responsible for deciding how services are designed and implemented within schools. Clinical programs can make general recommendations, but do not have adequate information to know how those recommendations might be carried out in a school district. For example, if a child has coordination challenges that are interfering with participation, the school might enhance the PE program, work on recess activities, add some classroom-level games, or engage a related service professional to support the teachers' efforts. It would not be appropriate for a clinical therapist to say, "Johnny needs OT twice a week to work on coordination"; rather he or she would say, "Johnny has challenges with coordination that seem to be interfering with his daily life. Including attention to this within his school program will be important."

Therapists who work with the same children and families from different agencies need to prioritize the families' needs and find ways to communicate in a collaborative way. Technology strategies (discussed below) can bridge the scheduling challenges so that all parties can share pertinent information. Visiting each others' programs to understand how services occur can reduce confusion and sends a clear message that we are all supporting families.

Communicating With Families

Communication is powerful and can make or break our relationships with children and families. When we listen and respond with empathy and compassion, we develop strong working relationships. Two essential components of best practice communication are using person-first language and emphasizing the child's strengths. These strategies make our respect for the child and family clear.

Person-first language means that every person is referred to by his or her name and not by his or her disability or diagnosis. When we talk about a child with a disability, we might say something like, "Joe has cerebral palsy." In the example, we refer to Joe as a person first and then state that he has a disability because knowing that Joe has cerebral palsy also informs us about his abilities and what kinds of questions to ask as we move forward in the intervention process. We do not say, "That boy next door who suffers from autism," but rather say, "Alex is a boy who lives next door." The children we serve are people first and not a diagnosis or label that may carry negative connotations.

A second feature of good communication is conversing in a way that reflects a strengths-based approach to service provision. As we discussed in Chapter 1, a strengths-based approach means that we regard the abilities and the strengths of the child and family and do not focus on the problems or deficits. We focus on building the capacity of families to support their children. This can be challenging for therapists, because, historically, we have been trained to share all the technical information about a diagnosis, prognosis, or impairments. In best practice services, we listen to what the family/teacher/person wants and needs for the child (or for themselves when children are older) and find out what they are good at.

Rush and Shelden (2005) recommend a method of reflective questioning that emphasizes using open-ended questions when conversing with a family about his or her child. Using open-ended questions means that the questions cannot be answered with a yes or no response, but rather require a thoughtful and evaluative response. They recommend a 4-tiered system of reflective questioning. We have examples of these questions in Chapters 8 and 9.

Awareness questions promote understanding and include questions that begin with phrases such as: What do you know about...? How are you currently doing...? What have you tried? How did that work for you? What happened when you...? How do you feel...? What supports were most helpful?

Analysis questions make comparisons and include phrases such as: How does that compare with what you did before? How is that consistent with what your goals are? How did you know you needed to change your plan? What do you think will happen if you....? How does that match with the standards?

Alternative questions promote one's ability to consider other options. Alternative questions begin with phrases such as: How could you find out about....? What else could you have done to....? What would it take for you to be able to...? What might make it work better next time? What other opportunities would be useful?

Action questions result in a plan with which to move forward and begin with phrases such as: How are you going to put that into place? What do you plan to do? What supports will you need? What will you do differently next time? Where will you get the resources you need? What option will get the best result?

Using a reflective questioning approach, Rush and Shelden (2008) teach that a conversation with a family should always end with an action plan so that the family has a direction to move forward as it relates to their child. The reflective questioning approach moves therapists out of the "expert" role and into the "coaching" role. With reflective questions, therapists do not presume they know the answers that will be just right for any family and embark on joint discovery of exactly how to solve the problem or meet the challenge with participation.

Rush and Shelden (2008) outline a strategy for explaining best practice early intervention to families. They suggest beginning with an introduction of the therapist and the organization the therapist represents when visiting the family. Following introductions, they outline the research that shows the importance of everyday learning opportunities and how to identify times convenient to the family and activities the family finds helpful or interesting. They discuss the parent's active role in problem-solving and the therapist's role in discovering what might work. They explain that the whole team will support the family throughout team meetings. They also provide a scenario for explaining the differences between traditional services and coaching; you can get a copy of these suggested scripts from www.fippcase.org. This Web site also contains other articles about evidence-based practices in early intervention; we will discuss other topics in other chapters. We can also use the reflective questions approach with teachers and other colleagues. You will see these possibilities discussed in Chapters 7 through 9.

Supporting Families to Have Health Literacy

(See National Network of Libraries of Medicine (2010, January 5). Health Literacy. Retrieved January 13, 2010 from nnlm.gov/outreach/consumer/hlthlit.html).

According to *Healthy People* 2010, health literacy is defined as, "The degree to which individuals have the capacity to obtain, process and understand basic health information and services needed to make appropriate health decisions." As occupational therapists, this means that we have a responsibility to ensure that families have a comprehensive understanding of their child's needs. It is often the case that families of children with special needs are bombarded and overwhelmed with unclear information in medical and legal terms.

To best serve families, we are perfectly positioned and trained to bridge some of the gaps between medical services and community programs by building the capacity of a family member to understand the information he or she receives. Therefore, another aspect of best practice communication is to check with families about their level of understanding about their child's condition and probable factors associated with that condition. By intersecting a strengths-based approach with health literacy, we can support families to focus on their children's positive and helpful qualities no matter what other information might also be available.

For example, when children have complex disabilities like Asperger syndrome, professionals may emphasize the communication challenges, rigidity, narrow interests, or lack of ability to understand social nuances. Although parents need to understand the criteria being used to make this diagnosis, we can use a strengths-based approach to point out how we might rely on what is considered a child's narrow interests to get detailed or obscure information. When the child's class is studying insects, if this child's "narrow interests" involve insects or species that use insects for food or the place of insects in the food chain, we can take advantage of his or her knowledge. Exploring possibilities for seeing the advantages of their child's quirky behavior maintains their strengths perspective.

Preparing Families for Medical Care Visits

With Ellen Pope, MEd, OTR

Routine visits for medical care can be challenging for families. These visits are reminders that something is "wrong" with their child and can be overwhelming. Community-based therapists can support families by preparing them for these visits and arming them with tools so the family feels "in charge" rather than victimized.

As you can see, communication will be critical in situations like this one. Table 5-2 provides sample comments and questions that a community team supported a family to develop as they prepared for a medical team visit. Preparing families prior to the

Table 5-2.

Strategy for Preparing a Family for a Medical Team Visit

Comments I Want to Make During My Medical Team Visit

I have confidence in my community team professionals; they know and understand my child.

We expect you to send them your reports and recommendations so we can decide about how your recommendations fit into our local plan of services.

We expect you to provide us with options and the evidence supporting those options.

We will not be deciding anything during the visit; we will need time to discuss your suggestions with our home team.

Here is what we want to accomplish during our visit: ______________________

We have three questions we want answered today: ______________________

We would like to see the following professionals when we visit: ______________

We do not need to see ____ services on our visit; we have other areas we would like to focus on for our visit, such as: ______________________

Questions to Prepare for My Medical Team Visit

What is your purpose for our visit?

What do you want to accomplish with our family?

Are there any new areas of concern about my child's health or well-being?

Are there safety issues I need to know about?

What should I be expecting to see in the next 6 months?

What is the best way for me and my home team to contact you if we need clarification or additional information?

How would you like to be involved as we plan my child's next IFSP?

When can we expect your reports?

When will we have a follow-up conversation so I can ask questions about things that are not clear?

visit helps them remember they are in charge of their child's care, and they get to lead the process. We recommend that you work with the family to create a written document that they can take to the visit. With comments and questions in hand, they will feel more prepared, and the service providers will see that they have prepared for the visit. The community-based team must also take responsibility to be sure the medical team gets the most updated reports prior to the visit so the parents do not have to provide this update "alone."

Prepare and practice a script with your families so they have a satisfying visit and get their needs met. Follow up with the medical team to integrate their information with the current interventions. If possible, attend clinic visits with families to demonstrate the strength and support in local services.

Using Technology for Communication

In recent years, the use of technology has exploded. Technology is widely used for personal and professional purposes. Before considering the use of technology with families, it is important to establish what, if any, types of technology a family has access to, is comfortable using, and their desire to use it as a mechanism for support. Using technology assumes that a person has sufficient resources to own or have access to equipment and has services needed to use the equipment. For example, in order to video conference with a family in a rural setting, the family must have a computer, a camera attached to the computer, internet service, and the desire to use the technology as one method of service delivery. We remember family-centered care when selecting communication methods.

E-mail is an efficient way to communicate a variety of topics because it is asynchronous. E-mail can be used amongst colleagues and with families. One can schedule and confirm appointments, provide follow-up resources, or ask questions that came up between visits. We must also take care to avoid emotional topics because nonverbal communication is unavailable, leaving the reader to make their own interpretation of the message. When emotional subjects come up, it is best to talk in person, by video conference, or over the phone. Whenever possible, keep e-mail short and succinct, perhaps address only one issue per e-mail. When e-mails are too lengthy and contain too much information, they can become overwhelming and important details are lost. Finally, remember to remove jargon in your communications just as you would in a written report or in a face-to-face interaction. Some organizations have strict rules regarding e-mail exchanges with clients. Some places do not allow e-mailing with clients, and some have encryption to protect privacy and confidentiality. Be sure to know what your employer's rules regarding e-mail are so as not to jeopardize yourself or your client.

Video conferencing is another type of technology that can be useful for teams and families who live in rural and remote settings; without this option, services have to be delayed or are not available at all. Live video provides additional information that cannot be gathered through e-mail or even on the phone. For example, if a family has a concern about their child's eating patterns, the parent can feed the child while the OT watches; the OT can provide suggestions in real time so they can see what happens. The therapist can watch a child playing or a student in the classroom and provide immediate guidance to adjust the activities and contexts to improve participation. This is most similar to a live face-to-face home visit in which the same chain of events would occur.

References

AOTA. (2009). Guidelines for supervision, roles and responsibilities during the delivery of occupational therapy services. *American Journal of Occupational Therapy, 63*(6), 797-803.

Bailey, D. (1984). A triaxial model of the interdisciplinary team and group process. *Exceptional Children, 51*(1), 17-25.

Bayona, C. L., McDougall, J., Tucker, M. A., Nichols, M., & Mandich, A. (2006). School based occupational therapy for children with fine motor difficulties: Evaluating functional outcomes and fidelity of services. *Physical & Occupational Therapy in Pediatrics, 26*, 3.

Bennett, F. (1982). The pediatrician and the interdisciplinary process. *Exceptional Children, 48*(4), 306-314.

Conner, F., Williamson, G., & Siep, J. (1978). *Program guide for infants and toddlers with neuromotor and other developmental disabilities*. New York, NY: Teachers College Press.

Dunn, W. (1988). Models of occupational therapy service provision in the school system. *The American Journal of Occupational Therapy, 42*, 718-723.

Dunn, W. (1990). A comparison of service provision models in school-based occupational therapy services: A pilot study. *The Occupational Therapy Journal of Research, 10*, 300-320.

Kemmis, B. L., & Dunn, W. (1996). Collaborative consultation: The efficacy of remedial and compensatory interventions in school contexts. *American Journal of Occupational Therapy, 50*, 709-717.

Lacoursiere, R. (1980). *The life cycle of groups*. New York, NY: Human Sciences Press.

Losen, S., & Losen, J. (1985). *The special education team*. Boston, MA: Allyn and Bacon, Inc.

Maher, C., & Bennett, R. (1984). *Planning and evaluating special education services*. Englewood, NJ: Prentice-Hall, Inc.

National Network of Libraries of Medicine (2010, January 5). *Health Literacy*. Retrieved January 13, 2010 from http://nnlm.gov/outreach/consumer/hlthlit.html.

Orelove, F., & Sobsey, D. (1987). *Educating children with multiple disabilities—A transdisciplinary approach*. Baltimore, MD: Paul H. Brookes, Publishers.

Rush, D., & Shelden, M. (2008). Script for explaining an evidence based early intervention model. *Family, Infant and Preschool Program, 1*(3), 1-5.

Rush, D., Shelden, M., & Hanft, B. (2003). Coaching families and colleagues: A process for collaboration in natural settings. *Infants & Young Children, 16*(1), 33-47.

Shelden, M. & Rush, D. (2005). Practitioner as coach: Our role in early intervention. *American Association for Home-Based Early Interventionists, 9*(3), 7-9, 11.

Sparling, J. (1980). The transdisciplinary approach with the developmentally delayed child. *Physical and Occupational Therapy in Pediatrics, 1*(2), 3-16.

Workgroup on Principles and Practices in Natural Environments. (November, 2007). *Mission and principles for providing services in natural environments*. OSEP TA Community of Practice-Part C Settings. http://www.nectac.org/topics/families/families.asp.

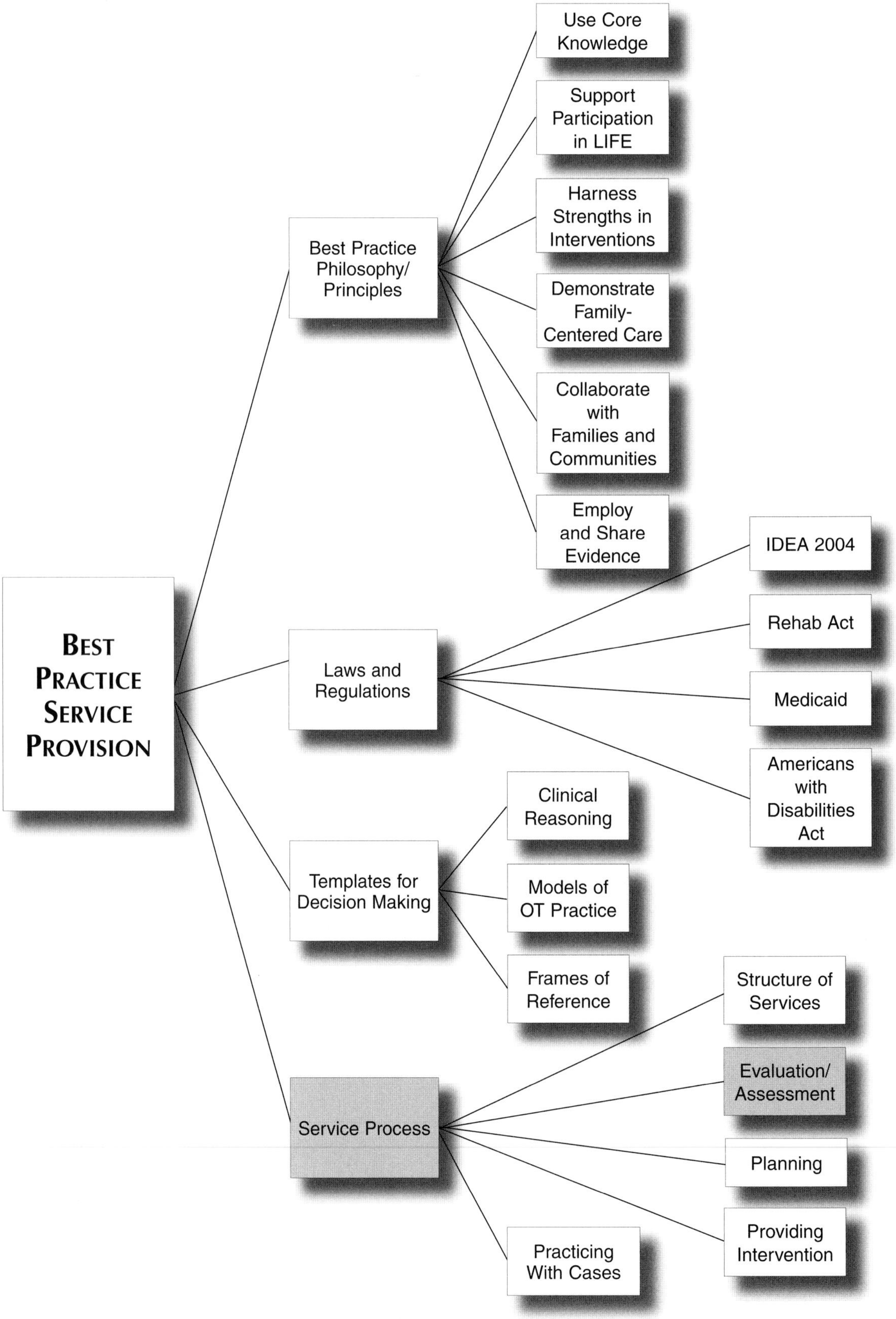
BEST PRACTICE SERVICE PROVISION
Best Practice Philosophy/ Principles
Use Core Knowledge
Support Participation in LIFE
Harness Strengths in Interventions
Demonstrate Family-Centered Care
Collaborate with Families and Communities
Employ and Share Evidence
Laws and Regulations
IDEA 2004
Rehab Act
Medicaid
Americans with Disabilities Act
Templates for Decision Making
Clinical Reasoning
Models of OT Practice
Frames of Reference
Service Process
Structure of Services
Evaluation/ Assessment
Planning
Providing Intervention
Practicing With Cases

CHAPTER 6

Best Practice Occupational Therapy Evaluation

Winnie Dunn, PhD, OTR, FAOTA; Becky Nicholson, MEd, OTR;
Jane A. Cox, MS, OTR/L; Ellen Pope, MEd, OTR;
and Louann Rinner, MS, OTR

Occupational therapists have a unique knowledge base and perspective to offer their teams; the evaluation process provides a way to employ that perspective on behalf of children and families. Teams use evaluation findings and interpretations to make a number of decisions about placement, programming, and service options, so skill and integrity are critical in this aspect of service provision. Tests and other assessment methods are powerful tools that must be used carefully in service to children and families; for example, certain assessments require specific training for administration, while others require broad-based knowledge for proper interpretation. The AOTA has provided standards that outline the appropriate use of standardized tests and other assessment techniques (see www.aota.org for more information). Professionals in general follow the American Psychological Association (APA) *Standards for Educational and Psychological Testing* (1999) (see www.apa.org/science/programs/testing/standards.aspx for additional information).

The various laws we have been discussing also have guidance about what is expected in evaluation processes. Table 6-1 provides an example of the IDEA 2004 guidance about evaluation for school practice. Look up these parameters for IFSP's and for Section 504 plans.

Defining Assessment and Evaluation

Evaluation is a comprehensive process through which professionals obtain information about a child and family. The term *evaluation* refers to the entire process of gathering information for decision-making. The term *assessment* refers to a specific strategy that a professional uses to gather data; we can use formal and informal evaluation methods as described below.

All team members participate in evaluation; the product of evaluation may be a diagnosis, determining eligibility, constructing an intervention plan, evaluating the effectiveness of an intervention (i.e., progress monitoring), or determining whether or not comprehensive services are still required. Any activity that constitutes data-gathering can be considered part of the evaluation, including records reviews, interviews, skilled observations (including by videotape), checklists, developmental or criterion measures, and formal tests. The goal of evaluation is to compile comprehensive information about a child's strengths and needs, thereby necessitating a team approach. The members of an assessment team

Dunn W. *Best Practice Occupational Therapy for Children and Families in Community Settings, Second Edition* (pp. 91-123)
© 2011 SLACK Incorporated.

Table 6-1.

Example of Regulations and Their Meaning for Occupational Therapy Evaluation

Evaluation Procedure	Federal Laws	Implications for Occupational Therapists
Pre-assessment process	300.304 Screening for instructional purposes is not an evaluation	Providing information to the teacher for educational programming as in the case of pre-assessment interventions is not considered an evaluation and does not require consent
Notice to Parents	300.304 (a) Public agency must give notice to parent of any evaluation procedure the agency proposes to conduct	Verify consent prior to conducting any evaluation procedures
Conduct Evaluation	300.304 (b) (1) Use a variety of assessment tools and strategies to gather relevant functional, developmental, and academic information about the child, including information provided by the parent, that may assist in determining (i) Whether a child is a child with a disability under 300.8; and (ii) The content of the child's IEP including information related to enabling the child to be involved in and progress in the general education curriculum (or, for a preschool child, to participate in appropriate activities); (2) Not use any single measure or assessment as the sole criterion for determining whether a child is a child with a disability and for determining an appropriate educational program for the child.	The occupational therapy assessment must include methods such as record review, observation in the context of the educational setting, interview of teacher and parent, and, if needed, formal assessment methods. The educational team determines if the child meets criteria for a child with a disability, and the occupational therapy evaluation will contribute to the development of IEP content. While scores from formal measures may be useful in determining the content of the IEP, evaluation of the child's performance cannot be based on the performance on a single measure.
Selecting Formal Methods of Evaluation	300.304 (3) Use technically sound instruments that may assess the relative contribution of cognitive and behavioral factors, in addition to physical or developmental factors. 300.304 (3) (c) (iii) Are used for the purposes for which the assessments or measures are valid and reliable. 300.304 (3) (iv) Are administered by trained and knowledgeable personnel; and (v) Are administered in accordance with any instructions provided by the producer of the assessments. 300.304 (3) Assessments are selected and administered so as to best ensure that if an assessment is administered to a child with impaired sensory, manual, or speaking skills, the assessment results accurately reflect the child's aptitude or achievement level or whatever other factors the test purports to measure, rather than reflecting the child's impaired sensory, manual, or speaking skills (unless those skills are the factors that the test purports to measure).	The occupational therapist who selects a formal measure as part of the evaluation process must review the technical properties of that measure to ensure that reliability and validity are at an acceptable level and that the therapist understands how to interpret the performance scores in the method intended by the test developer. In addition, the therapist must be confident in his or her ability to administer the measure appropriately. Many times, the team requests an evaluation by the occupational therapist to verify that there is a motor or sensory deficit that is interfering with performance. However, if the measure is not intended to identify a deficit, it is the therapist's responsibility to recognize when poor performance on a formal measure is the result of an underlying condition. If the therapist abandons the standardized procedure on an assessment in order to account for an underlying condition, the normative standards cannot be applied to the performance. Therefore, the results can only be interpreted in narrative form describing observations of the child's performance.

(continued)

Table 6-1. (continued)

Example of Regulations and Their Meaning for Occupational Therapy Evaluation

Focus of the Evaluation	300.304 (4) The child is assessed in all areas related to the suspected disability, including, if appropriate, health, vision, hearing, social and emotional status, general intelligence, academic performance, communicative status, and motor abilities; 300.304 (7) Assessment tools and strategies that provide relevant information that directly assists people in determining the educational needs of the child are provided.	The occupational therapist provides expertise in areas related to motor, sensory, and perceptual skills that impact motor performance. It is essential that the occupational therapist provide documentation of how educational performance is being impacted.
Determination of Eligibility	300.306 (a) General. Upon completion of the administration of assessments and other evaluation measures (1) a group of qualified professionals and the parent of the child determine whether the child is a child with a disability as defined in 300.8. in accordance with paragraph (b) of this subsection and the educational needs of the child; and (2) the public agency provides a copy of the evaluation report and the documentation of determination of eligibility at no cost to the parent.	The occupational therapist must provide an evaluation report that clearly describes whether or not the child is in need of occupational therapy services. Documentation must be provided to support how needs are being met if the expertise of the occupational therapist is not warranted. If occupational therapy services are needed, documentation of how the need to be addressed is directly related to the child's special education.

Resources for additional information:

www.wrightslaw.com/idea/law/FR.v71.n156.pdf

www.nichcy.org/idealist.htm

www.kansped.org/ksde/laws/idea04/idea04.html

http://dese.mo.gov/schoollaw/rulesregs/Inc_By_Ref_Mat/Special%20Education/IDEA%20Part%20B.html

www.nichcy.org/idealaw.htm

serving a child and family can include such professionals as a special educator, psychologist, speech pathologist, classroom teacher, physician, audiologist, social worker, occupational therapist/occupational therapy assistant (the official documents from AOTA contain "roles and responsibilities" for OTs and OTAs), and/or a physical therapist (along with the child, family, and/or other care providers). With each of these people engaging in unique "perspective taking," the team can conceptualize the child's overall performance patterns and identify possible supports and barriers to performance.

Conducting assessments as part of comprehensive evaluations requires various skills. Each assessment strategy or tool requires the professional to draw on particular abilities. Skilled observations and interviews require the professional to understand the possible reasons for performance strengths and difficulties (expressed in the referral or request), so that the professional can solicit (when interviewing) or notice (when observing) factors that will be informative to the decision-making process. Some formal assessments require special training because their administration is standardized or because advanced knowledge is necessary for proper interpretation.

Professional Knowledge and Skills for Best Practice Assessment

Professionals set the tone for the assessment and so must be prepared to create the optimal situation. First, the professionals must have the background and competence to conduct the assessment properly; this ensures that the team can count on the data to provide a reliable picture of the child's performance and on the therapist to report and interpret the data accurately.

Professionals must focus on establishing rapport with the child and family. The characteristics of good rapport building are empathy, genuineness, warmth, respect for children, and a sense of humor (Sattler, 2008; Sattler & Hoge, 2006). It is the professionals' responsibility to make everyone (the child, family, and teachers) feel comfortable; professionals must display an openness to information and an acceptance of the child's, family's, and teacher's perspectives to put them at ease. For new professionals, it is helpful to solicit feedback regarding rapport building; for example, you could have peers watch a video of several of your interactions to see what patterns are present, how different individuals respond, and the impact you have on the interaction as part of professional development.

During assessment procedures, professionals must be so skilled at their own recording and manipulation tasks that they are "transparent" to the child (i.e., they can get the information they need without distracting or interrupting the child's performance). Any feedback or encouragement from the professional must be of a benign nature and must avoid revealing any indication of the success of the performance (i.e., "You are really working hard on this," not "that was correct").

Practical Matters in Assessment

In the educational setting, evaluation provides information regarding diagnosis, eligibility, and program planning for the formulation of the Individualized Education Plan (Pierangelo & Giuliani, 2006). The evaluation process provides the foundation for each subsequent step an occupational therapist takes to understand what is supporting or interfering with participation. It is essential that evaluation decisions be firmly based in the evidence and employ clinical reasoning in order to construct an accurate picture of the child's performance.

There are many factors that can impede this process. As a pediatric therapist, it can be startling to realize that, although you dutifully administered a standardized measure, the 3 year old you are working with has no concern for your need to follow those standardized procedures. Very often, at the end of a testing session, we have a very clear picture of what a 3 year old might refuse to do, but have very little idea about his or her capabilities.

The community-based therapist also faces challenges of space availability, materials, and formal testing tools. However, despite these challenges, the community-based practitioner has several advantages in completing the evaluation process. Community-based therapists have the opportunity to evaluate the child within the natural environment. In addition, other professionals are available to provide insights about the child's performance rather than relying solely on the results of an assessment that measures performance on a given day. These advantages are emphasized within IDEA 2004; the law explicitly directs educational teams to use a variety of sources to evaluate the child's performance. The law requires that the educational team gather data that are relevant to educational participation and provide information regarding developmental level and specific academic performance, which are essential to program planning.

So, one of the first steps to developing an evidence-based approach to the process is to determine what evaluation methods will be most effective at providing the information needed to plan the best intervention program. As detailed by IDEA 2004, all sources need to be considered, including general education information and screenings, record reviews, interviews, observation, and formal evaluation methods. Furthermore, when the team determines that a formal evaluation tool is indicated, IDEA requires that the therapist administer evaluations that are valid and reliable in a standardized manner (see section 303.304 (1) iii of the law).

Although these guidelines would be familiar to most occupational therapists in a community-based practice, the interpretation of the guidelines may vary. For instance, if the therapist suspects that visual motor integration problems are interfering with the child's ability to complete schoolwork, the therapist may select an assessment such as the Test of Visual Motor Integration (Beery, 2004). As directed by

IDEA, the therapist may carefully practice administration and scoring of the test (i.e., give the test in a standardized manner). However, consistent with IDEA, the authors instruct anyone assessing visual motor integration to use the score as only a portion of evidence to indicate a delay and that observation and comparison of performance in daily activities is critical in determining a child's skill level.

For example, in many early childhood settings, the Peabody Developmental Motor Scales (Folio & Fewell, 2000) is the formal evaluation tool of choice. At face value, the use of a developmental assessment fulfills the requirement of IDEA to provide information regarding a child's developmental level. However, it is important to distinguish between the need to provide specific information regarding the child's mastery of developmental milestones when compared to same-aged peers and performing developmentally appropriate activities in the educational setting. A norm-referenced standardized test is designed to tell us whether or not the child's performance is within the typical range for the specific component skills measured by a particular test (Sattler & Hoge, 2006). While the Peabody test does provide the team with an objective measurement for these underlying skills, it does not provide information regarding the child's ability to function when performing daily tasks within the educational setting (Mulenhaupt, 2000). The Peabody Developmental Motor Scales (Folio & Fewell, 2000) is a norm-referenced, standardized measure that is widely used in our profession. It is a valid and reliable instrument for testing the developmental level for gross and fine motor skills. However, the use of a standardized assessment for children with autism is challenging given the language deficits and behavioral difficulties associated with the diagnosis (Tomchek & Case Smith, 2009).

To illustrate the impact of the choices made in the assessment process, we present three cases comparing performance component approach and participation-focused evaluation processes and the impact of these decisions on the child's program plan.

Case #1: Initial Planning Based on Performance Factors

The initial programming focused on increasing component skills related to fine motor performance (Table 6-2). The therapist gave Terrance the Peabody Developmental Motor Scales; he could not complete this assessment. The occupational therapist determined that there was a delay in fine motor skills and that occupational therapy services were needed to remediate these delays. When aspects of the diagnosis interfere with the administration of an evaluation, it may be difficult to determine when we are measuring a lack of certain abilities or when we are measuring a lack of understanding the directions.

There are several concerns for this initial approach. First, use of standardized procedures for a child with autism may not yield accurate results. There was not a focus on participation but rather on his skill development. There was also a lack of input on the part of school personnel and parents in the process. Collaborating with parents is critical to the assessment process to identify those areas that are a priority for families; parent interviews may provide unique insights into the strengths and abilities (Paikoff Holzmueller, 2005). While use of standardized assessment may be necessary during parts of special education services, in best practice services, we emphasize the child's strengths first, along with participation in authentic environments.

Planning Focused on Participation

The parent's number one priority for Terrance was that he would learn to eat independently. When we examined Terrance's program, the focus was on increasing coordinating and strength of fine motor skills. In using a developmental approach, the hypothesis would be that if we increased skills in strength and coordination, this would lead to increased function in activities such as eating. However, when we used observation and interview to evaluate Terrance's skills, we learned that he was able to take apart intricate pieces of toys and had the strength to pinch peers and teachers with great force. Many other observations provided evidence that strength and coordination were not the primary deficits that were interfering with performance even though he was not always able to demonstrate those skills on demand. At the time of the initial assessment, Terrance was eating lunch alone in his classroom to eliminate auditory distractions in the lunchroom.

When we conducted a file review and examined the Sensory Profile, Terrance did not appear to be overly sensitive to auditory stimulation. In addition, Terrance responded positively to certain visual and tactile cues. Using the sensory information in conjunction with a behavioral plan utilizing the Picture

Table 6-2.

Terrance's Plan

Case #1 Terrance. His parents want him to eat independently and socialize. Terrance has been diagnosed with autism.

Initial Assessment Procedures (age 4 years)	Initial Program Planning (focus on performance factors)	Alternative Assessment Procedures (age 6 years)	Best Practice Program Planning (focus on participation)
Peabody Developmental Motor Scales (Folio & Fewell, 2000) Sensory Profile Caregivers Questionnaire (Dunn, 2000)	Using the developmental frame of reference, the focus was on remediating grasp patterns, bilateral skills, and visual motor skills. A box of sensory toys was available in the classroom for sensory stimulation. A quiet area, recliner, and mat were available for a retreat area when overwhelmed.	File Review Observation Interview Parent/Teacher/Paraprofessional School Function Assessment (Coster, 1998)	Based on parent and teacher information interventions focused on increasing independence in eating skills and increasing opportunities to meet sensory needs so the student could participate with peers during class activities.

Exchange Communication System (PECS) (Charlop-Christy, Carpentar, Loc, LeBlan, & Kellet, 2002), Terrance began eating lunch in the lunchroom with typical peers as models. Currently, Terrance goes through the line with stand-by assist and eats finger foods independently and has been using a fork or spoon with increased success. Prior to this, he had not used utensils to eat and frequently would throw his food and grab others' food when eating, so parents were pleased with the improvements at school.

Recently, during an IEP meeting, the team discussed that, although eating behaviors had significantly increased at school, the family continued to struggle with eating at home. Terrance routinely throws food and refuses to use utensils during every family meal. The team decided to try strategies from a study on children with autism using social stories and video feedback for children with autism (Thiemann & Goldstein, 2001). The occupational therapist, teachers, and parents have initiated a collaborative effort to develop a more successful eating routine at home. Terrance was videotaped during a successful lunch period at school. The parents agreed to show Terrance the video after they read a social story with pictures representing positive lunchroom behaviors just before dinner time at home. In addition, the speech pathologist coached them about how to use a more consistent method of redirection using the PECS to communicate with Terrance during meals.

Case #2: Initial Plans and Findings

In completing a file review of previous developmental testing, professionals described Amanda's age equivalent for fine motor skills was that of a 10-month-old. Reporting an age equivalent score is not a recommended practice (Table 6-3). In Amanda's case, this is a misleading thing to report about her performance. Because she has cerebral palsy, we do not expect her to follow the same developmental trajectory as other children her age.

When we examined Amanda's skills on even these particular tests, we found that she was developing grasp patterns and was able to copy block patterns close to what we would expect for her age level. It is always essential to emphasize parent interviews and skilled observations, supplementing with any required standardized testing information so that we can provide an accurate picture of strengths as well as concerns. Observable, jargon-free descriptions of performance are not only a more accurate representation of a child's performance but are more respectful in discussing a child with the parents (Richardson, 2001).

Table 6-3.

Amanda's Plan

Case #2 Amanda. A girl whose parents want her to socialize with peers. She has a diagnosis of cerebral palsy.

Initial Assessment Procedures (age 3 years)	Initial Program Planning (focus on performance factors)	Alternative Assessment Procedures (age 9 years)	Alternative Program Planning (focus on participation)
Peabody Developmental Motor Scales (Folio & Fewell, 2000) Test of Visual Motor Integration (VMI) (Beery, 2004)	Provide strategies to increase hand use, eye-hand coordination, and manual dexterity	File Review Parent/Teacher Interview Skilled Observation School Function Assessment (Coster, 1998)	Focus on strategies to increase Amanda's opportunity for social interaction, increase independence in daily life activities

DO NOT USE AGE OR GRADE EQUIVALENT SCORES

The American Psychological Association and the American Educational Research Association (1999) recommend the use of standard scores rather than age or grade equivalent scores. Age and grade equivalent scores are misleading because the increments of time (e.g., 6 months) do not reflect the same increments of growth in different parts of development. For example, the amount of growth from 2 years 6 months to 3 years 0 months does not represent the same amount of change as 10 years 6 months to 11 years 0 months. Similarly, the amount and type of changes in first grade is not equivalent to the changes in fourth grade.

School-Based Team Planning

In interviewing Amanda's mother, she discussed the fact that Amanda was a twin and the twin was typically developing. Amanda often played with her twin and other children in the neighborhood; in this context, Amanda had many skills socially and was very motivated to participate with typically developing children. Increasing Amanda's time with typically developing peers was paramount to this parent. With this information, the team decided to complete the School Function Assessment (SFA) on Amanda to gain information about her level of participation in non-academic activities in the school setting. Interpretation of the SFA revealed that Amanda received a high level of assistance for many physical tasks in the school day, and there were currently few adaptations in place. The team began to focus on methods to reduce the amount of physical assistance by an adult.

In addition to increasing time with typically developing peers, the mother also wanted to increase emphasis on independence in toileting behaviors and the activities that Amanda performs within the regular classroom. Participation and activity performance of students with cerebral palsy were affected by the amount of environmental barriers in both self-contained and fully included settings (Schenker, Coster, & Parush, 2004). These authors recommended examining the environment and identifying barriers that may prevent activity performance and interfere with participation in daily activities.

Following an observation in her regular classroom, the therapist identified a number of missed opportunities for participating in the classroom routine. The team is currently negotiating on methods to increase participation that will work into Amanda's classroom routine. The occupational therapist provided Amanda with some individual coaching to improve her independence in toileting.

Table 6-4.

Malcom's Plan

Case #3 Malcom. A boy who needs support to participate throughout the day. He has been diagnosed with autism.

Initial Assessment Procedures (age 9 years)	Initial Program Planning (focus on performance components)	Alternative Assessment Procedures (age 10 years)	Best Practice Program Planning (Focus on participation)
Children's Rehabilitation Unit Gross and Fine Motor Evaluation	Increase fine motor skills, bilateral skills, and prevocational skills. Increase ability to write his name.	File Review Parent/Teacher Interview Observation Sensory Profile Sensory Profile School Companion	Identify opportunities to meet sensory processing needs throughout the school day so he can participate in learning activities with peers.

Case #3: Initial Program Planning

Previous testing focused on measurement of developmental milestones based on a locally compiled developmental checklist. There are several issues that would prevent us from basing our planning on this type of assessment. The age range for this particular assessment is birth to 6 years of age. At the time of testing, Malcom was 9 years, which is 3 years beyond the range for this evaluation (Table 6-4). In addition, there is no published information regarding the reliability or validity of this evaluation tool.

Planning Focused on Participation

At the time of the re-evaluation period, Malcom was in a self-contained special education classroom and had a teaching assistant throughout the day. Observation of classroom activities revealed that Malcom primarily worked on tracing and matching activities during seatwork. Teacher interview indicated that she wanted Malcom to be more independent in classroom activities; she was also concerned with his inability to concentrate when multiple activities are going on in the classroom.

The therapist administered the Sensory Profile (Dunn, 2000) and the Sensory Profile School Companion (Dunn, 2006). Both questionnaires indicated that Malcom is highly attentive to visual stimulation. Malcom seeks movement throughout his day, which may be why he is fidgety with items and is constantly getting up. Malcom also seeks out tactile input, which is enjoyable and may be calming to him. For example, during skilled observations, the therapist noticed that Malcom rubbed on the lining of his jacket when there was more activity in the classroom. Malcom is very sensitive to auditory stimuli. He often becomes distressed with loud, unexpected noises, and when there is increased environmental noise, he covers his ears. This response to noise may create difficulties in his ability to attend to auditory directions. Malcom often copes with noise by humming, talking, or singing.

His mother reports that he likes the texture of liquids, sand, and paper. She also reports that he likes fuzzy, soft fabrics. He avoids social situations and activities that involve interactions with others. He demonstrates a need for routine and experiences difficulty with transitions, which is consistent with the teacher's experience as well. His need for order and routine combined with the increased noise during transition periods seems to be contributing to these challenging times of the day.

Table 6-5 outlines some of the suggestions the therapist made to improve Malcom's participation in his classroom. The OT and teacher examined the school routines and found appropriate adaptations within each learning setting to support Malcom.

Table 6-5.

Adaptations for Malcom's Day

School Routine	Adaptations to Support Participation in School Routine	Observations to Indicate Malcom's Participation is Improved With This Support
General suggestions within classroom	Create a Visual Schedule so Malcom can see what is coming next Create a program for Malcom to walk laps between work periods Provide hand lotion that he can easily access Place velcro under his desk for him to touch	Increase in work efficiency
Morning Routine with class	Speak in a calm quiet tone when giving directions	Malcom remains with the class
Class instruction followed by small group support as needed	Provide written instructions for directions for daily tasks Allow Malcom to do work in various positions (e.g., let Malcom complete his math standing at the white board)	Malcom completes work assigned in time provided
Seatwork time	Provide a quiet work space with limited noise (e.g., allow him to work in the library when possible) Have Malcom get up to put finished assignments in a mailbox or folder Provide a ball chair or air cushion on his chair so he can stay at his seat and get movement while working	Malcom continues to work during the seatwork period Malcom completes at least 75% of work
Social Studies/ Geography/Life Science (combo of large, small group, and individual work)	Use bump paper to provide a tactile cue to increase attention to detail Write on varied surfaces, different textured paper, sand paper, slick surfaces Provide models of written work to be copied	Malcom completes his work within the time period provided
Get ready to go home	Use headphones to help regulate noise when in louder environments (can be just muting the noise or playing soft music)	Is ready with belongings when others are ready to go
Go to the bus	Let Malcom use an mp3 player on the bus with preferred music	Successfully rides home without incident

So, with these examples highlighting a best practice approach, let's examine the details of these processes.

Parameters for Best Practice Assessment

Occupational therapists are concerned with participation in daily life. This focus needs to be evident throughout the occupational therapy process, but is particularly important during evaluation because evaluation sets the stage for all subsequent intervention and follow-up activities. The primary focus of best practice occupational therapy assessment is to identify what the person wants and needs to do. The second focus is to identify the daily life contexts for participation because best practice services are set in the authentic contexts for participation. After these two issues are addressed, the occupational therapist employs additional assessment methods that identify person, task, and environmental variables that seem to be supporting and creating barriers to participation; this is the data from which we build best practice intervention recommendations.

When designing best practice occupational therapy assessment, the occupational therapist organizes the work by beginning with participation in authentic contexts. As you will see, assessment of person variables only occurs as this information is needed to understand the performance issue more clearly.

Law, Baum, and Dunn (2005) provide reviews of assessments of person factors, environmental factors, participation factors, and assessments that evaluate interactions of these factors.

Strengths-Based Assessment

When children are struggling in a particular area of life, it is easy to focus on the difficulties and how to fix them. However, in best practice, we remember to focus on the child's strengths as well. By examining how a child is successful, we can learn what factors are necessary to support success. For example, if a student gets more seatwork completed when going to the library to work, we might hypothesize that the walk down the hall, the quiet of the library, and the solitude away from peer pressure are supporting the student's performance. The teacher or librarian may have insights about which hypothesis is correct; armed with information about what it takes to create success (e.g., the walk down the hall gives the student a movement break), we can use this information to create more successful learning experiences. In a strengths model, we ask, "What does it take for this student to be successful?" Even though we will also examine what is interfering with performance, knowing the student's strengths keeps us focused on successful outcomes.

Occupationally Focused Assessment

The referral concern provides the best guidance about the participation focus for assessment. A parent may be concerned about how to play with the child, a teacher might be concerned that a student with severe disabilities needs to develop eating skills, or a school-to-work coordinator may want assistance in selecting a well-matched job for an adolescent. These statements about performance needs indicate both what the child needs to do and where the child needs to participate; occupational therapy assessment will uncover what is supporting or interfering with these activities.

The most common strategies for assessing occupation are skilled observation and interviewing (in the next section, we describe these in detail). These two techniques provide a means for understanding why this performance is a priority, the factors that may be supporting and creating barriers to performance, and what would constitute satisfying performance. Therapists also need to characterize the child's current approach to the task of interest; sometimes, children approach performance in an unusual, but successful manner (i.e., they are satisfied with how they do it), but others may wish for the child to conduct themselves differently or believe that a different approach would solve the performance problem.

For example, it is common for teachers to want children to have a mature tripod grasp of writing utensils for classroom work; because this is how most children write the best, they believe this grasp is related to completing schoolwork efficiently. However, some children will hold the writing utensil in a different, but functional way while working (just as many adults do, look around your class!). In addressing performance, the occupational therapist can determine the need, utility, and feasibility of changing the grasping pattern. The therapist will use clinical reasoning to determine whether the current grasping pattern is efficient for the child in completing schoolwork and whether the grasping pattern presents any risks for malformations, skin breakdowns, or joint deformities (which would ultimately interfere with schoolwork performance). The therapist can also consider whether it is possible for the child to use a different grasping pattern and, if possible, the length of time it would take for the child to change and regain efficiency. The therapist will also be thinking about adaptations to using the writing utensil in consideration of all possibilities for functional written communication in schoolwork. This example illustrates how consideration of person and task factors can affect performance, while remaining focused on the performance itself (i.e., completing schoolwork).

There are several assessment tools available to characterize overall occupational performance in context. Table 6-6 provides some examples for you; to get more details, refer to Law et al. (2005).

Contextually Relevant Assessment

It is also important to consider assessment of the environment. This information is helpful for placement decisions (i.e., is this or that setting a better match for the child) and for resource acquisition (i.e., what will it take to make this environment user-friendly or accessible to the child). For example, the Home Observation for Measurement of the Environment (HOME) measures the content, quality, and responsiveness of home environments (Caldwell & Bradley, 1978). Other scales measure the service setting environment (e.g., the Early Childhood Environment Rating Scale and the School Age Care Environment Rating Scale, see Law et al., 2005, for more details). Other contextual measures consider the relationship between the person and the environment (see Table 6-6).

Measurement Options in Best Practice Evaluation

There are several options for gathering data during evaluation. Each option gives professionals a specific way to understand the factors that might be contributing to or interfering with participation. Occupational therapists focus attention on the referral concern to construct the overall evaluation plan because the referral provides an indication of participation needs. Knowing evaluation options enables the therapist to select a combination of data collection methods that reveal both the child's participation strengths and needs and possible underlying factors that are supporting or interfering with participation.

Because we are concerned about a child's participation, it is appropriate to organize evaluations to discover participation strengths and needs early in the process and then move toward other methods to discover what might be supporting or interfering with participation. We can use a range of strategies and will outline their contributions here.

Review the Records

Records review is a preliminary step to provide background information. When we receive referrals, it is common that other team members have gathered information about the child. This can include history (including birth history, age, family structure, developmental milestones reached, and achievement test history), referral concerns, or even some initial testing. When children are older, their files can contain previous testing and school records as well. It is prudent as part of evaluation for the occupational therapist to review the available records. This review can provide a background for the child's needs, avoid duplication of questions for the family or teacher, and guide choices for further assessment procedures. If another professional has already given a particular measure recently, it is appropriate to use these data in your assessment interpretation rather than administering the evaluation or asking questions again. Some therapists think they must administer each evaluation so they can observe the child themselves; this is not an effective use of the child's or therapist's time. It is best practice to glean whatever we can from the records and then proceed with other assessment strategies.

Identify the Participation Strengths and Issues

Because participation is of prime interest to occupational therapy, we must remain focused on what the child, family, and teachers want and need for

Table 6-6.

Examples of Assessments That Capture Occupational Performance and Contextually Related Performance

Assessment	Use as an Occupationally Focused and Contextually Relevant Assessment*
Canadian Occupational Performance Measure (COPM) (Law, Polatajko, Pollock, McColl, Carswell, & Baptiste, 1994)	Solicits the child (if appropriate), family, and/or teacher to identify performance issues in activities of daily living, productive activity, and leisure. The COPM also asks the person to characterize the level of competence and rate satisfaction of that performance competence. One of the most interesting things about the COPM is that it supports the idea that less than perfect performance is still satisfying and therefore acceptable. Intervention planning and goal setting emerges from the COPM in relation to those performance areas that are not satisfying to the person, family, or teacher. (See Tammy, Chapter 9, for an illustration.)
School Function Assessment (SFA) (Coster, Deeney, Haltiwanger, & Haley, 1998)	Teachers complete the form, rating the child's level of function in 14 performance areas at school; they report whether the child needs accommodations or assistance to complete the school tasks of interest. (See Peter, Chapter 9 for illustration.)
The Vineland Adaptive Behavior Scales, Second Edition (Vineland-II) (Sparrow, Cicchetti, & Balla, 2005)	Measures the child's ability to engage in functional interaction with people, objects, and situations. Typically, the rater characterizes the child's ability to perform the functional life tasks, including functional communication, self help, socialization, and motor skills. (The Web site indicates that a professional needs specialized skills to use the Vineland; occupational therapists are considered appropriate professionals to use this assessment.)
The Coping Inventory (Williamson & Szczepanski, 1999)	Characterizes a person's responses to internal and external forces and the person's ability to manage in consideration of these forces, with the recognition that there is a level of stress that is motivating to act and a level that interferes with performance. (See Peter, Chapter 9 for an illustration.)
Transdisciplinary Play-Based Assessment II (Linder, 2009)	The team works collaboratively to identify children's performance issues while observing the child playing. Everyone learns about the others' perspectives while conducting the assessment; additionally, the child is more comfortable in this assessment setting because the activities can be familiar.
Pediatric Evaluation of Disability Inventory (PEDI) (Haley, Coster, Ludlow, Haltiwanger, & Andrellos, 1992)	Provides a method for recording the impact of the child's disability on function within their living environments.
The Sensory Profile, Infant Toddler Sensory Profile, Sensory Profile School Companion, Adolescent Adult Sensory Profile (Dunn, 1999; 2002; 2006; Brown & Dunn, 2002)	Solicit the caregivers' or self-perspective on how sensory events in the daily living environment, including home, community, and school, affect performance. Sensory processing patterns are considered as they may support or interfere with everyday life activities.

*See Law, Baum, & Dunn (2005) for additional assessments, reviews, and references.

this child to do. Sometimes, the records will give us clues, but then we need to follow up with additional assessment methods to confirm or reject our initial hypotheses. Typically, therapists conduct interviews and skilled observations to get a clear picture of participation strengths and needs. We want to create an "occupational profile" and history that informs us about the child's life.

Interviews

Interviewing is an artful task in which the professional is seeking information from an informant (e.g., the teacher, the parent, a sibling or friend, and/or the child being evaluated). Although this is a data-gathering tool, interviewing is also a time for establishing rapport. The comfort (or discomfort) a person feels will influence the amount of information he or she feels comfortable providing.

There are a number of ways to conduct an interview, and each needs to be selected based on the information needed and the comfort level of the interviewee. Parents may feel more comfortable in their homes or may wish to get away for a little while and be interviewed at a coffee shop. Some teachers will select the teacher's lounge at school, while others will find this environment less private than they like and will choose another location. Most of the time, a face-to-face interview is better, but there may be situations in which the person will suggest a phone interview (usually related to time or distance restraints). With technology options available, video phone options also exist if this is available and comfortable for both parties. There are also occasions when the therapist will send a questionnaire along ahead of time so the person has time to formulate his or her thoughts before the interview; as with other techniques, it is important to invite the person to help you decide what is best. You can say, "Would it be helpful for you to receive some questions ahead of time, or would you prefer to just chat with me when we meet?" This gives the person an opportunity to participate in the process in the most comfortable way.

Interviewing requires the therapist to be very focused on both the information needed and what the person is relaying in the conversation. Some interviews require very explicit information (e.g., developmental milestones), while others need to be more open-ended to elicit descriptive information (e.g., "tell me about mealtime"). For example, we might ask a parent to discuss their specific concern and then branch to other issues as the parent talks. Or we might ask the parent to describe his or her home life and work toward specific concerns.

When formulating interview questions, it is important to ask mostly open-ended questions that do not indicate a right or wrong response. We use words like *describe* to encourage the person to elaborate on the issue. Questions that require only a "yes" or "no" response do not encourage elaboration. We reviewed the reflective questioning approach in Chapters 5 and 8; it invites the person to elaborate and share ideas about what he or she thinks behaviors and concerns mean. This open strategy for interviewing provides the therapist with much more information to use as a basis for program planning.

It is helpful to reflect back to the person what he or she has just said to make sure that you clearly understand his or her perspective and to indicate that you are listening actively to what he or she is saying. Additionally, it is important to use positive nonverbal communication, such as eye contact, open postures, leaning forward, and facial expressions, to indicate involvement in the conversation. Therapists can also take notes during the interview to indicate their interest in the person's comments. All of these strategies increase the likelihood that the informant will share his or her perspectives and concerns candidly and therefore increase the possible insights into the performance situation.

Determine What Is Supporting or Interfering With Participation

When you have an idea about the child's participation strengths and needs, it is then important to consider what might be supporting or interfering with participation for this child. Frequently, we get initial ideas about supports and barriers from our interviews; these ideas guide us toward particular hypotheses. The next step involves gathering more information to confirm or reject these hypotheses. Having an accurate picture of the child in context contributes to more precise intervention planning. Occupational therapists conduct skilled observations, ecological assessments, and activity analyses to gather this more detailed information. We only use formal testing using standardized or criterion-referenced measures to anchor our evaluations with evidence or to provide data for other reporting requirements.

Conduct Skilled Observations

Skilled observation is the most critical assessment tool available to occupational therapists. Because occupational therapists are trained to notice and interpret behaviors in a particular manner (based on our knowledge and skills), we call this process "skilled observation." Skilled observation enables us to capture the nature of the behavior in its natural context and therefore reveals what might be supporting or interfering with the desired participation. Skilled observation is also the most difficult assessment method because it requires the therapists to bring all of their knowledge to bear (e.g., all practice model knowledge, clinical reasoning skills) on the moment-by-moment interaction between the child and the child's activity and environment.

We can construct a plan for observation, complete a questionnaire, or engage the child in a set of activities to identify participation strengths and needs. We might design a list of questions for the teacher to respond to regarding the child's behaviors in the classroom or ask the teacher's aide to collect data on a particular behavior for a period of time to get a record of the patterns of performance. Sometimes, there are informal tools that have been designed in a particular work setting, and all the therapists in that setting use the forms as part of their agency's assessment process.

When the referral concern is about a particular area of participation, the therapist might work with the child during that activity, changing aspects of the activity to see how the child responds. For example, if a teacher states that the child is having trouble with math worksheets, the therapist might first observe the child during math seatwork to form some initial hypotheses and then make suggestions about how to adjust the environment (e.g., where the student is sitting) or the activity (e.g., enlarging the math problems to make more room for writing in the answer). The teacher would keep track of the student's math success as a method for determining whether these adjustments were effective. In this example, the therapist is contributing to the "Response to Intervention" process used in regular education to identify ways to support students in their natural context. We will be discussing this process a little later in the chapter, and there are more detailed examples in the case studies (see Chapter 9).

Performance Skills Assessment

Through skilled observation, we determine a child's use of sensory, motor, cognition, regulation, communication, and social skills within daily life participation. We identify what environmental stimuli enable a child to focus or what might be distracting. We see the process the child uses to solve problems and how the child selects to engage when not being directed by others. All of these aspects of participation can be tested in isolation, but we do not know whether they are interfering with performance until we conduct a skilled observation in the natural context.

For example, perhaps the therapist observed that the child took a longer time to gather materials for the reading group than the other children, or perhaps the mother described the child's frustration when trying to find his or her favorite toy. Both the mother and the therapist provide skilled observation data. From these observations, the therapist hypothesizes that there may be a visual perception problem and so decides to administer the Test of Visual Perceptual Skills to test this hypothesis. The score profile indicates that the child has visual figure ground perception difficulties (when compared to the norm group), thus verifying the hypothesis and linking visual figure ground perception to difficulty with participation at home and school. This formal test score merely verifies the interview and observation hypothesis that visual figure ground perception is interfering with participation in actual daily life situations.

The most artful part of best practice occupational therapy assessment is recognizing the performance skills and difficulties as they present themselves during performance in daily life. With appropriate training and practice, anyone can administer a formal test. However, it takes clinical reasoning skills to use skilled observation to glean information from everyday activities. In this section, we will consider some ways to recognize the performance skills (i.e., sensory perceptual, motor and praxis, emotional regulation, cognitive, communication, and social skills) in children's daily performance.

The best way to become proficient in skilled observation is to practice. Watch others perform, and identify the "performance skills" aspects of the performance. View videotapes with your peers and talk about the performance skills that you see in the people's behaviors. Make this aspect of your clinical reasoning part of the fabric of your everyday thinking. Use the *OT Practice Framework* (www.aota.org) as a guide to structure your observations.

PRACTICE SKILLED OBSERVATIONS

Identify a video from the internet illustrating a person/people doing something in everyday life. Working with peers, conduct individual skilled observations of the clip with particular attention to "performance skills." Then, have a discussion about what you documented compared to others. Create a more comprehensive list of observations, and apply them to a new clip. Each time, discuss with others to improve your proficiency.

As we discuss in another section, there are formal tests of performance skills available. These are only used when we need to verify a child's status or validate the source of participation challenges.

Skilled Observation of Sensory Perceptual Skills

Team members count on occupational therapists to know how sensory perceptual skills affect performance. The applied science literature about the impact of sensory processing originated in the historic work of A. Jean Ayres, who was an occupational therapist and researcher. As we discussed in Chapter 4, sensory processing is a practice framework that is considered the special expertise of our discipline; others expect us to be a resource on sensory processing and its impact on life.

Sensory information forms the basis for our brain's ability to recognize and derive meaning from the world. Children can have difficulty receiving sensory information due to a structural defect in the sensory organ itself (e.g., with visual and hearing impairments), or they can have difficulty deriving meaning from the sensory information they receive (Dunn, 1997; Kandel, Schwartz, & Jessell, 2000). To discriminate these functions, we look for any signs of noticing stimuli. For example, even premature infants will have autonomic nervous system (ANS) responses to stimuli when they notice them (e.g., eyes dilating). Children with nonfunctioning sensory organs will not have ANS reactions because their nervous systems have not taken in any information.

Recognizing the sensory processing features of a child's performance is a unique gift that occupational therapists give their teams and families. No other discipline studies sensory processing in their entry preparation; this perspective enriches the discussion of performance needs, and it is the occupational therapists' responsibility to provide guidance and leadership regarding this perspective. There are many resources that provide detailed information about sensory perceptual observations (e.g., Dunn, 2007, 2008).

Perception is a cognitive ability to interpret the sensory information the brain receives. There are many types of perception, based on the many ways that the brain receives and makes sense out of the information available. Perceptual difficulties can interfere with many aspects of daily life; as occupational therapists, we are concerned about perceptual difficulties as they impact living. Although there are formal tests of perceptual skills, these scores are irrelevant if the child is functioning successfully at school

PRACTICE OBSERVING SENSORY PERCEPTUAL SKILLS
(also see Dunn, 2008)

- Does the child react to sensory events like the other children? Is it bigger/smaller than others?
- In a busy context, what does the child notice? Is the child distracted/oblivious to stimuli?
- What food choices does the child make?
- Does the child engage in behaviors to increase sensory experiences (e.g., tapping pencil, humming, getting up a lot)?
- Does the child engage in behaviors to decrease sensory experiences (e.g., hands on ears, moving to a more isolated area)?
- Review references that provide guidance about how to interpret behaviors (e.g., Dunn, 2007, 2008).
- Work with colleagues to identify behaviors you can document about the integrity of the sensory and perceptual systems (e.g., looking at video clips together).

and at home. Table 6-7 contains a list of perceptual terms, their definitions, and an example of when this perceptual ability is used in daily life.

Application of Sensory-Perceptual Skills

Skilled Observation of Motor and Praxis Skills

When observing children's motor skills, knowing what to expect developmentally creates a scaffolding for knowing what to document. It isn't that all children need to follow milestones, but rather that we have ideas about what to look for and to imagine whether the movements you see will support the child to be successful within a peer group and in activities expected of children in a particular age group. For example, coordination skills between the two body sides will look different for a 4-year-old and a 14-year-old; coordination is important to participation in both ages, but the demands will be different.

Praxis is the cognitive process of conceiving and planning new motor acts. When motor sequences become familiar, they no longer require praxis (Ayres, 1979). For example, if a person gets on a bike and has not ridden one for years, the person will be a bit rusty at first, but the motor schemas to support this activity are still available and will support bike riding in a short time. This is very different from a person who has never ridden a bike before. Although this second person may have the balance, bilateral integration, and postural control needed, the person has never before put them together into a schema for bike riding. Therefore, to develop the new schema called "bike riding" would require praxis.

There are 2 primary areas of difficulty in praxis. First, children can have difficulty with "ideation," or coming up with the ideas needed to explore the environment and engage in discovery (Ayres, 1979). During skilled observation, these children appear uninterested in play and may sit quietly even in an enticing environment, or they may engage in a repetitive movement (e.g., opening and closing a door) without changing the pattern. They lack the ability to retain or develop play patterns that they can build on for increasingly complex play. When you watch, it is like they don't have any "ideas" about what to do; that is a way to remember this kind of praxis.

Second, children can have difficulty with "planning," or constructing the way to move to act out one's ideas (Ayres, 1979). These children are active and engaging, but their movements are ineffective and clumsy. They understand what they want to do, but have difficulty making their bodies do the correct patterns (enacting the idea). When you are observing, these children display signs of frustration; they

PRACTICE OBSERVING MOTOR SKILLS

- Watch a group of children the same age and see how many different ways they exhibit the same motor skills.
- Watch children on a playground so you see different ages at the same time; notice what the children select to do and how they move their bodies at different ages.
- Watch how children manipulate objects, including balls or pencils, and how they use objects to accomplish a task (e.g., wiping off the counter with a sponge).
- While observing, consider the relationship between particular motor skills and the child's successful participation. Do children keep trying, do they get frustrated, do they refine their movements as they go?
- Consider some specific observations too:
  - Are there some movements that are easier or harder for children?
  - Do some muscle groups appear more predominant in functional tasks than others?
  - Does the child "lock" joints when moving as if to stabilize the body?
  - What grasp pattern does the child use during tasks? How does the grasping pattern help or interfere with the task?
  - What base of support is the child using during the task?
  - Is there a balance of stability and mobility during the task?
- Work with colleagues to identify behaviors you can document about the integrity of the motor systems (e.g., looking at video clips together).

Table 6-7.

Perceptual Terms and Examples in Daily Life

	Definition	Everyday Life Example
Visual	Being able to take information in through the eyes and make sense of it for learning.	A preschooler finds the green crayon in the crayon box. The children put a puzzle together. The child helps mom find the spatula in a crowded kitchen drawer.
Auditory	The ability to take in information through the ears and make sense of it for learning.	A child hears his name being called on a crowded busy playground and stops what he is doing to attend to the voice of his mother. An adolescent is more efficient doing homework with background music. A student works better in the quiet library.
Proprioceptive	The ability to know where one's body is in space.	A student understands how much force is needed to push the classroom door open. A preschooler knows how much pressure to place on the cup to pick it up and drink from it. An adolescent prefers wearing tight jeans and a backpack.
Tactile	The ability to know about things that come in contact with the skin.	A child prefers to wear loosely fitted clothing. A child is bothered by crowded areas because he gets unintentionally bumped by other children. An adolescent refuses to eat "slimy" foods.
Olfactory	The ability to interpret smells.	A student notices when the teacher has a new air freshener on her desk at school. An adolescent objects to scented soaps.
Gustatory	The ability to interpret tastes.	A child prefers to eat foods that have a specific flavor. (e.g., prefers to eat only salty food).
Vestibular	The ability to know where your head is in relation to gravity.	A child enjoys swinging on the playground or riding a roller coaster at the amusement park. A child does not mind tipping her head back under the water to rinse her hair while bathing.

understand the plan and their inability to "do it right" can be upsetting. Children with difficulty planning may refuse to try new things or may direct others to do things for them to avoid the failure from trying it themselves (remember, they understand what is supposed to happen). You may observe or hear from interviews that these children are destructive (their incoordination can lead to breaking toys). We must be careful to consider difficulty with praxis when we see these behaviors and not assume they reflect psychosocial difficulties.

Skilled Observation of Emotional Regulation Skills

We observe emotional regulation skills throughout the child's day. We can actually obtain a lot of information from parents, teachers, or employers because these people spend a lot of time with the child. Although we can make specific observations at given points in time, emotional regulation occurs across time. Our skilled observations at one point in time can only provide partial information that has to be combined with other information for a complete picture.

PRACTICE OBSERVING EMOTIONAL REGULATION SKILLS

- How does the child react to other people's emotional reactions?
- How does the child behave when facing something frustrating?
- What emotions does the child exhibit in a particular situation, and how does this reaction match with the circumstances?
- What is the range of emotional reactions? Is it a typical range? Does it match other children's reactions?
- How does the child calm self? What upsets the child?
- Work with colleagues to identify behaviors you can document about the integrity of the emotional regulation systems (e.g., looking at video clips together).

Skilled Observation of Cognitive Skills

Other disciplines consider cognition along with occupational therapy; teachers focus on learning, psychologists evaluate cognitive subskills. Our unique contribution involves determining how cognitive skills occur during everyday activities. We may not be the team member who tests cognitive skill components, but we will offer perspectives about the child's use of cognitive skills. During skilled observation, we might document the behaviors that seem to indicate a child's attention or memory. For example, an adolescent may not look at the teacher, but we observe that the adolescent complies with the teacher's instruction, indicating the adolescent is paying attention and processing the information. If a child has technical skills (e.g., adequate memory based on a memory test), but cannot call on those skills when the situation demands it (e.g., doesn't remember homework assignments), we might ask ourselves the relevance of the memory test score.

PRACTICE OBSERVING COGNITIVE SKILLS

- How does the child organize objects/ideas while working to solve a problem?
- What categories does the child use to name things (e.g., "doggie" for all 4-legged animals")?
- How does the child sequence the task so he or she has success? Does the child self-correct during tasks?
- Does the child place objects in relation to each other for tasks (e.g., putting the cheese on the bread to make a grilled cheese sandwich)?
- What behaviors might indicate that the child is generalizing skills to new situations?
- Consider some specific observations, too:
  - o Does the child use visual cues to keep on track during activities (e.g., looking at other children to see what to do next)?
  - o Is the child able to follow oral directions like peers?
  - o Does the child find ways to complete a task when appropriate tools are not available (e.g., pour batter into two smaller pans)?
- Work with colleagues to identify behaviors you can document about the integrity of the cognitive systems (e.g., looking at video clips together).

Skilled Observation of Communication and Social Skills

As with cognition, other disciplines consider communication and social skills along with occupational therapists. Social workers make sure children and adolescents can broker their social skills within appropriate community contexts. Speech language pathologists address all components that comprise communication and share our interest in how children use their communication skills to get their needs met. We want to make sure that communication and social skills support children's occupational pursuits, including friendships, learning, work, family life, and personal interests. When conducting skilled observations in this performance skill area, document the child's actual behaviors, the context within which you are observing, and how the target child's performance compares to other children in the same context. Not all children have to communicate or socialize in the same ways; some children will be quiet while others may be very interactive. It is whether the child feels successful within the given context that matters; use this filter to decide what your observations mean.

PRACTICE OBSERVING COMMUNICATION AND SOCIAL SKILLS

- Does the child engage in similar behaviors within a particular context (e.g., take turns in a game)?
- Does the child use eye contact, gestures, intonation when interacting with others?
- How does the child respond to others' nonverbal communication?
- How does the child use personal space/acknowledge others' personal space?
- Work with colleagues to identify behaviors you can document about the integrity of the communication and social skills systems (e.g., looking at video clips together).

Remain Part of the Background While Observing

When conducting a skilled observation, the therapist must be careful not to interfere with the natural course of events being observed. This means that we must remain in the background of the activity and not become the person directing the activity or creating reinforcement by responding to the child directly. When a therapist becomes overly engaged, he or she becomes part of the activity and loses the vantage point that facilitates good data recording. For example, the therapist who gets too involved in a conversation with a child during the skilled observation may miss the directions from the teacher to the class or may not notice the other children's responses to the target child. We must make sure that we are available for all possible opportunities to notice what might be supporting or interfering with performance.

Notice the Role of Environmental Features

Factors in the environment can support or interfere with participation. Initially, the therapist records objective statements about the environment and then later can consider the impact of these environmental features on the child's participation. The therapist must record information about all aspects of context as outlined in the AOTA Practice Framework (see www.aota.org) (i.e., physical, social, cultural, and temporal features). Some aspects of context may remain stable during a skilled observation (e.g., physical room layout) and form the backdrop, while other aspects of context may be fluid and interact with the child's performance (e.g., the teacher giving directions and the children following along) and must be recorded along with the child's responses. By recording the facts, the therapist can review and interpret the information later, remaining open and available to observe during the session.

Document the Interaction Among the Child, the Environment, and the Task

Examining the interaction among the child, the environment, and the task is critical to best practice evaluation in occupational therapy; it provides the backdrop for the child's performance. Children's performance skills and challenges are only relevant in the natural context; we cannot know the impact of person factors on participation without also knowing about environmental features. Sometimes, the environment is helpful to the child (e.g., the toothbrush and toothpaste on the sink cues the child to brush teeth). Other times, the environment is interfering (e.g., when there is too much clutter on the sink to see the toothbrush). Ecological assessment (i.e., observing behavior within authentic settings) is dynamic so that the professional can capture the interaction among person, task, and context factors.

We frequently conduct these assessments with other discipline colleagues. Figure 6-1 illustrates a method for adapting environments and activities to support children in their natural context. In this strategy, we consider both what the typical child in the situation does and what the target child does; this comparison helps the team to figure out possible adaptations to support the child.

Define Behaviors in Observable and Neutral Terms

Skilled observation requires therapists to record the actual behaviors that have occurred, without interpreting the meaning of the behavior or generating hypotheses. This is an important skill when working on a team because colleagues from other disciplines might interpret a behavior differently than we do from an occupational therapy perspective. If we only record our interpretations, it is difficult to get others' perspectives about the meaning of the core behavior. We might even interpret the meaning of a behavior differently based on what frames of reference we are using.

For example, "an infant squirms, cries, and pushes away from the care provider when she tries to pick the child up from the bassinet" is a description of a behavior. A sensory processing interpretation might be that the child is having difficulty organizing the vestibular input provided when moving from supine to upright. A psychoanalytic interpretation would focus on the child's difficulty attaching to a person other than the mother. A behavioral interpretation might address the child's association of this care provider (e.g., the developmental "work" to come). If the occupational therapist records, "the child is hypersensitive to movement" (i.e., the interpretation of the behavior from a sensory point of view, not the behavior itself), then the other possibilities offered by the other perspectives become unavailable to the team for consideration. To have the best possible chance for accurate interpretations of our assessment data, we must stay open to possibilities. The quality of our intervention plans is dependent on the accuracy of our observations and our willingness to consider alternative interpretations of behaviors.

Activity Analyses

Along with skilled observation in authentic environments, activity analysis is a hallmark of occupational therapy practice. In the *OT Practice Framework*, we consider the "activity demands." The purpose of activity analysis is to identify the features of the task (i.e., demands of the task) so that we can change some aspects when needed to support more efficient and satisfying task performance. We are trying to find out what conditions will be necessary to ensure the child's successful participation.

For example, when analyzing the task of completing seatwork, the therapist considers the child's sitting posture and position, the grip on the pencil, the type of materials (e.g., paper, workbook, textbook), the cognitive demands of the task, and the length of time required for a typical child to complete the task. The therapist would assess the contribution or barrier created by each feature as part of the activity analysis. This information leads directly into intervention planning (e.g., if the child is writing too randomly on the page, the therapist might suggest lined paper or might even enhance the lines with a marker to make them more obvious to the child). If the task is too hard for the child, the therapist might suggest smaller amounts to complete at a time or the use of a peer tutor.

Activity analysis is a strong tool that occupational therapists bring to their teams; it is part of our core knowledge for the discipline. We understand the nature of task performance (i.e., what it takes to be successful and satisfied when doing things). We also have scientific reasoning information regarding the individual's capacity to perform, the characteristics of objects and materials, and the cognitive and psychosocial features of the actual task performance. We therefore recognize how to make things harder or easier, simpler or more complex by changing some

Analysis of Participation in Authentic Contexts

Context: preschool classroom during snack time
Student: Tommy (+ comparison child for observation)

Activity: drinking juice, eating snack
Date:

General description of the activity setting: Teachers announce that it is snack time and walk toward the snack area/table. They provide extra prompts to children who do not respond to requests to come to snack time.
Table is appropriate size, and chairs are arranged around the table.

Events That Occur in This Activity Setting	Comparison Peer's Behaviors in This Activity Setting	Target Child Observations: Responses That Support Participation	Target Child Observations: Responses That Interfere With Participation	Possible Ways to Adapt the Activity	Possible Ways to Adapt the Context
Teachers call the children to snack time	Moves to snack table and sits down	Tommy looks up when teacher calls	Tommy does not move to the snack table	Teacher stands near Tommy and touches him while giving instruction to the group	Give Tommy an activity at the snack table prior to snack time
Teachers pass out napkins, plates, utensils, food	Takes items as they are offered	Takes first item offered	Doesn't notice other items offered	Ask Tommy to hold the stack of items for the teacher	Have Tommy's place set already
Teachers pour juice	Holds cup to steady it while teacher pours	Sees another student hold cup, so he holds his cup		Make sure Tommy isn't first to be served so he has a model to follow	
Teachers sit down and model eating snack	Eat snack and drink juice	Drinks juice, doesn't eat snack	Spills some juice on face and table	Provide an adapted cup with either straw or sippy lid	If it is important for Tommy to eat, only make cup available after eating something
Teachers wait for requests for more juice, snack	Asks for more juice, snack	Follows peer by asking for more juice	Gets up from table to walk around		Place Tommy's chair in the corner so he cannot get up so easily
Teachers model and ask students to clean up snack area	Picks up dishes and puts them in sink; throws trash away	Follows peer in throwing trash away	Leaves area; returns with teacher prompt and picks up dishes	Make sure he has peer models; cue him to "do what xxx is doing"	Set up the ending so dishes have to be handled before the trash

Figure 6-1. Sample portion of an ecological assessment for a young child in a preschool setting.

aspect of the situation. Other team members may recognize the nature of the problem, but have not been trained in the art of recognizing the features of tasks, performance, and environments and how to make adjustments in all of these features to support performance.

Norm-Referenced Measurement

Norm-referenced measures (also called standardized measures) have been designed to evaluate particular behaviors; the developers collect data on typical individuals as a comparison group (i.e., the normative group). Because we are comparing the person we are testing to a comparison group, we must use the same directions and procedures for testing each time. We cannot compare performance of the person we are testing to the comparison group if we allow the person to perform in a different way.

Most norm-referenced measures yield specific score results that are translated into standard scores in order to easily compare performance against the comparison group. Figure 6-2 illustrates the relationship among the most common types of standard scores and the bell curve. The bell curve is the pictorial representation of a normal distribution of scores on any test (Sattler, 2008). The shaded area in the center represents the range of scores that are considered the "normal range." Scores above this area are better than the norm group, and scores below this area are worse than the norm group.

It is important to note that percentile scores do not distribute evenly across the bell curve as other scores do. The percentile score reflects the ratio of people who scored at or above a certain level. If a person obtains a 70% score, this means that the person performed as well as or better than 70% of the people in the norm group. Because the bell curve does not evenly distribute the scores (the middle of the bell contains 68% of the people, while the edges contain only 2%), the percentiles are more densely represented in some parts of the bell curve than others.

Teams frequently use norm-referenced measures to establish a child's performance status (e.g., level of intelligence, level of motor performance). Remember, a status measure only records the child's current capacity in an area; the nature of the standardized task does not lend itself to intervention planning. Norm-referenced measures establish a child's status or eligibility; you need other measures to gather data for program planning. Frequently used status measures are plotted on Figure 6-2 so you can see the comparison of a standard score on each of them. For example, an IQ score of 85 on intelligence tests is comparable to a score of 40 on the Bruininks-Oseretsky Test of Motor Proficiency. You can see what other scores would be comparable to any score by drawing a vertical line on the figure.

USE OF STANDARDIZED TESTS

Typically, there are very clear parameters for acceptable use of standardized measures, including an acceptable age range, type of disability, and intelligence level. If a professional uses a standardized tool with an individual outside of the parameters, then the professional cannot calculate scores for this performance and must limit assessment remarks to observations.

Criterion-Referenced Measurement

Criterion-referenced measures compare a person's performance to a previously established standard of performance. In norm-referenced testing, we are comparing the person to other individuals, while, in criterion measures, we are comparing him or her to a performance standard (Sattler, 2008). We use criterion measures to investigate mastery, readiness, and skill acquisition, so this information enables the team to plan programs. These are only suggested procedures for testing with criterion measures. Table 6-8 contains a summary of the features of criterion measures in comparison to norm-referenced measures.

Many developmental tests are criterion measures. Developmental tests include skills that we have come to believe represent particular age levels (e.g., when a child can stand on one foot for 10 seconds, how many 1-inch cubes the child can stack). When we determine that a child can do certain behaviors and not others on the criterion list, we hypothesize about the child's developmental level. There are more difficult items beyond the child's performance on criterion measures; these form the structure for designing the intervention process and ultimately provide the structure for charting progress. We need to be careful about developmental criteria; even children without disabilities have variations from developmental criteria. When we consider children with particular disabilities, we need to remember that they will never reach typical milestones. They will have their own unique trajectories.

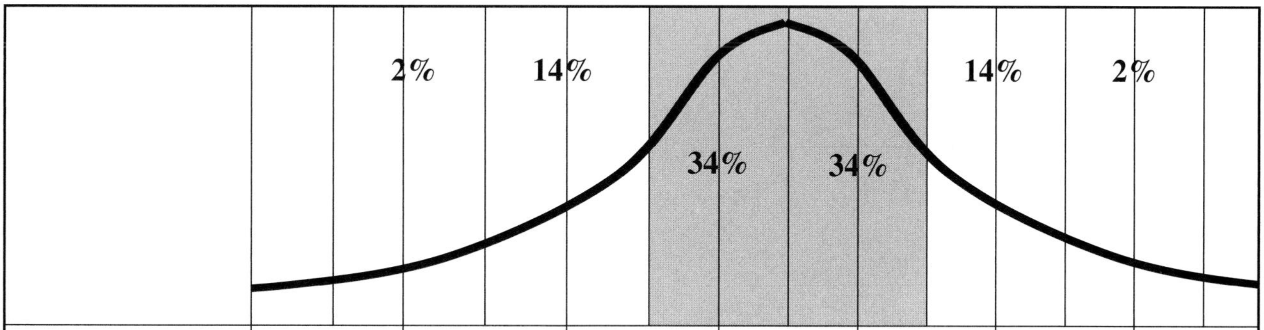

Standard Deviations	-3.0	-2.0	-1.0	mean	+1.0	+2.0	+3.0
Cumulative Percentages	0.1%	2.0%	16%	50%	84%	98%	99.9%
T scores	20	30	40	50	60	70	80
IQ Composite Scores (Wechsler scales)	55	70	85	100	115	130	145
Bruininks-Oseretsky composite scores	20	30	40	50	60	70	80

Figure 6-2. Relationship among frequently used standard scores to the bell curve. Use the last three rows to add your own tests to the figure: the middle box contains the mean score; add (to the right) and subtract (to the left) the standard deviation to complete the boxes appropriately.

A WORD OF CAUTION WHEN USING FORMALIZED MEASURES

Some criterion- and norm-referenced measures report age or grade equivalent scores. They are calculated by finding the average score for children of the specified age (i.e., in years and months) or grade (i.e., in grade and tenth of a grade level). The American Psychological Association (1999) strongly urges that we discontinue using age or grade equivalent scores because they are misleading. The units of measure between age and grade equivalents are not equal and can vary dramatically between each raw score. The number and type of skills in the 6th year are not the same as those we associate with the 13th year. The equivalent scores are merely the average age of the child who received that raw score.

Table 6-8.

Comparison of Criterion- and Norm-Referenced Tests

Norm-Referenced	Criterion-Referenced
Compares a subject's performance to a normative sample. It is essential that the characteristics of the subject are similar to those of the normative sample.	Compares the subject's performance to a level of mastery for a specific domain rather than comparison to the normative sample.
Used to determine if the subject's performance falls within the average range or how far from the average the performance falls. In other words, it provides comparison to how similar or different the performance is from the average (Asher, 2007).	Used to determine what skills the subject can and cannot perform within a specific domain. These skills have generally been designated as critical to performance by expert opinion (Asher, 2007).
May be useful in providing guidance in determination of services when documenting performance outside the average range is required.	May be useful in program planning. Interventions focus on remediating skills that are essential to mastery and identifying methods to facilitate participation.
Norm-referenced tests are not sensitive enough to be used to measure progress. They are intended to document differences from the average population (Mulenhaupt, 2000).	Criterion-referenced tests are generally sensitive enough to be used to measure progress in performance. They are intended to provide guidance in changes for program planning (Mulenhaupt, 2000).

Asher, I. E. (Ed.) (2007). *Occupational therapy assessment tools: An annotated index* (3rd ed.). Bethesda, MD: AOTA Press.

Mulenhaupt, M. (2000). OT services under IDEA 97 decision-making challenges. *OT Practice, 5*(24), 10-13.

Other Factors Associated With Evaluation

Occupational therapists are also involved in other processes associated with the evaluation process, including screening, referrals, and the Response to Intervention process (RtI). Let's review each of these briefly here. We will illustrate these factors in cases (see Chapter 9).

The Screening Processes

As occupational therapy becomes more integrated within community service systems, colleagues and team members solicit our participation in population-wide services. Population-wide services are those activities that survey the needs of cohort groups (i.e., groups that share features, such as their age and interests), provide guidance for service exploration, and construct preventative strategies to support children's successful performance within natural contexts.

Many times, screening is the first contact the family has with the service system. During this initial contact, it is very important that the family receives accurate and helpful information. When screening tools meet the same standard as other measures, we can feel safer that the decision we make based on screening results will be correct. Screening tools must also be simple to learn, administer, and interpret; many screening programs have some volunteer staff supporting them. There must be cost-effectiveness in the screening program as well, including costs of materials and supplies, personnel, and space to conduct the program. Community-based screening programs for children are typically directed at younger children in an effort to identify the potential difficulties early and provide supports for improved outcomes.

There must be additional services available after the screening (i.e., assessment procedures to evaluate the problem in more depth than the screening and intervention services to address the problem). Best practice dictates that communities have a cascade of services and professionals available to families. It is inappropriate to use community and family resources to conduct and participate in screening programs if there will be no follow-up activities for families whose children are at risk. The essential nature of screening is to identify potential needs and issues that can be minimized or resolved if dealt with efficiently; it is inappropriate to give parents feedback about difficulties without offering guidance about what to do next.

Screening is reserved for those performance features that are prevalent and/or have serious (negative) impact. Early community screening programs are designed to locate those children for whom early intervention will improve their overall outcomes. Although theoretically we may think that we should screen all children for all possible issues, this is not a good use of community resources or family time and resources. For example, there are enough developmental issues that impact school performance to justify early school screening. We also want to screen everyone for problems that may be rare but which have a very negative impact; for example, all infants are screened for phenylketonuria (PKU) in the hospital. Very few children have this condition, but we have a very effective treatment, and the early intervention prevents severe retardation. Therefore, the cost/benefit makes this type of screening worthwhile. On the other hand, it may not be cost-effective to conduct community screenings for foot size because it does not typically impact overall performance.

The Referral Process

Referral is the process of either receiving a request from or making a request to others in a child's and family's interest. We use the referral process to provide the family or care provider with additional resources for problem-solving (i.e., to broaden the perspectives in an attempt to understand the needs more clearly). Occupational therapists can receive referrals or make referrals and, therefore, need to understand how to use this process effectively.

The most common sources for referrals are team members from early intervention, preschool, and school-based programs. These individuals might make a referral to the occupational therapist as a result of population screening, RtI processes, or as part of comprehensive assessment for special education services. We might also receive referrals from physicians who have particular medically related concerns with daily life or from parents who need guidance in supporting their children at home. Some states require particular documentation of referrals as part of the licensing or registration laws; be sure to check these regulations in your state.

Novice therapists may be hesitant to make referrals, fearing that they are making poor judgments about a situation (either too leniently or too strictly). It is always good to use a more experienced professional to guide these early decisions about referrals, because, many times, this brings up the availability of resources that the novice would not know about and provides a mechanism for learning the system while providing services.

It is also appropriate for occupational therapists to make referrals to others who may support the child and family. When we have medically related concerns, we make referrals to physicians or nurse practitioners. We might see that a related discipline such as social work, physical therapy, speech pathology, or psychology needs to be involved in a case. It is also appropriate to make referrals to other occupational therapists with expertise that the family needs. For example, a school-based occupational therapist is not likely to be skilled at fabricating splints, even though he learned it in college. If a child needed a splint, this therapist would make a referral to another therapist with splinting expertise to ensure that the family receives the best possible services.

We also make referrals to other community agencies if their mission and resources will be supportive to the family. Community referrals can also include resources such as karate classes, swimming, scouts, and activity or support groups. To be effective as a community service provider, therapists must familiarize themselves with the options available.

Response to Intervention

RtI was originally designed for literacy programs and has now expanded to apply across all of early intervention, early childhood, and public education as a structure for problem solving. RtI is a model for early identification of potential barriers to learning, which then offers tiers of support to make sure that children are successful within their natural contexts (Fox, Carta, Strain, Dunlap, & Hemmeter, 2009). RtI has grown out of the No Child Left Behind (NCLB, 2001) initiative,

Academic & Behavioral Systems Characteristics		Response to Intervention Tiers
Intensive, Individualized Assessment-Based Longer Duration Durable Procedures	Tier 3	
Targeted Groups Efficient Rapid Achievement	Tier 2	
Core Instruction All Students All Settings Prevention Intervention	Tier 1	

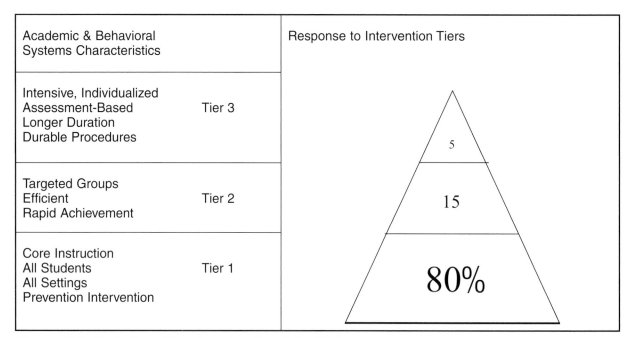

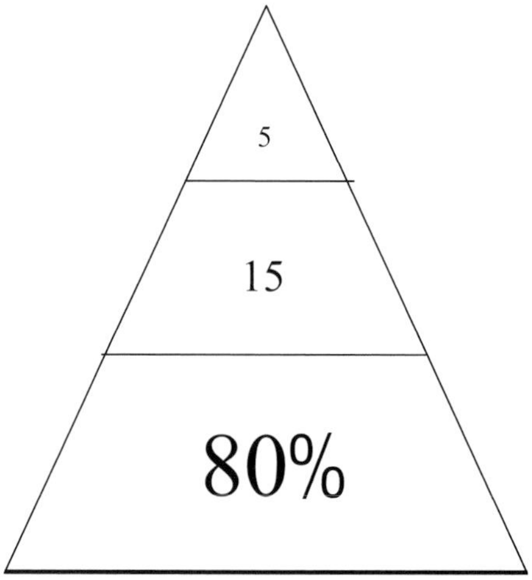

Figure 6-3. Illustration of the characteristics of the RtI tiers.

which requires education personnel to employ evidence, thus professionals are expected to use evidence-based practices and establish data-collecting methods to evaluate whether a particular practice is contributing to the desired educational outcomes. RtI is also designed to reduce the number of children who need to be referred to special education services by finding methods to support a child's learning within authentic contexts. From an EHP point of view, RtI employs a prevention intervention approach to services.

RtI is built on the beliefs that professionals can find ways to effectively teach all children, especially if we begin before the children are failing. RtI implements problem-solving methods supported by evidence to design effective plans for learning. There is also a belief that assessment and intervention require a multipurpose approach to meet all learners' needs (Griffiths, Parson, Burns, VanDerHeyden, & Tilly, 2007).

Buysse and Peisner-Feinberg (2009) outline 5 critical features of RtI for educational programs. First, professionals must screen all students to see if they are making sufficient progress and to identify which students might be at risk for making sufficient progress without additional supports. Second, RtI expects professionals to monitor progress so that a student can be identified quickly if learning is not keeping pace with expectations. Third, there is an expectation that in addition to the core curriculum, education programs have both modified core curricula and individualized methods that will support children to be successful in the core curricula. Fourth, professionals must use data-based decision-making to determine progress and make adjustments as needed. Finally, professionals routinely check the fidelity of their practices to make sure that interventions are consistent with both the evidence and the plans developed for that student.

Evidence is emerging about the effects of RtI. For example, students who were at-risk improved in early reading (O'Connor, Harty, & Fulmer, 2005). Other reports indicate a reduction in referrals and placements in special education (Bollman, Silberglitt, & Gibbons, 2007). Researchers have also reported that on-task and task completion has improved with RtI supports (Buysse & Peisner-Feinberg, 2009; Kovaleski, Gickling, Morrow, & Swank, 1999).

There is a 3-tiered model for RtI (Fox, Carta, Strain, Dunlap, & Hemmeter, 2009; NASDSE/CASE, 2006), which can address both academic and behavioral issues that may be interfering with successful participation. Figure 6-3 illustrates the components of this tiered system.

RtI has gained popularity for a number of reasons. People have been unsatisfied with the current system in which we take action when children are already unsuccessful. To change the focus from corrective action to prevention, the educational system has to create a more integrated approach to serving children's learning (NASDSE/CASE, 2006). In this new paradigm, education professionals acknowledge that the general education system contains effective methods that already employ problem-solving approaches when children are not learning effectively and challenges the notion that children must have a label to be eligible for supports. People also begin to question the wisdom of separate systems (i.e., regular education and special education) as the best approach for everyone's learning. So, professionals begin to construct an education system that continuously checks in on learning, provides access to strategies to adjust learning experiences, and involves everyone in creating successful educational experiences (NASDSE/CASE, 2006).

This is good news for occupational therapy both in our roles as related service professionals and in our core philosophy to support participation. In the current system, children are already failing as learners when we are invited to help. In the RtI system, we can actively participate early in the process of supporting children in their regular education experiences (e.g., offering seating alternatives during Tier 1). Occupational therapists have many strategies that are helpful to children within their regular classroom, and, often, these strategies are implemented much later in the process, after the child is receiving special education services. When we can contribute to the early problem-solving process in a child's regular education experiences, we have the possibility to generate success quickly and prevent further frustration for the child, teacher, and family.

> Up to 15% of special education funding can be used to support RtI activities. Thus, it is completely appropriate for occupational therapists to participate in the tiered process of interventions. Because we want to support children's participation in their natural environments as a best practice approach, advocating to work in Tier 1 provides a way to use our knowledge in a best practice way.

The RtI process is similar to the occupational therapy process. Assessment provides information for intervention planning and includes screening to identify children quickly and ongoing assessment of progress to determine whether interventions are having the desired impact (i.e., progress monitoring). Intervention planning and implementation is based on available evidence; everyone participates in the process to ensure the best possible plans are implemented. We expect that nearly all children will have successful outcomes because we are keeping close tabs on their learning and the effectiveness of our choices.

There have been misconceptions about RtI; knowing these misconceptions and the facts arms you with information when RtI topics come up in conversation. Table 6-9 provides you with talking points for these inevitable discussions. (See the NASDSE Web site for the most current information; this table reflects myths from 2006.) Additionally, each state has its own RtI guidance and may have a distinctive name, so be sure to find out what is going on where you practice. For example, in Kansas, we call the RtI system "Multi-Tiered System of Supports" (MTSS). It is always a good practice to access your state's Department of Education Web site to obtain the most current policies and practices within your state.

So as a member of the school team, occupational therapists play a key role in RtI. In a sense, we are working toward a "universal design" (see Core Principles of Universal Design in Chapter 5) of regular education to support more students to be successful (for more information about universal design concepts in learning, see the National Center on Universal Design for Learning, www.udlcenter.org). Many of the strategies we have recommended under special education can be applied in RtI to support students to remain in their regular education classrooms. Table 6-10 contains some examples; brainstorm your own examples or interview a school-based OT to find out more ideas. The case studies in Chapter 9 also contain some RtI examples.

Example of RtI Teamwork

Let's consider an example. Donald is a second grade student. His teacher has begun to notice that Donald is slow to complete his seatwork, drops his pencil a lot, continues to reverse letters, and produces messy papers. She had tried to support Donald by giving him more time, but this did not help his work product. She met with the members of the RtI team to outline her concerns.

The occupational therapist at Donald's school serves on the RtI team. They meet every other week to review concerns filed by classroom teachers. The team decides that, for Donald, the occupational therapist is the best person to provide support in

Table 6-9.

Some Misconceptions About RtI; Facts and Implications for OT

Misconceptions	Facts About RtI	Implications for OT
RtI identifies learning difficulties that feed into special education services.	RtI provides methods to support students so they can remain in regular education. RtI is designed to broaden the options for learning in regular education. Special education strategies might be used as RtI tools within regular education.	Adaptations that we might have used only for students in special education can be employed in RtI to support students to remain in regular education.
Tier 3 RtI is actually special education services and can operate as "pre-referral" for special education.	Although Tier 3 interventions are more intense and may be ideas harvested from special education literature, they are employed in regular education to support learners. We are trying to prevent students from being segregated from their regular education context.	We are not limited to simple adaptations when working within RtI in regular education.
We continue to conduct comprehensive assessments to test for eligibility.	RtI moves teams away from traditional testing for eligibility to the development of a cadre of data collected in the regular education classroom that can be used for planning.	Occupational therapists must design data collection methods that match desired outcomes of learning, not those focused on intervention methods alone (see section on monitoring progress/goals writing for examples).
There are time limits to each tier, and the time counts as part of required special education time limits.	There is not a specific formula; the team must make this determination while planning. RtI is not part of special education services, so this time does not count.	Occupational therapists will need to be aware of the literature on effectiveness to make good estimates for RtI.

Table 6-10.

Occupational Therapy Interventions Within RtI

Academic and Behavioral Systems Characteristics of RtI		Examples of OT Interventions Applied in RtI	Your Ideas about RtI Interventions: (Refer to case studies in Chapter 9 to get you started)
Intensive, individualized assessment based longer duration durable procedures	3	Design a behavioral prompting and reinforcement system to keep a student on track during group instruction	
Targeted groups Efficient Rapid achievement	2	Rearrange the furniture in a classroom to create a quieter, less distracting place so the teacher can provide direct instruction for a small group who needs targeted help in math, reading	
Core instruction All students All settings Prevention intervention	1	Make adjustments to seating to facilitate attention during instruction	

the classroom. They decide that an 8-week period of observation and intervention trials will provide enough time to review progress data and make further decisions. The teacher and the occupational therapist agree on a meeting schedule and times for the therapist to observe in the classroom during the pre-assessment period. The occupational therapist also gave the teacher a handout about adaptations that are appropriate for the classroom and asked her to review it before their meeting.

After two observations and one meeting with the teacher, they decide to try several strategies. The therapist gets a pencil grip for Donald's pencil to stabilize his grip and suggests using unlined paper for a while to see if the decreased "pressure to be inside the lines" will reduce Donald's frustration. The teacher and therapist also designed a data collection strategy for these interventions so they could monitor Donald's progress.

After 3 weeks, the teacher reported that Donald was demonstrating less frustration (i.e., he had only been in one "altercation" with a peer) and had only thrown away 3 papers. He was not dropping his pencil, but was fidgeting with it a lot, so the therapist provided the teacher with 3 other types of grips to try. After 6 weeks, Donald seemed more comfortable with one of the grips and asked to keep that one. When they went back to the pre-assessment team, everyone agreed with the teacher that Donald did not require further assessment.

Terminating Services

Professionals conclude their services when the children and/or family they are serving have the skills and/or supports they need to live a satisfying life. This does not mean that we have "cured" the disability, but that we have provided all the strategies that enable the child and care providers to support functional performance. For school-aged children, this means that they have the supports and strategies to be a successful student. For young adults transitioning to community living and work, it might mean that we have supported a job search, placement, and the probationary period and have set natural supports in place (e.g., a supervisor or peer to help).

There are a number of strategies for conducting assessment to terminate services. The most efficient method is to have designed the intervention program with functional and measurable goals related to the child's performance so that, when the child reaches the goals, it is clear to everyone that services are no longer needed. The COPM is an excellent tool for concluding services because it is a reflection of the child and family's priorities and expectations about performance.

Sometimes, families and teachers have come to rely on the occupational therapist and feel uncomfortable without these professionals to support themselves (on behalf of the child). Communication is critical to the process so the families and teachers feel supported; with good rapport, the therapist can also anticipate the source and features of the anxiety and can incorporate supports into the transition planning process. Therapists must also keep in mind that it is important to provide support without making boundaries unclear. Therapists provide a professional service and need to avoid codependence that will hamper the child, family, or teacher's progress and competence to handle future situations. We design probe assessment strategies to ensure that our "departure" was not premature and continue to address the other care providers' concerns.

For example, a parent might be worried that her third-grade daughter will "slide" back into poor social engagement patterns when the therapist is no longer supporting her. In this case, we would find out exactly what the parent fears will happen, and we set a transition goal related to the concern (e.g., "Karen will talk with a peer at lunch at least three times a week," or "Karen will play with a group of two to four children at least three times a week during recess"). The team then agrees that if there ever is a week in the next quarter that Karen does not meet this criterion, the occupational therapist would immediately re-enter Karen's educational program and collaborate with the teacher regarding this event. At the end of the quarter, the team and the parent can celebrate Karen's success. We have demonstrated Karen's ability to sustain performance and have been respectful of the parent's concerns all in one strategy.

There may also be times that we terminate services at one point in a child's life and will need to re-enter the child's life a little later when task demands change. Many times, if children have received consistent services in preschool and elementary school,

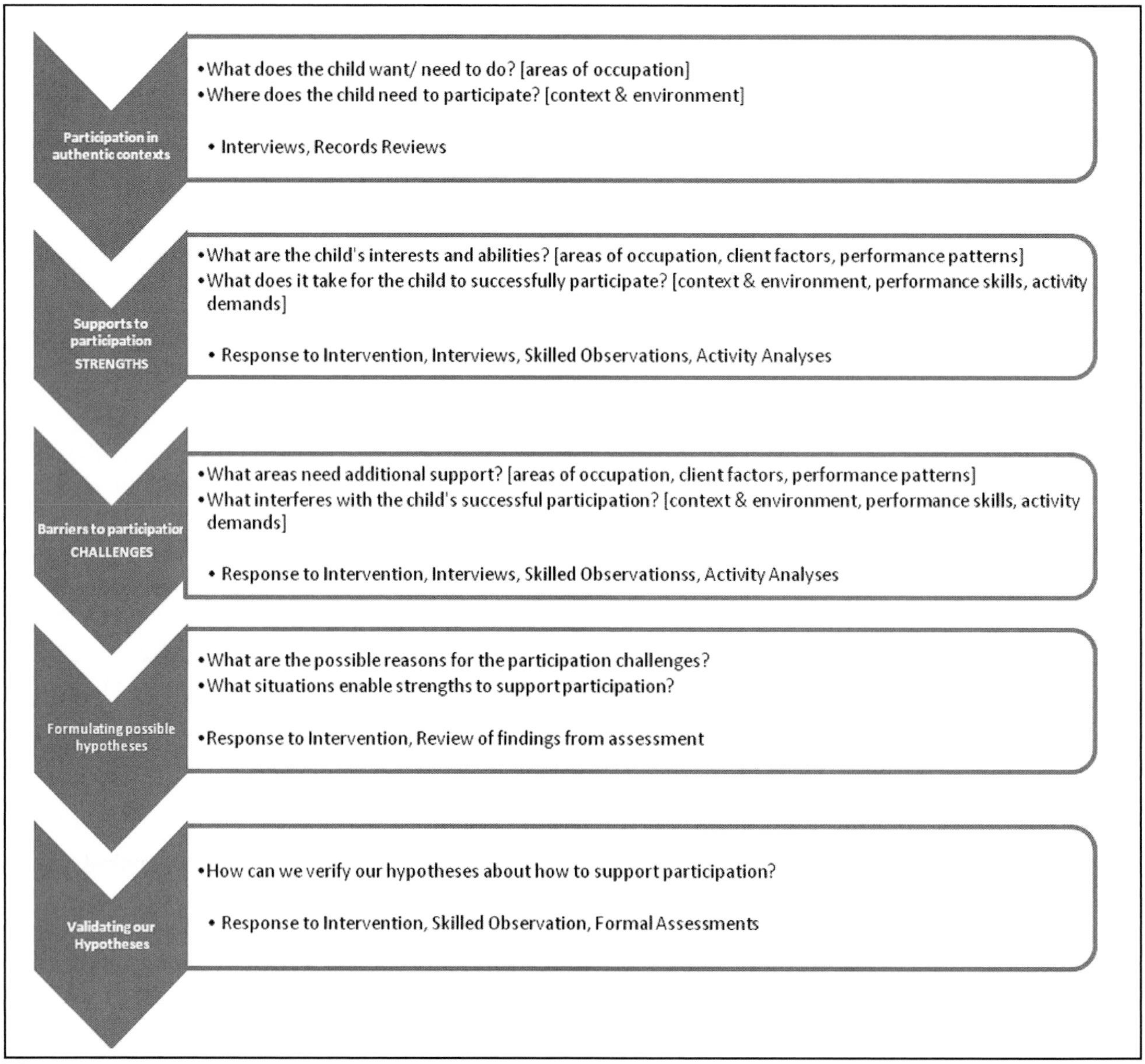

Figure 6-4. Best Practice Evaluation Planning Guide.

they will not need services in the pre-adolescent period. This same child may need occupational therapy support in the transition to high school or in career and life planning. It is completely appropriate to move in and out of children's lives.

Template for Best Practice Occupational Therapy Assessment

Sometimes, the assessment process can seem overwhelming to a novice who wants to be sure to conduct a complete assessment in the most efficient manner. Figure 6-4 contains a template for planning a best practice assessment strategy. As you see, we begin with occupational performance in authentic contexts, and then we move to identifying strengths so we can build on them to support the child. Finally, we examine potential barriers so we can minimize their impact on participation. You will notice that the template only includes formal assessment for times we need to anchor our work in evidence and to validate our hypotheses. Chapter 9 contains cases that illustrate the evaluation process as it leads to planning and intervention.

Summary

Best practice assessment is a complex process that draws on all of one's professional expertise. We must be able to construct a set of experiences that reveal the child's strengths and barriers to performance and form hypotheses about how to change the situation to support more successful performance. In this chapter, we reviewed all the features of comprehensive assessment and offered methods for constructing a best practice assessment program.

References

American Psychological Association (1999). *Standards for educational and psychological testing*. Washington, DC: APA.

Asher, I. E. (Ed.) (2007). *Occupational therapy assessment tools: An annotated index* (3rd ed.). Bethesda, MD: AOTA Press.

Ayres, A. J. (1979). *Sensory integration and learning disorders*. Los Angeles, CA: Western Psychological.

Beery, K. E. (2004). *Developmental test of visual motor integration: Administration, scoring, and teaching manual* (5th ed.). Minneapolis, MN: NCS Pearson, Inc.

Bollman, K. A., Silberglitt, B., & Gibbons, K. A. (2007). The St. Croix River education district model: Incorporating systems-level organization and a multi-tiered problem-solving process for intervention delivery. In S. R. Jimerson, M. K. Burns, & A. M. VanDerHeyden (Eds.), *Handbook of response to intervention: The science and practice of assessment and intervention* (pp. 319-330). New York, NY: Springer

Brown, C., & Dunn, W. (2002). *The adult sensory profile*. San Antonio, TX: Psychological Corporation.

Buysse, V., & Peisner-Feinberg, E. (2009). Recognition and response: Findings from the first implementation study [on-line] from http://randr.fpg.unc.edu/sites/randr.fpg.unc.edu/files/KeyFindingsHandout.pdf

Caldwell, B. M., & Bradley, R. H. (1978). *Home observation measurement of the environment*. Little Rock, AR: University of Arkansas Center for Child Development & Education.

Charlop-Christy, M. H., Carpentar, M., Loc, L., LeBlan, L. A., & Kellet, K. (2002). Using the picture exchange communication system (PECS) with children with autism: Assessment of PECS acquisition, speech, social-communication behavior, and problem behavior. *Journal of Applied Behavior Analysis, 35*(3), 213-231.

Coster, W. (1998). *The school function assessment manual*. San Antonio, TX: The Psychological Corporation.

Coster, W. J., Deeney, T., Haltiwanger, J. & Haley, S. M. (1998). *School function assessment*. San Antonio, TX: The Psychological Corporation/Therapy Skill Builders.

Dunn, W. (1997). Implementing neuroscience principles to support rehabilitation and recovery. In C. Christiansen and C. Baum (Eds.), *Occupational therapy: Enabling function and well-being* (2nd ed.). Thorofare, NJ: SLACK Incorporated.

Dunn, W. (1999). *Sensory profile: user's manual*. San Antonio, TX: The Psychological Corporation.

Dunn, W. (2000). *Best practice occupational therapy in community service with children and families* (2nd ed.). Thorofare, NJ: SLACK Incorporated.

Dunn, W. (2002). *The infant toddler sensory profile*. San Antonio, TX: Psychological Corporation.

Dunn, W. (2006). *The sensory profile school companion manual*. San Antonio, TX: Psychological Corporation.

Dunn, W. (2007). Supporting children in everyday life using a sensory processing approach. *Infants & Young Children, 20*(2), 84-101.

Dunn, W. (2008). *Living sensationally: Understanding your senses*. London: Jessica Kingsley Publications.

Folio, M. R., & Fewell, R. R. (2000). *Peabody Developmental Motor Scales* (2nd ed.). San Antonio, TX: Psychological Corporation.

Fox, L., Carta, J., Strain, P., Dunlap, G., & Hemmeter, M. L. (2009). *Response to intervention and the pyramid model*. Tampa, FL: University of South Florida, Technical Assistance Center on Social Emotional Intervention for Young Children.

Griffiths, A., Parson, L., Burns, M., VanDerHeyden, A., & Tilly, W. D. (2007). *Response to intervention: Research for practice*. Alexandria, VA: National Association of State Directors of Special Education, Inc.

Haley, S. M., Coster, W. J., Ludlow, L. H., Haltiwanger, J. T., & Andrellos, P. J. (1992). *Pediatric evaluation of disability inventory: Development, standardization, and administration manual, Version 1.0*. Boston, MA: Trustees of Boston University, Health and Disability Research Institute.

Kandel, E., Schwartz, J., & Jessell, T. (2000). *Principles of neural science*. New York, NY: McGraw-Hill Companies.

Kovaleski, J., Gickling, E., Morrow, H., & Swank, H. (1999). High versus low implementation of instructional support teams: A case for maintaining program fidelity. *Remedial and Special Education, 20*, 170-183.

Law, M., Baum, C., & Dunn, W. (2005). *Measuring occupational performance: Supporting best practice in occupational therapy* (2nd ed.). Thorofare, NJ: SLACK Incorporated.

Law, M., Polatajko, H., Pollock, N., McColl, M. A., Carswell, A., & Baptiste, D. (1994). Pilot testing of the Canadian Occupational Performance Measure: Clinical and measurement issues. *Canadian Journal of Occupational Therapy, 61*(4), 191-197.

Linder, T. (2009). *Transdisciplinary play-based assessment 2*. Baltimore, MD: Paul H. Brookes Publishing.

Mulenhaupt, M. (2000). OT services under IDEA 97: Decision making Challenges. *OT Practice, 5*(24), 10-13.

National Association of State Directors of Special Education and Council of Administrators of Special Education (NASDE/CASE). (2006). Response to intervention white paper. Retrieved from www.nasdse.org/Portals/0/.../RtIAnAdministratorsPerspective1-06.

O'Connor, R. E., Harty, K. R., & Fulmer, D. (2005). Tiers of intervention in kindergarten through third grade. *Journal of Learning Disabilities, 38*, 532-538.

Paikoff Holzmueller, R. L. (2005). Therapists I have known and (mostly) loved. *American Journal of Occupational Therapy, 59*(5), 580-587.

Pierangelo, R., & Giuliani, G. (2006). *Assessment in special education: A practical approach* (2nd ed.). Boston, MA: Allyn and Bacon.

Public Law 107-110: the No Child Left Behind Act of 2001. [NCLB].

Richardson, P. K. (2001). Use of standardized tests in pediatric practice. In J. Case-Smith (Ed.), *Occupational therapy for children* (4th ed.) (pp. 239-240). St. Louis, MO: Mosby Inc.

Sattler, J., & Hoge, R. (2006). *Assessment of children: behavioral, social, and clinical foundations* (5th ed.). La Mesa, CA: Sattler Publishing.

Sattler, J. (2008). *Assessment of children: cognitive foundations* (5th ed.). La Mesa, CA: Jerome M. Sattler, Publisher, Inc.

Schenker, R., Coster, W., & Parush, S. (2004). Participation and activity performance of students with cerebral palsy within the school environment. *Disability and Rehabilitation, 27*(10), 539-552.

Sparrow, S., Cicchetti, D., & Balla, D. (2005). *The Vineland Adaptive Behavior Scales* (2nd ed.) (Vineland II). San Antonio, TX: Pearson.

Thiemann, K. S., & Goldstein, H. (2001). Social stories, written text cues, and video feedback: Effects on social communication of children with autism. *Journal of Applied Behavior Analysis, 34*, 425-446.

Tomchek, S., & Case Smith, J. (2009). *Occupational therapy practice guidelines for children and adolescents with autism.* Rockville, MD: AOTA Press.

Williamson, G., & Szczepanski, M. (1999). Coping frame of reference. In P. Kramer & J. Hinojosa (Eds.), *Frames of reference for pediatric occupational therapy* (2nd ed.) (pp. 431-468). Baltimore, MD: Williams & Wilkins.

Additional Web Sites

www.aota.org

www.apa.org/science/programs/testing/standards.aspx

www.wrightslaw.com/idea/law/FR.v71.n156.pdf

www.nichcy.org/idealist.htm

www.kansped.org/ksde/laws/idea04/idea04.html

http://dese.mo.gov/schoollaw/rulesregs/Inc_By_Ref_Mat/Special%20Education/IDEA%20Part%20B.html

www.nichcy.org/idealaw.htm

www.udlcenter.org

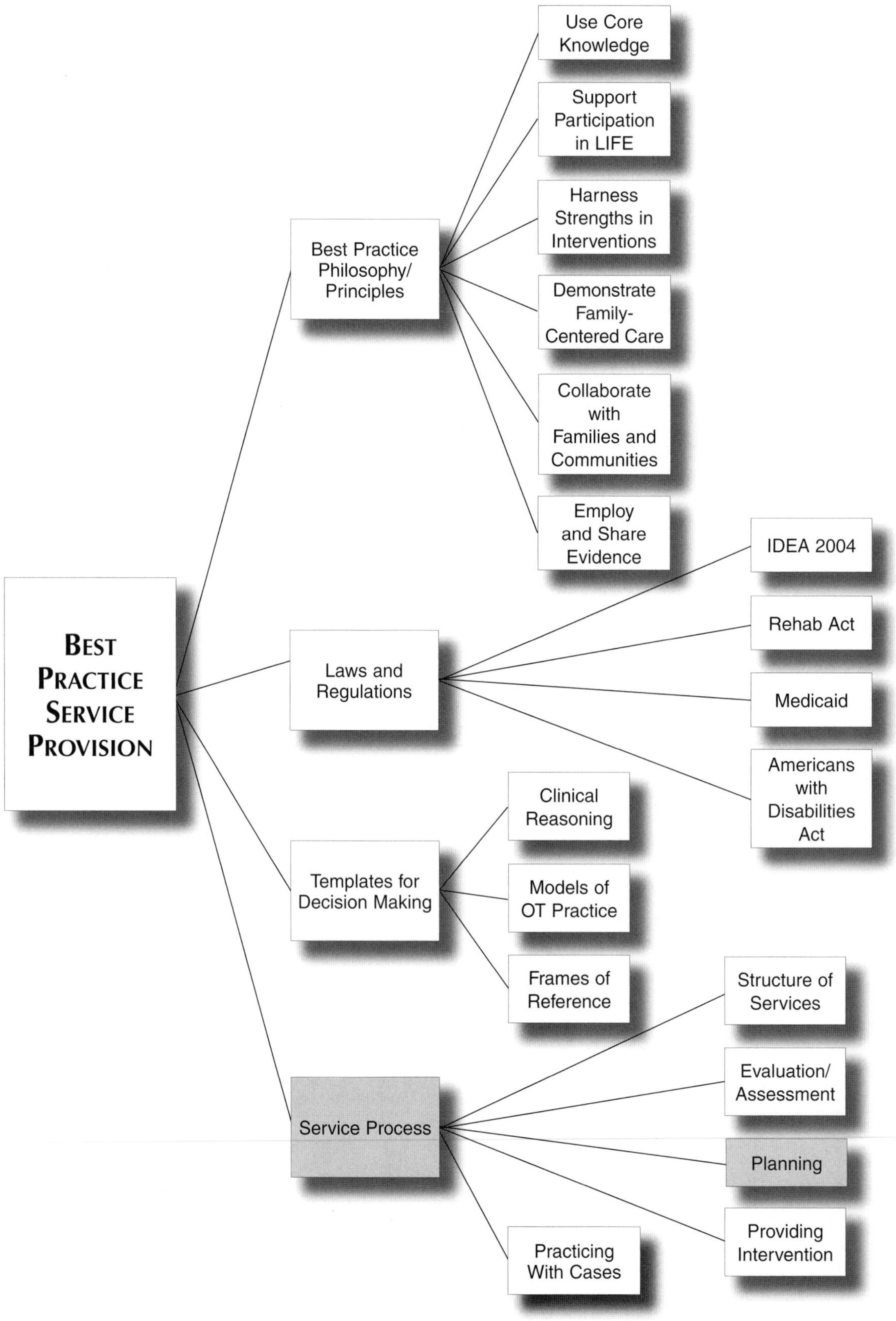

Best Practice Service Provision
Best Practice Philosophy/ Principles
Use Core Knowledge
Support Participation in LIFE
Harness Strengths in Interventions
Demonstrate Family-Centered Care
Collaborate with Families and Communities
Employ and Share Evidence
Laws and Regulations
IDEA 2004
Rehab Act
Medicaid
Americans with Disabilities Act
Templates for Decision Making
Clinical Reasoning
Models of OT Practice
Frames of Reference
Service Process
Structure of Services
Evaluation/ Assessment
Planning
Providing Intervention
Practicing With Cases

CHAPTER 7

Developing Intervention Plans That Reflect Best Practice

After the evaluation process and before the actual implementation of interventions, there is a sacred space in which we pause to plan our course of action. Because we are trained to provide interventions, these ideas come brimming to our minds throughout the RtI process and during evaluation. It is important however, to pause and make sure we plan in a systematic way to be of the best possible service to the children, families, teachers, and systems within which we serve.

The *OT Practice Framework* provides structure for the planning process, but this is not the only place we turn to for guidance about planning. Most community-based agencies operate based on state and federal legislation, which outlines the requirements for services, including the planning process. There are a lot of resources that provide up-to-date information about particular requirements and expectations, so be sure to use these resources to support your work. Table 7-1 provides some of these resources with current internet addresses. Look up something on each Web site to acquaint you with what each has to offer.

Laws and Regulations Provide Guidance for Planning

As we discussed in Chapter 2, many of the community services we provide are founded on federal, state, or local legislation and regulations. At the beginning of our careers, it is hard to imagine being interested in legal or administrative issues; we want to practice! However, those who thrive in community practice take time to understand how regulations influence organizational and policy decisions. When a professional understands the requirements and restraints of particular laws, it is easier to creatively apply discipline knowledge in service to the children, families, and systems we serve. In this section, we will review some of the key factors to consider when using laws as guidelines for planning. We will use the IFSP, IEP, and Section 504 processes as our examples. If you encounter other regulations in practice settings, you can use this same format to think through how you will operationalize your practice within that structure. Effectiveness of occupational therapy within a particular system is in large part judged by how the services fit into the system requirements. Being

Dunn W. *Best Practice Occupational Therapy for Children and Families in Community Settings, Second Edition* (pp. 125-155)
© 2011 SLACK Incorporated.

Table 7-1.

Resources to Assist With Planning Programs and Services for Children and Families

Name of Agency Resource	Current Internet Address
Wrightslaw Provides parents, educators, advocates, and attorneys with accurate, reliable information about special education law, education law, and advocacy for children with disabilities.	www.wrightslaw.com
National Early Childhood Technical Assistance Center (NECTAC) Provides resources for professionals and families regarding best practices services.	www.nectac.org
National Dissemination Center for Children with Disabilities (NICCHY) Provides resources about disabilities, evidence, services for professionals and families.	www.nichcy.org
Kansas Inservice Training System (KITS) Provides professional development materials and resources for early childhood professionals and families.	www.kskits.org
IFSPweb Provides online assistance to support families and professionals develop best practice IFSPs.	www.ifspweb.org

smart about this aspect of planning provides leverage for increasing your leadership and impact.

Planning With Individualized Family Service Plan Regulations

With Ellen Pope, MEd, OTR

The Individualized Family Service Plan (IFSP) is a required document when we are serving infants, toddlers, and their families (called Early Intervention, EI). This document provides a template for all the things the team needs to include in their planning process; it becomes the documentation of the decisions and plans for each family and child. Table 7-2 summarizes some key excerpts of IDEA 2004, part C regarding the IFSP process, along with explanations and examples.

Laws are operationalized with regulations; the regulations provide guidance about how to do what the law says. It is important to understand the key regulations that go with federal laws because states base their decisions on how to set up their programs based on these regulations. Table 7-3 summarizes some of the key aspects of the law related to EI services, associated regulations, and for illustration, how these regulations play out in Kansas. We are also leaving a blank column so you can find out what is relevant in your state.

It is challenging to address unexpected issues that arise during planning. Families can have questions that you did not prepare for; team members can have unexpected findings, or your findings are surprising from evaluation. Table 7-4 outlines some frequent occurrences and some suggestions about how to handle them. You will notice that many of the strategies reflect the process of accommodating individual differences within situations and activities.

When you enter EI practice, colleagues on your service team, families, or other agency personnel will guide your practice. Sometimes, professionals who have been in an area of practice for a while will have patterns in their practices; these patterns may or may not reflect best practice and may or may not meet the spirit of the laws that govern EI services. Table 7-5 outlines some common myths about EI practice, along with the facts. Following up, the information box contains frequently asked questions about the IFSP process. You can also access the www.IFSPweb.org Web site for current information.

Table 7-2.

Translating the Individualized Family Service Plan Law Components

Excerpts From the Law and its Regulations	What This Part of the Law Means	Examples of This Aspect of the Law in Practice
"...a multidisciplinary assessment of the unique strengths and needs of the infant or toddler..."	Of the 16 identified professionals, at least two from different disciplines must conduct the assessment	OT and Early Childhood Special Educator conduct the eligibility evaluation
	We must identify the strengths as well as needs of this child	We report that the child does better in quiet places
"...a statement of the natural environments in which early intervention services will appropriately be provided..."	We must provide services and supports in the environments in which the child would be if the child did not have a disability (e.g., home, childcare, parks, library, shopping areas)	We plan to visit the family at the time they typically have a meal We join them at the park for their play time
"...including a justification to the extent, if any, to which the services will not be provided in a natural environment..."	Under those rare circumstances that might require services outside the child's everyday life, we must document clearly why we must provide services in a more restrictive (e.g., clinical) place	The child is at risk for infections due to aspiration; the therapist arranges for a feeding evaluation at the children's hospital The child needs an orthotic device, and the clinic has tools for constructing it
"...appropriate early intervention services are based on scientifically based research..."	Professionals must have evidence that meets professional standards to support their decisions	Primary provider goes to discount store with mom and child to work on management strategies (based on Principle 1: children learn best through everyday experiences... in familiar contexts—see Chapter 1) Therapist establishes a Goal Attainment Scale to chart improvements in social interaction during bath time

Table 7-3.

State Implementation of Part C of IDEA 2004

Excerpt From the Law and Its Associated Regulations	How Kansas Implements This Regulation (Procedural Manual)	How YOUR STATE Implements This Regulation
"...a multidisciplinary assessment of the unique strengths and needs of the infant or toddler..."	"...the evaluation team must consist of at least 2 professionals from different disciplines, but can include as many members as necessary based on the child..."	
"...a statement of the natural environments in which early intervention services will appropriately be provided..."	"...Early intervention services must be provided in natural environments to the maximum extent appropriate, including the home and community settings in which children without disabilities participate. The decision is made by the IFSP team based on the child's outcomes identified in the IFSP..."	
"...including a justification to the extent, if any, to which the services will not be provided in a natural environment..."	"...Early intervention services may be provided elsewhere only when early intervention services cannot be provided satisfactorily for the infant-toddler in a natural environment as determined by the parent and the IFSP team. A justification of the extent to which an early intervention service will not be provided in a natural environment must be provided..."	
"...appropriate early intervention services are based on scientifically based research..."	"...The IFSP must include a statement of the specific early intervention services, based on peer reviewed research (to the extent practicable), that are necessary to meet the unique needs of the child and the family to achieve the results or outcomes identified..."	

Table 7-4.

Strategies for Handling Challenging Situations With Part C

What Might Happen During Planning	Strategies for Handling the Situations
The family wants to take their child to center-based services.	This is an opportunity to explain EI mandates, which include service provided in natural environments. We can also make sure they know that this regulation is based on evidence about what works best for families and children. We also let them know that they are free to access center-based services in addition to EI services if they wish.
The family wants to start an intervention program you know to be controversial or that does not have adequate evidence to support its use.	We "coach" the family through this decision by asking what they know about the intervention and what they hope to gain from using this intervention with their child. We help the family craft a short-term goal from using this practice, so they have tools to decide whether it is helpful. This opens the door for discussing the fact that they will encounter many ideas and gives them strategies for making decisions about each new idea that comes along. We ask to share what we know about that practice and offer resources that would provide additional information. We can also reiterate what we have to offer, so the family knows we are not going to reject them for making this decision.
The family thinks they are getting fewer services when there is a primary provider model being used.	Actually, families get the same or more intervention supports because the whole team will review their services and supports quarterly, or more frequently if needed. They have access to any team members any time, if they feel this need to support outcomes for their child and family.
The family wants their child to be like everyone else, when the team doesn't feel this is realistic.	We always write the family's desired outcome down (e.g., to be like everyone else) because that is what matters to them right then. In planning together, you then determine what the first step would be from the family's point of view to move in that direction. The process of problem-solving also provides instruction and insight as the family learns about their child's individual development.
A team member says you are violating discipline boundaries by asking for guidance about an aspect of the child's development.	With team members, we want to engage in a conversation so we can understand each others' point of view. We would use a "coaching" approach to this situation to gain clarity about what the team member is precisely concerned about. We could also have a discussion about each practice act, which are quite broad. This is also an appropriate time to talk about trust on the team to know what boundaries are and to know when to seek help from each other.

Table 7-5.

Myths and Facts About the Individualized Family Service Plan Process

Myths About the EI Practice	Facts About EI Practice
We have to conduct formal standardized assessments to "qualify" a child for EI services.	Each state determines the eligibility criteria for infants and toddlers as well as the methods and instruments to determine eligibility.
Children have better outcomes in center-based programs.	The current evidence does not support this belief. Interdisciplinary evidence supports what the laws and regulations state: that children learn better in their daily life routines (see Chapter 1, Principle 2).
It is a violation of a practice act to coach another discipline with your knowledge and expertise.	Every discipline has expertise that the team relies on for planning. We are not practicing another discipline when we take advantage of another discipline's wisdom and insight. By receiving appropriate guidance from another (or providing it), we are enhancing each practice. We continue to provide services from our discipline's point of view. For example, if you are providing information to a colleagues about how to structure activities to reduce the impact of a child's sensitivity to touch, that colleague will use that information in the context of their own discipline. A dietitian is still working as a dietitian, but may select different food options based on knowing the child's sensitivity to certain textures.
All that is required for family-centered care is to be in the family's home.	You violate the core principles of best practice if you enter a family's home and then segregate your practice outside of the family's routines. It is not sufficient to be present in the natural contexts. We must also engage in the family's priorities and style, and must support them to choose the options that fit into their life.
Each discipline has to write their own goals or objectives.	The IFSP are everyone's outcomes. Because they are based on the children's participation, everyone works toward the same goals. Individual disciplines contribute their expertise to meeting this participation goal.

FREQUENTLY ASKED QUESTIONS ABOUT THE IFSP PROCESS

* *Do we really have to write down exactly what the family says for an outcome? Some families aren't realistic.*

YES. In a strengths-based approach, we believe that the family has the best interests of their children in mind. It is up to the professional to help quantify the family's outcome so that it is measurable. For example, the family wants Eve to play happily with her brother while mom is trying to make dinner. We would need to find out what "happily" means to the mom and get a sense of how long "making dinner" takes. In our planning, we would also want to explore what Eve and her brother's common interests are so we can design activities that will keep their interest.

* *If a physician prescribes a specific therapy, does that automatically become a service on the IFSP?*

NO. The IFSP team is responsible for the services with the child and family. Families are always free to obtain additional professional services, but that does not mean it is part of the EI services. While the physician is always invited to participate on the IFSP team, no one member can make decisions about what services are appropriate, including how those services will be delivered.

* *We keep hearing that we should "front load" services. How can we do this when the state data system asks for a specific amount of time per week?*

"Front loading" means that we see families a lot at the beginning to get them started and then taper our visits/contact as they feel more capable of handling the situation themselves. The law actually says that the family and the team must be INFORMED about and understand how the family's services will happen; Kansas regulations (for example) also state it must be free of jargon or other professional terminology and be sensitive to the family. The law also states that we must provide the most appropriate services for the family's needs and priorities. So, we cannot let a restrictive data system keep us from meeting the spirit of the law, which is to provide the best possible plan. In these cases, we provide an attachment, note, or some other addendum to the report that states the exact pattern of services, rather than try to squeeze the services into an artificial number. In fact, reporting a number when this misleads the family would be a violation of the law.

* *How can I be part of the IFSP process when we cannot be funded to attend the meeting?*

When professionals find themselves in this situation, it is incumbent upon them to explore options within their state systems to support their participation in the team meetings. For example, in Kansas, local programs have the state's support to include funding the meetings in their budgets. Frequently, professionals pass along "folklore" about how procedures are handled, and people become misinformed. Sometimes, contract services include billable time that includes meetings, either through the base charge or through explicit language in the contract. The IFSP is a process, not a meeting, so professionals would actually be involved along the way.

Planning With Individualized Education Plan Regulations

With Becky Nicholson, MEd, OTR and Jane A. Cox, MS, OTR/L

The Individualized Education Plan (IEP) is a required document when we are serving preschoolers and school-aged students. This document provides a template for all the things the team needs to include in their planning process; it becomes the documentation of the decisions and plans for each student. Table 7-6 summarizes some key excerpts of IDEA 2004 regarding the IFSP process, along with explanations and examples.

Laws are operationalized with regulations; the regulations provide guidance about how to do what the law says. It is important to understand the key regulations that go with federal laws because states base their decisions on how to set up their programs based on these regulations. Table 7-7 summarizes some of the key aspects of the law related to school-based services, associated regulations, and, for illustration, how these regulations play out in Kansas. We are also leaving a blank column so you can find out what is relevant in your state.

Table 7-6.

Meaning of Part B of IDEA 2004

Excerpts From the Law	What This Part of the Law Means	Examples of This Aspect of the Law in Practice
"...a multidisciplinary team uses a variety of assessment tools and strategies to gather information about the child that may assist in determining whether a child is a child with a disability..."	The parents along with other qualified professionals complete the evaluation process. Must identify the disability and services needed to benefit from education.	The parent, teacher, psychologist, speech and language therapist, and the occupational therapist review records and complete formal and informal assessment procedures. The team determines that the child needs specialized instruction for reading and needs increased opportunities for movement.
"...to the maximum extent appropriate, children with disabilities are educated with children who are nondisabled... removal of children with disabilities from the regular educational environment occurs only if the nature and severity of the disability is such that education in regular classes... cannot be achieved satisfactorily..."	We are obligated to provide supports within the regular education in an effort to allow the child to remain in the least restrictive environment.	The occupational therapist provides services during recess to improve socialization skills and enable the child to participate in physical activity on the playground.
"...Development of the IEP, the team must consider the strength's of the child; the concerns of the parents... most recent evaluation findings, and academic, developmental, and functional needs of the child..."	We must clearly outline the abilities of the child and the areas that are interfering with the child's participation in the educational setting.	The speech and occupational therapist collaborate with the classroom teacher in order to use the child's ability to communicate using a voice output device during a science lab. The occupational therapist modifies the tools to use in the experiment.
"...improving ability to perform tasks for independent functioning if functions are impaired or lost..."	The team documents that the child has difficulty using tools such as scissors and crayons in a manner expected for his age.	The occupational therapist provides adaptations within the regular art class so that the child with physical challenges can participate with regular peers.

Table 7-7.

State Implementation of Part B

Excerpt From the Law	How Kansas Implements This Regulation (Kansas statutes)	How YOUR STATE Implements This Regulation
"...a multidisciplinary team uses a variety of assessment tools and strategies to gather information about the child that may assist in determining whether a child is a child with a disability..."	"...the first activity the evaluation team should conduct is a review of the existing data. The evaluation team needs to consider all data that [are] currently available..."	
"...to the maximum extent appropriate, children with disabilities are educated with children who are nondisabled... removal of children with disabilities from the regular educational environment occurs only if the nature and severity of the disability is such that education in regular classes... cannot be achieved satisfactorily..."	The IEP must include an explanation of the extent, if any, that the child will NOT participate with children without disabilities in general education classes AND in extracurricular and other nonacademic activities (K.S.A. 72-987 (C) (5)). The general education environment encompasses general education classrooms and other settings in schools such as lunchrooms and playgrounds in which children without disabilities participate.	
"...Development of the IEP the team must consider the strength's of the child; the concerns of the parents... most recent evaluation findings, and academic, developmental, and functional needs of the child..."	"...In developing each child's IEP, the IEP team shall consider (1) the strengths of the child and the concerns ..." (Note: Sometimes, states use the exact language from the federal mandates.)	
"...improving ability to perform tasks for independent functioning if functions are impaired or lost..."	"...paraeducator services, speech/language pathology services, and any other related services, if it consists of specially designed instruction to meet the unique needs of a child with a disability; (3) occupational or physical therapy and interpreter services for deaf children if, without any of these services, a child would have to be educated in a more restrictive environment."	

It can be really challenging as a novice to confront new and unexpected issues as you plan. Teachers and administrators ask questions that you do not know the answer to without more research, or team members can report what seems to be conflicting findings. Table 7-8 outlines some frequent occurrences and suggestions about how to handle them. You will notice that many of the strategies reflect the process of accommodating individual differences within situations and activities.

When you enter school-based practice, colleagues on your service team, families, or other agency personnel will guide your practice. Sometimes, professionals who have been in an area of practice for a while will have patterns in their practices; these patterns may or may not reflect best practice and may or may not meet the spirit of the laws that govern school-based services. Table 7-9 outlines some common myths about school practice, along with the facts. Following up, the information box contains frequently asked questions about the IEP process. You can also access www.nectac.org for current information.

Planning With Section 504 Regulations

With Louann Rinner, MS, OTR

The "504" Plan is a required document when we are serving students who do not meet the criteria for special education, but who require some accommodations to be successful students. This document provides a template for all the things the team needs to include in their planning process; it becomes the documentation of the decisions and plans for each student. Table 7-10 summarizes some key excerpts of Section 504 of the Rehabilitation Act regarding the planning process, along with explanations

FREQUENTLY ASKED QUESTIONS ABOUT THE IEP PROCESS

* *Should there be separate goals on the IEP dedicated to OT and/or PT so that the team and family know what the specific contributions of the OTs and/or PTs will be?*

No. Discipline-free goals facilitate more of a collaborative effort from the IEP team. In most situations, OT and PT services should support the accomplishment of the child's educational goals. Any teacher, paraprofessional, or parent should be able to read and understand the IEP. Goals are not assigned to one particular service provider or discipline. (From Frequently Asked Questions for Occupational and Physical Therapy in Kansas; go to: www.ksde.org/default.aspx in the search box on the right top of the site, type 'occupational therapy' and the PDF link comes up. Click on the link and you get the PDF file.)

* *Can OT and/or PT services stand alone as specialized instruction?*

OT or PT can stand alone as a special education service if the student has a disability and the service consists of specially designed instruction to meet the unique needs of the child, or if without the service, the child would have to be educated in a more restrictive environment. This may occur, for example, for a student with a disability who doesn't need the assistance of other special education service providers, but may need the services of an OT or PT. In most districts, if the OT or PT is the only provider, he or she will have the responsibility with the IEP team to develop the IEP and manage the required documentation. (Source: 2001 KSDE Special Education Process Handbook, Chapter 5.)

* *We are getting a lot of referrals for fine motor delays and handwriting. It seems that these skills are part of the curriculum for everyone. What is the best way for an OT to support this part of the curriculum without diverting limited resources to a topic that can be implemented in the regular education curriculum?*

OTs may devote time collaborating with teachers and staff to recommend strategies to meet student needs within the general curriculum. It is imperative that the OT identify opportunities for these strategies to be effectively implemented throughout the school day. Evaluation includes information about how the fine motor and handwriting challenge is impacting important outcomes (e.g., work product, attention, and group participation). OTs are discouraged from providing direct services for the sole purpose of implementing a handwriting program (Dunn, 2000).

(See also the Kansas Department of Education web site for FAQs for OT and PT services; go to: www.ksde.org/default.aspx in the search box on the right top of the site, type 'occupational therapy' and the PDF link comes up. Click on the link and you get the PDF file.)

Table 7-8.

Strategies for Handling Part B Situations

What Might Happen During Planning	Strategies for Handling the Situations
The team demands that you use a test that is inappropriate for the student's situation.	Provide evidence for the decision to use an alternative measure. Identify the educational need and how the measure tool you will use will provide information about that educational need. Refer to evaluation requirements in IDEA.
All referrals from a teacher are for "sensory issues."	Collaborate with the teacher to identify the areas of difficulty in functional performance that may be impacted by sensory issues. Emphasize the need and provide the appropriate sensory opportunities throughout the day rather than attempt to change sensory patterns.
Your team thinks you are the "fine motor therapist."	Provide the team with information regarding the parameters of our practice as is outlined in the OT Practice Framework; use children in their school to point out what supports you could provide throughout the routines of the school day.
Your caseload consists of students receiving 2 x 30 minutes/week services, so the team expects this recommendation.	Provide literature that supports a variety of service delivery patterns, including consultation, integrated services, and services provided one time per week (Dunn, 1990; Baranek, 2002).

Table 7-9.

Myths and Facts About the Individualized Education Plan Process

Myths	Facts
Each discipline that works with a student has to have their own goals for the student.	The IEP goals reflect the student's outcomes in the appropriate settings. Related service team members (which include OT) make intervention plans that are relevant to these student outcomes, thereby being "related" to the student's education.
There must be goals about every aspect of the student's performance at school.	The team has the responsibility to prioritize student outcomes. When the team identifies a need that is interfering with the student's participation in the educational setting, this must be documented in the present levels of achievement and academic performance (PLAAP). The team must address this need on the IEP but it does not have to be addressed with a goal (e.g., providing movement opportunities throughout the day could be described as a modification).
OTs can only serve students who are on IEPs and receiving other services.	Occupational therapists can be involved with screening and developing strategies for improved performance as part of the RtI process before a special education referral has been made. In addition, OT can be the only service provider on the IEP if it can be documented that, without OT services, the child would have to be placed in a more restrictive environment.
Only formal assessments that provide comparisons to normative data provide objective determination for eligibility for OT services.	There is no requirement in IDEA regarding the use of standardized, norm-referenced tests. There is no score that qualifies a child for occupational therapy services. Related services are to be provided when the team determines that the child requires those services in order to benefit from their educational placement. A norm-referenced test is not designed to provide that information. The occupational therapist will assist in the evaluation process to determine if the expertise of an OT is needed by examining the child's ability to participate in school-related activities.

Table 7-10.

Explanations of the Section 504 Regulations

Excerpts From the Law	What This Part of the Law Means	Examples of This Aspect of the Law in Practice
"No otherwise qualified individual with a disability… shall be excluded from the participation in, be denied the benefits of, or be subjected to discrimination…"	People are deemed "qualified" for education, work, housing, and other services based on meeting the requirements, and having a disability cannot be the reason someone is rejected.	A person who is a wheelchair user and meets the prerequisites for a college program must be considered equally to other candidates.
"…under any program or activity receiving Federal financial assistance…"	If a company, school, or community agency receives any money from the government, they are accountable for the rules under the Rehab Act.	A public school receives federal funds for IDEA 2004 implementation, and so must also comply with Rehab Act requirements, e.g., in making sure the education experiences are accessible to all children.
"Small providers are not required by subsection (a) to make significant structural alterations to their existing facilities for the purpose of assuring program accessibility, if alternative means of providing the services are available…"	The government is acknowledging that some changes are very costly and so provide a way for small programs to make adjustments that are still accommodating, but represent adjustments to other aspects of their services.	A rural program does not have to install an elevator to get a student to the second floor classrooms, but they do have to move the class to an accessible place so the student can participate.

and examples (www.access-board.gov/enforcement/rehab-act-text/intro.htm).

Laws are operationalized with regulations; the regulations provide guidance about how to do what the law says. It is important to understand the key regulations that go with federal laws because states base their decisions on how to set up their programs based on these regulations. Table 7-11 summarizes some of the key aspects of the law, associated regulations, and, for illustration, how these regulations play out in Kansas. We are also leaving a blank column so you can find out what is relevant in your state.

There are always unanticipated issues to confront during the planning process. Learning settings can change, or people can have misconceptions about what the law requires. Table 7-12 outlines some frequent occurrences and some suggestions about how to handle them.

Within school-based practice, colleagues on your service team, families, or other agency personnel will guide your practice. Sometimes, professionals who have been in an area of practice for a while will have patterns in their practices; these patterns may or may not reflect best practice and may or may not meet the spirit of the laws that govern 504 plans. Table 7-13 outlines some common myths about 504 plans, along with the facts. Following up, the information box contains frequently asked questions about the IFSP process. You can also access www.specialresolutions.com for current information.

Planning Transitions With Regulations in Mind

Some of the most challenging points in time for children, families, and professionals are the times when children are transitioning from one service setting to another. These are times of ambiguity; service providers are changing, the systems have different requirements and expectations, as you can see from the discussions above, and children themselves are changing their interests and focus as well. Two of the most critical transitions are transitions from early intervention to school-based services and the

Table 7-11.

State Regulations Related to Section 504 Expectations

Excerpt From the Law	How Kansas Implements This Regulation (www.kcdcinfo.com/index.aspx?NID=224)	How YOUR STATE Implements This Regulation
"No otherwise qualified individual with a disability... shall be excluded from the participation in, be denied the benefits of, or be subjected to discrimination..."	"It is important to note that the Rehabilitation Act and IDEA 2004 are completely separate federal laws. Thus, a student who receives protection through Section 504 and has a 504 plan created by a school or school district cannot receive special education services through IDEA 2004 at the same time..."	
"...under any program or activity receiving Federal financial assistance..."	"...Depending upon the needs of a student who has a Section 504 plan, the student and parents may be wise to seek assistance through other sources such as community resources, but the student will not likely receive transition services unless [he or she receives] special education services under IDEA 2004."	

FREQUENTLY ASKED QUESTIONS ABOUT THE 504 PLANNING PROCESS

(See also http://ed.gov/about/offices/list/ocr/504faq.html.)

* *Why do we need the 504 process when we have the IEP process already?*

Some students need some accommodations to support learning, but would not qualify for specialized instruction. As we get better at using the RtI process, the need for Section 504 plans is likely to reduce.

* *If the team goes through the IEP process and determines the student does not need specialized instruction, does he or she automatically qualify for a 504 plan?*

No. The need for specialized instruction is different from the need for there to be accommodations to support learning. The current trend to use the RtI process to find ways to support learning is likely to reduce the need to consider 504 plans in the future.

* *Does every student who has received special education in the past automatically become a 504 candidate because of the identified disability?*

Educational accommodations under Section 504 indicate that students must have a current substantial impairment for learning to qualify, so a past record is insufficient to qualify for a 504 plan.

Table 7-12.

Strategies for Handling Challenging Situations Related to Section 504 Implementation

What Might Happen During Planning	Strategies for Handling the Situations
There is ambiguity about who is responsible for carrying out the 504 plan.	Be sure to add a "who is responsible" section to the goals and plans documents. It is also helpful to have a 504 resource person identified in a building or district, so everyone has a person to help him or her with difficult decisions and plans that arise.
People do not understand how often 504 plans need to be reviewed/updated/ changed.	They need to be updated at least annually. Plans need to indicate student progress expectations, and based on the student's progress, 504 plans would need to be updated to reflect current needs. For example, if a student no longer needs a particular strategy to support learning, then the revision needs to reflect this.
The team/district does not understand how the 504 plan will be funded.	Teams need to consider how RtI strategies can be used to support students, and these are part of the school routines already. As a civil rights law, Section 504 might be funded any number of ways and is not restricted to special education funding.
Families question whether you have appropriately determined eligibility and made accommodations.	The school's responsibility is to follow consistent procedures for determining whether a student is eligible, and, if eligible, what services/supports are needed to ensure learning occurs. The family can contact the Office of Civil Rights if they feel that the school is not making appropriate accommodations, but if the school has been consistent in its application of the regulations, the school's decisions will not be over-ridden.
Someone on the team suggests there is no consequence for not following through on a 504 plan (the IEP process does have consequences).	Families can contact the Office of Civil Rights to investigate. There is also case law regarding Section 504 claims; districts have had to make monetary awards and implement plans imposed by others from these case findings.

Table 7-13.

Myths and Facts About Section 504 of the Rehabilitation Act

Myths	Facts
You have to have a physical impairment to qualify for a 504 plan.	Because Section 504 addresses issues that substantially limit learning, not all students with physical impairments would qualify.
Every student who has ADHD needs a 504 plan.	A diagnosis of a condition is not sufficient to constitute a disability according to the Section 504 regulations. Students only need a 504 plan if the behaviors associated with the diagnosis substantially limits learning.
Every student on medication needs a 504 plan.	Not every student taking medication needs a 504 plan. These students may need a health plan to monitor their medications. Students only need a 504 plan if the illness substantially limits learning.
The student is not performing up to his or her potential (i.e., making Bs and Cs), so he or she needs a 504 plan to meet his or her potential.	The identified condition must be substantially limiting the learning for the student to qualify. These students are learning.

transition from school programs into community supports. Children and families certainly experience many more transitions than this; like all families, they must deal with adolescence, moving, and having siblings. We can also support families during these changes in their family life by using good OT practices. With a focus on successful participation, we can always be available during life transitions.

Planning Transition From Early Intervention to School-Based Service

This transition most often occurs when children turn 3 years of age. Some states allow children to remain in the EI program through their third birthday if a later transition time better meets the needs of the child. At this time, it is appropriate for children's worlds to expand and include their peer group, so programs with groups of children meet their evolving developmental needs. Families get attached to their service providers during EI services, so changing to a new team can be traumatic for the parents and the children. Parents gain a sense of safety and trust with their first team members, so changing providers represents a vulnerable period when they must worry that someone will not understand them or their children, or that someone will judge them negatively for what they have or have not done for their child. Because the world is expanding to include peers, this transition also exposes the children's differences from peers, which can make the families feel vulnerable or defensive.

A common concern for parents is that their children will be "abandoned" from care. For example, parents might perceive that providers must see their children the same amount to be getting the same quality of services. We must be sensitive to these underlying feelings and engage families in ways that reassure them. For example, instead of stating the "facts" about how services will change during this transition, we can emphasize the positive impact that EI services had to prepare the child to be more independent in school and that being more independent is a great long-term goal.

For the first time, parents may be sending their child to a school where they may feel disconnected and not as engaged as when the supports and services were provided in their home. Both the EI providers and the early childhood providers have a responsibility to make sure this transition is successful. Going with the EI provider to visit the family prior to the transition can be helpful in sending the message that you are working together. Inviting the family to visit the preschool program can also be helpful to reassure the family that their child is ready to enter this bigger world. As with all planning, asking the family what they want to accomplish in this next section of their child's life sets the stage for planning that is relevant to their priorities and interests. Linking families who have made the transition with families who are getting ready to enter early childhood services can also provide a vehicle for asking questions and feeling secure that this change is going to be beneficial for growth.

This transition also marks a change for the families because the funding sources for their services changes from Part C (EI services) to Part B (school services) of IDEA 2004. Paperwork, procedures, and expectations change, which can feel unsettling for families who have gotten used to a routine in EI services. Best practices involve working with both teams to make this change as seamlessly as possible. For example, the early childhood team can receive the assessment and planning documentation from the EI program and work from these materials rather than insisting that they "start from scratch" to make plans.

Planning Transition From School to Community

Another critical transition period occurs when young people are in high school and are beginning to plan for life and work in the community. As with all transitions, this one marks some important milestones for all young people, not just those who have particular needs. Students are interested in their social relationships so go out with friends or join clubs, are trying out different part-time jobs, and are thinking about going to college and where they will live when they leave home. When students need additional support for these life activities, it can add another layer of stress on both the student and family.

Funding sources for services change during this transition as well. Depending on the circumstances, some students will be eligible for funding under new agencies, while others will not. For example, some students will qualify for vocational rehabilitation supports to assist with living and working. It will be important for you to work with your school administration and special education leadership to identify appropriate sources of support for the students and their families.

Traditionally, occupational therapists have worked with younger children in school-based services. This is important, but it should not be to the detriment of transitions to community for older students. Occupational therapists are uniquely suited to identifying settings and activities that will be a good match for a young person. Knowing the young person's strengths, we can identify jobs that take advantage of these strengths.

For example, we served a young man who wanted to work after recovery from his head injury. He was very social, and everyone liked him; however, he would stand too close to people for a little too long, so it made others uncomfortable. He had tried a couple of jobs unsuccessfully because of his "visiting" and making people uncomfortable. In looking at his strengths (which included his motivation to work and socialize, his independence in moving about), we identified a job that took advantage of his strengths: he became a bagger at the local grocery store. The counter provided a natural barrier between him and others, so he could not get too close and make people uncomfortable. His interest in socializing was considered a strength in this context; people loved coming to his line because he was so pleasant while they were checking out. Another advantage of this job was that his interactions with customers had a natural ending point (i.e., when they completed checking out). The occupational therapist's ability to see the advantages of his behavioral repertoire rather than his "dysfunction" made it possible for him to meet the goal of transitioning successfully into work.

Families need help mapping their future during this time. They may have difficulty seeing their children as successful, independent adults because of their lifelong experience receiving supports. Another aspect of this transition is helping families plan and dream for the long-term. Young people need a voice, and this might be a new role for the young person and parents who have been caretakers. We might serve as a mediator in discussions about where to live, how to navigate transportation, etc. We can guide these discussions with "coaching" questions, such as, "So you want your own apartment; How about we make a list of what you and your parents think you will need to be able to do to manage your own apartment." Coaching like this helps families stay calm and focused.

The best approach to preparing students and families for transition to community is to begin early. Because there are many skills needed for transition to adulthood, planning time for practicing along the way will improve the success of the transition. This is an area that occupational therapists need to increase time and commitment to; our ability to see the possibilities in a student's capacities and how to match them to just the right activities and settings makes us uniquely qualified to support families with this important life-planning activity.

Team Meetings as a Forum for Planning

Team meetings can be times we look forward to or that we dread. Everyone on the team needs to take responsibility for making sure that meetings are productive and efficient. Families are legitimate team members, so it is not appropriate to exclude them from planning. Every agency has its own way of conducting team meetings; however, here are some tips to keep in mind to make your meetings *great*:

- **Be prepared.** Time is of the essence, so everyone must be a good caretaker of the meeting time. Review your materials prior to the meeting, and know what points you want to make.
- **Ask the parents what they want, and listen to what they have to say.** We can get caught up in our professional activities and forget that we are not in charge of this child's life. The family gets to set the priorities. By beginning here, the team sets a tone that parents are important members. Using reflective listening (i.e., repeating back the parents' priorities) ensures everyone understands the framework for planning.
- **Frame all comments in relation to the parents' priorities.** After listening to the parents' ideas, it is helpful to use their priorities and goals as the framework for our comments. For example, if parents say they want their child to learn to read, then we attach our comments to the goal of learning to read. We might say, "I observed Eric during individual reading time. He squirmed in his desk and fell out once. He seems to be struggling to focus on practicing his reading." Even though there are many ways to frame this behavioral observation, because the parents are focused on reading, this is what we talk about. By linking to the parents' priorities, we help them see the relationship among all the component behaviors and the outcome behaviors.
- **Emphasize the "so what" part of your reports.** Everyone on your team believes that you have a particular expertise, and they trust you to bring that wisdom to the table. No one wants to hear you recite test scores or developmental levels; besides, everyone has some of these! In one or two sentences, state how you collected your data (e.g., "I interviewed the teacher, observed Polly in class, and conducted some follow-up testing..."). Then, spend the rest of your time *interpreting* your findings. What does it *mean* that Polly was out of her chair during group instruction? What did you discover that might be *interfering* with Polly's seatwork completion?
- **Make recommendations that are linked to outcomes.** Many times, team members have strong recommendations based on evidence, but if they are not explicitly linked to the family's priorities, it can be unclear to other team members why this recommendation matters. For example, if we recommend that Eric stand at a counter to do his work, someone might think this is a punishment. However, if we say that Eric may be able to focus on his reading better if he stands so he is getting more input to his body and more stability from the counter, then our recommendation is anchored in the overall plan.

Coordinating Plans With Other Community Services

Children and families have many agencies that may serve their needs within a community. As has been discussed earlier, each agency has a mission, and occupational therapists who work within those agencies have a responsibility to carry out that mission in their own work. Planning services gets complicated when families need services from multiple agencies; professionals have the responsibility for

Table 7-14.

Best Practice Philosophy Principles	How It Looks During Planning Across Agencies	
	What It Does Not Look Like	**What It Looks Like**
Professionals have a knowledge base that represents their profession and enables them to derive particular meaning from situations; individuals expect professionals to provide services that reflect the expertise of their discipline.	Agencies have protocols that they select for each "diagnosis" or "condition." Disciplines have prescribed roles so there is no "encroachment."	Teams reflect the depth of their expertise from all disciplines by designing plans that address all areas of need the family identifies.
Individuals have the right to participate in daily life activities of their choosing; communities have the responsibility to provide reasonable access to these activities.	The professionals dictate to parents what they will receive and who will provide their services. Agencies/professionals pressure families into using their services.	Families access services based on family priorities and needs. Professionals discuss needs with families and help them consider options for getting needs met.
Professionals who serve children and families have the responsibility to provide family-centered care, i.e., to honor the family's priorities and style in designing and implementing intervention plans.	The agencies tell families what services they will get, with no flexibility. Families who don't "comply" with methods do not get services.	Professionals seek to understand family needs and priorities. Professionals tailor their plans to meet family needs.
Individuals have characteristics that support their participation; professionals have the responsibility to focus on these strengths as the foundation of service programs and satisfying outcomes.	Each agency conducts its own standard assessment protocols to identify deficits; planning addresses remediating deficits and are independent of each other.	Professionals describe strengths as a central part of reporting and employ these strengths in their integrated intervention planning.
Professionals and families have the mutual and reciprocal right and responsibility to involve each other in the organization and structure of services within community-based systems.	Agencies have prescribed "clinics," "units of time," or "protocols" that are available.	Professionals collaborate with families to tailor just the right services to meet the family's needs. Professionals are flexible in scheduling supports to fit into family schedules.
Individuals have the right to consider options and choose interventions; professionals have the responsibility to provide information regarding the effectiveness of the options we offer as potential solutions.	Agencies state what they offer, and families either get this plan or do not get services at that agency.	Professionals at all agencies collaborate with families to identify which services will meet a family's stated needs. Professionals support families to decline services.

supporting families so that all the services they need can be coordinated.

Sometimes, families feel placed in the middle between service agencies when they receive what seems like conflicting messages. Best practice service planning principles are critical here. Let's examine the core philosophical principles from Chapter 1 and see how they are and are not implemented in planning across agencies (Table 7-14).

Projecting Outcomes as Part of Planning

Many times, we are all feeling pressure about the child's current struggles and focus our attention to meet immediate needs. Although this is a primary focus, the team also needs to look into the future and consider longer term outcomes as well. Professionals and families consider what they "dream" and "fear" the child will be doing in adulthood. Long-term projections can include living, working, and social situations. The team discusses skills and supports for living a satisfying life; when children are older, they can participate in this process themselves. Two widely used approaches are the COACH model (Giangreco, Cloniger, & Iverson, 1990) and the MAPS process (Vandercook, York, & Forest, 1989); be sure to find out about your setting's strategies and participate in them.

For example, if we are serving a kindergartner, we automatically think about the kindergarten curriculum. However, we also need to think about later primary grades and consider what we might need to put in place during kindergarten and first grade that will be useful for fourth or fifth grade. A student might forget directions; we anticipate this will interfere with remembering assignments in fifth grade. Although remembering assignments is not a kindergarten issue, because the teacher provides a lot of cues, if we see a student forgetting directions, we might anticipate these other challenges arising from this behavior in the future. We review the student's strengths; he remembers better when he sees what to do. So part of our intervention plan will include making sure the student and teacher have visual supports (a picture, a model, someone to demonstrate) when giving directions. We will also teach the student that he does better with visual cues (e.g., "Dan, here is a picture to help you remember what to do," or "Dan, if you watch someone else, it will help you remember better"), so as Dan grows, he learns to recruit his own strengths during tasks.

Projecting outcomes also provides clarity about what might be appropriate or inappropriate for current intervention plans. For example, if the team of a young child projects that the child will use an augmentative communication system as an adult, they can begin working on this outcome immediately. This projected outcome might guide the occupational therapist to work on adaptations for optimal positioning of the device and on reaching and pointing to activate the device. The speech language pathologist might address vocabulary and phrasing for programming the device. The occupational therapist and speech pathologist might explore augmentative devices and switch options that lead to an adult setup. There would be a low demand for addressing oral control for talking, and so this would not be a priority for this child's plan (although there may be a need to address oral motor control for eating in another aspect of planning). The occupational therapist might decide not to emphasize head control, opting for biomechanical support, so that the child can spend more time interacting with the augmentative device for talking and socializing.

We must also be sensitive to the family's coping abilities when projecting outcomes. In Case #1 (see Chapter 9), David is a very young infant; his mother is distressed due to David's highly aroused state and her inability to cope with his behavior. You will see in reading the case materials that the mother is resistant to therapist involvement at first; this is probably related to her inability to see past the day-to-day challenges she faces in caring for David. The therapists and the community nurse express their confidence in David's ability to learn to play and interact, and the mother eventually experiences some successes with David herself. During the initial distress period, the mother would not have been able to participate in a process to project outcomes for herself and David. However, as she began feeling more competent, this would be a good time to begin the projecting outcomes process.

When we serve adolescents, we project towards college, independent living, getting a job, and having a social life. We bring up the future and give parents a forum for discussing their dreams and fears about their children's futures. Parents worry about whether their vulnerable children will be successful on their own or what supports they will need to be independent. Sometimes, we are better equipped to imagine a hopeful future because we have studied behavior across the lifespan and understand resilience. Parents also have dreams for their children; they want them to be happy, safe, and productive citizens. Our expertise as occupational therapists makes us uniquely qualified to find ways for these dreams to happen. By simply having this conversation while children are young, we open the doors to a wider view of planning our current programs with those long-term outcomes in mind.

For example, many parents of children with complex disabilities worry that there will be no one to care for their child when they grow older or die. It is important to provide an environment that supports the family members to express concerns such as these; the team can only address issues that are expressed. When parents are silently worried about a concern such as this one, it can contaminate current intervention planning (e.g., "what's the use...," or "we must provide everything possible so my child is 'cured' before I get too old..."). When the team projects long-term life outcomes, it becomes easier to determine what is relevant for current planning. In this example, knowing that the parents are thinking about independent/supported living guides the team members to discuss issues in relation to the child's functional skill development for independent living. The team can also introduce the family to community supports that they might learn about so they feel ready for various transitions they will face.

Projecting outcomes is an emotional process, and professionals must be prepared to deal calmly with the situations. When families project outcomes, they also must mourn the loss of the "child they dreamed they would have," regardless of how much they love the child that "is." It is appropriate for people to be sad, angry, despondent, and even hopeful when they hear the dreams projected by the more informed members, such as the occupational therapist who has scientific reasoning knowledge to recognize the possibilities.

Documenting Best Practice Plans

Documentation is the key to communicating all aspects of occupational therapy services to other professionals, the family, the child (if appropriate), and involved agencies. As occupational therapists participate in the processes of referral, assessment, planning, implementation, and re-assessment, they collect an immense amount of information that must be reported efficiently and effectively. The therapist also continually manages additional information (e.g., results from other professional team members, the family's concerns, third-party payer inquiries, or medical and educational issues). Records must reflect the quality of the intervention taking place. In a very real sense, documentation represents the quality of one's professional work; recording one's information, decision-making, and outcomes demonstrates the professional's willingness to be accountable for the work (Hopkins & Smith, 1993).

It is not only the plan itself that we document; we need to document everything that supports the plan and demonstrates how we will track the children's progress. Therefore, we create written documentation of our work to meet several purposes. First, we want to provide a *comprehensive record* of the child's performance, programs, and changes across time. Professional records create a history of what has happened; this information can help us understand the trajectory of changes and what was or was not helpful, and may provide clues about planning. This comprehensive record also *fosters communication* among professionals, families, and community-based services that contributes to the child's care. When everyone has access to the assessments, plans, and outcomes in a child's history, we can plan effective future programs and supports as well.

Documentation can also reflect a *professional's problem-solving processes* that led to decisions about what plans have been appropriate or effective for a child. Assessment documentation frames the child's strengths and challenges and how these characteristics seem to be affecting life activities. We generate hypotheses and design initial plans from assessment data. Sometimes, professionals only report the facts about their findings; this strategy leaves others to figure out what the facts mean. In the interest of transparency, explaining how facts link together and what hypotheses might be generated from these facts lets the reader know *how* conclusions and recommendations are associated with the initial referral concerns. When occupational therapists take responsibility for explaining how we came to a decision, we make it possible for others to understand our reasoning and offer alternative interpretations.

Finally, documentation reflects *progress and goal achievement*. We write measurable goals that reflect the children's participation in everyday life. Part of this aspect of documentation includes graphs, counts, checklists, scales, or whatever the team creates to keep track of the children's behaviors.

Professional, agency, and governmental standards and regulations dictate the type of documentation and the time frames required for services. Chapter 2 summarizes pertinent laws. It is the responsibility of the occupational therapist to know and meet those requirements. However, each therapist must select what is relevant to report from a vast amount of data collected about the child, activities, performance, and context variables.

We must also consider the audience for which the documentation is intended (Hopkins & Smith, 1993). The type of documentation necessary for school-based therapy is not the same as required for a referring physician, a concerned parent, or a third-party payer. The occupational therapist must clearly understand the purpose of the documentation and communicate in an appropriate manner to those consumers. Documentation in all settings may include evaluation reports, intervention plans, record of contact, progress notes, discharge summaries, parent consent forms, and, when applicable, physicians' orders and billing records (Lewis-Jackson, 1994).

Documentation as Respectful Written Communication Among Professionals, Agencies, and Families

Regardless of the regulatory or standards requirements, professionals must follow basic communication principles when recording findings, decision-making, plans, and effectiveness of services. The same communication principles from oral communication apply to documentation. These are a sense of respectfulness, clarity, and reciprocity in the communication process.

Respectful written communication involves using words that everyone will understand so that they will not need a "translator" to decipher comments. As discussed in Chapter 5, when professionals use jargon in reports, it creates a barrier between themselves and others without this expertise, including professionals from other discipline as well as families. Instead of saying, "The child demonstrates vestibular hypersensitivity," the therapist can report, "Sam cries after swinging a very short time and refuses to participate in tumbling in physical education class, suggesting that he is very sensitive to movement experiences." Using everyday words also contributes to reciprocity of written communication. When the reader understands, it is easier to formulate comments and questions.

As stated in Chapter 1, "person-first" language also contributes to respectful written communication. Therapists say the child's name whenever possible and say "the child" or "the student" when needed. We refer to the child's limitation or disability only when absolutely necessary for clarity of communication. It is not necessary to include the child's disability in statements about other functions (e.g., "The child with cerebral palsy will participate in the reading group"). We reserve comments about a child's disability when we need to communicate about the impact of the condition on performance (e.g., "Sam needs a wedge for sitting to minimize the impact of his spasticity on getting his seatwork completed").

Professionals use active verbs in written communication to establish clarity. This means that professionals construct sentences in the following manner: "who did it," then "what did they do."

In passive form #1, one must infer who did the evaluation; in passive form #2, one finds the "actor" imbedded in the sentence. Both active forms state who the "actor" is immediately, providing a context for the action to come. Some professionals and some settings prefer the more formal "the occupational therapist" rather than using a more personal reference (i.e., "I"); both active forms are acceptable for best practice documentation.

Several things contribute to reciprocity in written communication. As stated above, writing respectfully and clearly provides the opportunity for discussion about the reports and plans. Occupational therapists also generate a reciprocal communication when we relate all of our comments to the performance

PASSIVE FORM SENTENCE	ACTIVE FORM SENTENCE
The child was evaluated for cognitive abilities.	The occupational therapist evaluated the child's cognitive abilities.
The child was evaluated by the therapist for cognitive abilities.	I evaluated the child's cognitive abilities.

concern and explain meanings and decisions in this context. When individuals solicit occupational therapy services, they want our professional expertise, but they primarily want their problem solved. If we communicate our expertise but do not link our insights to the original problem, we leave our communication partners to wonder what our insights have to do with anything that is relevant to them. It is inadequate to say, "Jackie has a postural control problem." Instead, say, "The teachers have been concerned that Jackie cannot complete her seatwork in a timely manner. I observed Jackie during seatwork and found that her trunk muscles are not strong enough to hold her up in her chair so she can complete her work."

Documentation That Outlines the Problem-Solving Process for Intervention Plans

The team designs the intervention based on information from the functional assessment (including observation in the environment, interviewing significant individuals, conducting ecological assessments, reviewing records or collected data, and, when necessary, evaluation results; see Chapter 6). Intervention planning, implementation, and monitoring is a clinical reasoning process in which the professional conducts hypothesis-testing procedures. There is no way to guarantee that a particular intervention plan will succeed. Using clinical reasoning skills, the therapist forms several hypotheses as possible explanations for the child's performance difficulty. The intervention plan is an effort to test these hypotheses.

To design the intervention plan, the team identifies hypotheses, generates as many ideas as possible, then chooses strategies that are feasible and acceptable. We include all aspects of the strategies (i.e., the special materials or equipment needed, frequency, setting, model of service, and people responsible for carrying out the plan) and include the parameters for monitoring the effectiveness of the intervention (i.e., the goal, criterion for success, measurement strategy, and decision-making rules).

Documentation to Chart Progress and Goal Achievement as a Method to Establish Accountability

Occupational therapists are accountable for the services that they provide. The only way to make professional decisions and outcomes available for scrutiny is through the documentation process. Best practice dictates that when we design and implement intervention strategies, therapists must produce sufficient evidence to demonstrate that their efforts actually increased or improved the desired outcomes. Accountability for improved results is a major emphasis of IDEA 2004. The questions to be answered are simple, yet can become challenging if one does not collect the appropriate data to answer these questions convincingly. Are the children we care for making progress in areas of priority to families? Does occupational therapy intervention make a difference in the daily lives of children with special needs and their families? Through ongoing assessment and documentation, those questions can be answered.

For example, a practitioner may have tried various intervention strategies and reported the child is "doing significantly better than the previous 4 weeks." One is then forced to ask which intervention strategy was most effective and specifically how much improvement the child made in the performance area of interest. In best practice, the therapist would have recorded the strategies and responses and would have observed the impact of the strategies on the performance of interest, so that she could report, "Andrew can participate in 5 minutes of the reading group when the staff provides touch cues during the discussion. He participates for 1 minute in the reading group when the staff provide oral cues for paying attention." In the second scenario, the therapist is reporting what the team tried and the impact of that trial strategy on the performance of interest (i.e., participating in reading group).

Ongoing assessment and documentation of progress toward identified goals makes therapists accountable for the right thing—improved participation in children's daily lives. Documentation of outcomes also allows agencies to be accountable and to satisfy a community's reasonable question on how the system is performing (e.g., Are the children making progress? Is this service worth the dollars it costs?).

There are essential procedures for designing and implementing a systematic approach to monitor children's progress toward participation goals. This process simultaneously allows the team, system, and discipline professionals to take responsibility for their work because an ongoing assessment process yields objective data describing the child's rate of progress and level of performance in goal areas. The data collection and analysis system can be used to document a child's improvement or lack of improvement, and the team can then make decisions about the relative effectiveness of a therapeutic intervention and the need to change strategies to meet the goals. Fuchs (1989) cites studies that have demonstrated that ongoing progress monitoring is associated with effective special education practices and improved outcomes for students.

Systematic Approach to Ongoing Data Collection

Outcomes for the child are based on the family's priorities; data from the team's comprehensive assessment inform us about why certain areas of participation might be challenging. From this initial picture of the child and the participation need, the team defines targeted behaviors and establishes measurable goals and individualized interventions that they believe will support attainment of the target behaviors. Best practice directs teams to use this systematic approach so that there is a useful database for making service modifications, program modifications, and decisions to end therapy.

It is necessary to write specific goal statements to communicate a clear understanding of the desired outcomes and to be able to make judgments about the child's progress. Goals enable the team to determine the relative effectiveness of an intervention. Goal statements emerge from functional assessment data and have a direct relationship to the identified behaviors of concern. The team considers both the child's current level of performance as well as the intended outcome after intervention when developing a goal.

Goal statements have predictable parts. We always use the student's name, rather than using terms like "student" or "worker." Goals then must describe the *conditions for the behavior*. We might include the timeline, settings for the behavior, prompts provided and/or equipment/materials needed. For example, we could say:

Timeline	*...in 6 weeks...*
Settings	*...during snack time...*
Prompts/supports	*...with a maximum of two verbal prompts...*
Equipment/materials	*...use a weighted spoon and bowl of oatmeal...*

We state the functional behavior that we expect of the child. This targeted behavior must be observable, measurable, and specific and must reflect participation in the child's daily life. It is a description of the task to be performed. The behavior must be stated in a positive way so that the team and the child know what is expected (e.g., "Lou will eat oatmeal," rather than "the student will not spit out the food"). When trying to reduce a negative behavior, it is better to record what the desirable behavior is that will replace the current negative behavior.

Finally, we state what level of the behavior is acceptable. When setting the criterion, remember to be ambitious, yet realistic. Research cited in Fuchs and Shinn (1989) indicates that the ambitiousness of the goal was associated with better growth in skills. The goal takes into account the child's current levels of performance and reflects a level of improvement that would reduce or eliminate the performance problem. Professionals can use various performance standards to establish the appropriate criterion, including peer performance (child's behavior approximates a typical peer in the setting), criteria for next environment (what the child has to master to participate in the program of interest), teacher or therapist judgment, or the school district's expectations. In the example we have been building, we might say, "...five spoonfuls of oatmeal." So our example would be:

Lou will eat at least five spoonfuls of oatmeal with her weighted spoon during snack time with a max of two verbal prompts (per meal) by 6 weeks from now.

Monitoring the Effectiveness of the Intervention

Progress monitoring as an essential aspect of best practice plans. We collect performance data on a regular basis to provide objective data regarding the individual's progress toward the goals. As with writing the goals, having a systematic plan for progress monitoring is an important part of the plan. The team has to decide how frequently data will be collected;

Figure 7-1. Kim's Goal Attainment Scale for riding the bus.

-2	-1 current	0 goal	+1	+2
Kim has to be pulled out of bus line and have parents pick her up	Kim pushes and bumps people while going to the bus	Kim gets to the bus w/o incident	Kim gets to the bus and seated w/o incident	Kim gets positive reports about bus ride after getting on the bus w/o incident

generally, data need to be collected frequently (at least once a week for most behaviors) to be a good tool for making decisions about the effectiveness of our interventions. The more frequently data are collected, the sooner decisions can be reached regarding the success of the intervention. The data collection methods must be simple, cost-effective, and sensitive to small changes in the child's performance.

The team makes decisions about the child's progress based on a review of the data. There are 3 options for data-based decision making: (1) continue with current intervention; (2) modify intervention or criteria; and (3) discontinue current intervention or services. We have illustrated these options within Signe's and Geoff's progress monitoring plans (these cases will be discussed later). Signe's plan had to be adjusted to support her progress, while Geoff continued to make adequate progress. In standard practice, team members can become frustrated with the rigidity of intervention plans that are only linked to the IEP process, because these are designed for annual review. In best practice, therapists design data collection procedures along with intervention plans so that there is a continuous flow of information throughout the year.

In best practice, the team identifies the criteria for the child's successful participation. These criteria are documented as part of the intervention plan (as described here). Service modifications, program modifications, and decisions to discontinue services are based on these specific criteria. Many times the team will anticipate a child's readiness to move into more independent work (e.g., in the regular classroom without supports) and will include criteria about the stability of the child's behaviors in inclusive settings to ensure success across time. Therapists must make systematic decisions when considering modifications or discontinuation of the child's intervention program. The team must review all the information available and collect any new information that might aid in the decision-making process. We must make decisions about the nature of the changes and then design and implement a plan for implementing the changes.

Including progress monitoring in a program plan ensures that the team is taking responsibility for making sure they will be checking in on the child's responses to interventions regularly. It is unacceptable to wait for an annual review to find out that a child is not achieving outcomes.

(Tables 7-15 and 7-17 later in this chapter contain two examples of goals a team wrote using these standards and the data collected about these goals and plans.)

Setting Clear Behavioral Markers of Progress

Another systematic strategy for charting progress is the Goal Attainment Scale (GAS). In GAS, we describe the child's current behavior in context and then describe progressively improved versions of the behavior to move toward the goal. Finally, we describe what the behavior would look like if it got worse than current performance. The increments become the GAS, or the measure of progress during intervention. Figure 7-1 contains an example of a GAS for riding the bus. GAS is an effective way to measure progress in practice and research programs (Mailloux et al. 2007). Typically, the therapist interviews the parent, teacher, or child to identify the priority behaviors and to get a description of more and less desirable versions of the behavior. The process of operationalizing the exact behavior that will serve as the marker of progress is in itself a helpful process; it seems to focus everyone's attention on the most important participation issue(s). Some hypothesize that the process of composing the GAS is itself an intervention in the sense that it creates mindfulness for everyone about what the interventions are aiming to change (e.g., Rodger, 2010; Chapparo, 2010).

Recording Data Using Graphs

Although there are many ways to record data, a graphed, visual presentation of data is frequently easier for community-based teams because they can review a lot of data very quickly and see the relationships between the interventions and the impact on performance simultaneously. When time is of the essence, reading lengthy reports can be cumbersome.

A chart or graph is a visual method that allows the professionals to display a large quantity of data in a systematic manner. This allows the viewer to analyze actual student performance and compare this performance to the expected student performance. It promotes decision-making, because the viewer can easily determine if the intervention is promoting student performance. When data indicate that interventions are not supporting change, the team can modify the intervention immediately. The most important graphing decision is to determine how to display data on the chart or graph so team members can easily make decisions.

We will illustrate two methods for displaying data in this chapter. This will enable the novice to begin and then branch out to more complex graphing strategies when needed. In the first method, we recorded the rate of behavior. In the second method, we recorded the acquisition of the various sub-skills of the goal behavior.

Method 1: Graphing Increasing Time

Signe needs to participate in group time in her classroom. Table 7-15 illustrates her Progress Monitoring Plan, and Table 7-16 contains the data graph that the teacher completed each day during the intervention. As you can see, we set up the graph with seconds and minutes on the vertical axis and days/weeks on the horizontal axis. The teacher graphs the actual time on the graph.

During comprehensive assessment, the occupational therapists observed that Signe ran around the room during the teacher's direct instruction time at the beginning of the day. Signe's peers were able to stay in the group time, which was about 5 minutes per day. During goal setting, the team decided that they wanted her to remain with the class for this 5-minute period after 6 weeks. You can see from the progress monitoring plan that the therapist designed a series of strategies to support Signe and her teacher.

Look at the graph; you see a diagonal line. This line represents the time criteria Signe must meet each week; when the teacher charts the time, the time needs to be higher than this diagonal line. The team agrees that any week Signe does not pass over this line, it will indicate that the intervention plan needs to be adjusted. The teacher and therapist agree to meet each week to check in about Signe's progress.

The teacher plots Signe's performance each week; at the end of week 3, Signe does not make adequate progress. The therapist and teacher discuss the intervention plan and decide that Signe needs more intense movement input than the "move and sit" cushion provides. They implement a new plan (see Table 7-16 at the bottom), and Signe gets back on track to meet her goal by 6 weeks.

Method 2: Graphing Acquisition of Skills

Geoff is a young adult with a developmental disability. He wants to be more independent and asked to start with ordering food at a restaurant counter so he can hang out with his friends. Tables 7-17 and 7-18 contain the Progress Monitoring Plan and the data graph. The team has outlined the sub-skills that Geoff must master to meet his goal of selecting, purchasing, and eating a meal without help from his coach.

The team and Geoff identified 6 sub-skills, or milestones, to be mastered over a period of 6 weeks in order for Geoff to purchase a meal independently. This technically means that in order for Geoff to meet his goal, he will have to master one additional sub-skill each week. The team writes down the sub-skills on the graph and agree to document whether physical or verbal prompting is needed to complete the sub-skills.

Geoff's graph illustrates that he needed a lot of physical and verbal prompts at first. The graph also shows that Geoff achieved the sub-skills in varying

Table 7-15.

Sample Progress Monitoring Plan for Signe

Components	Signe's Plan
Behavior	Signe is a 5½ year old who runs around the room during group instruction time.
Goal	Signe will participate in group time by remaining within the carpeted area while the teacher is providing instruction (approximately 5 minutes).
Hypothesis for observed behavior	If Signe's behavior is due to her body's need for additional sensory input, then providing her with movement opportunities during instruction will enable her to pay attention to instruction.
Intervention plan	1. Review Signe's sensory processing patterns with teacher and aide, and explain the impact of her "seeking" pattern for movement on her classroom behavior. 2. Discuss options for Signe to get movement input while also participating in group time, e.g., use of "move & sit" cushion, opportunity to stand/walk at the perimeter of the group, using Signe to gather materials needed from other parts of the room. 3. Teacher selects option that fits her classroom, talks to Signe about it. 4. Collect data to see if Signe's participation increases (which at this time is simply to be present in the group; later, we will work on her contributing to discussion and repeating back instructions).
Measurement strategy	Teacher will start a timer as she starts group time and stop it if Signe leaves the group; teacher will chart the time on the graph each day.
Criteria	By 6 weeks, Signe will remain with group time for the full 5 minutes at least 3 days per week. To meet this goal, Signe has to improve approximately 10 seconds per day; during any week that this intermittent goal is not met, the therapist and teacher will meet to discuss adjustments to Signe's intervention plan.

Table 7-16.

Signe's Progress Monitoring Data Collection Graph

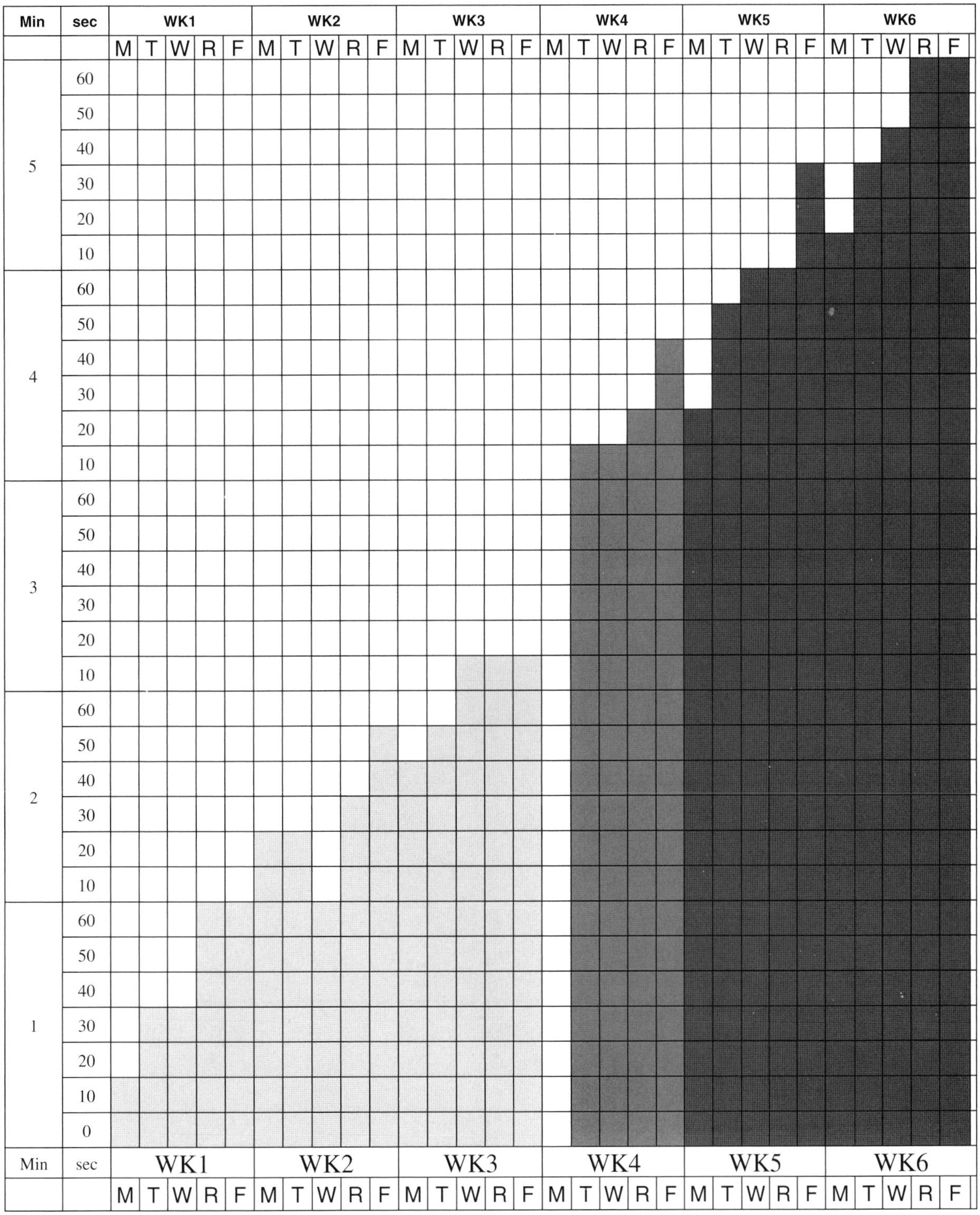

INTERVENTION PLAN A: Signe sits on a "move & sit" cushion on the carpeted area for group time.

INTERVENTION PLAN B: Signe stands at perimeter, hands out materials, and points for teacher.

Table 7-17.

Sample Progress Monitoring Plan for Geoff

Components	Geoff's plan
Behavior	Geoff needs a helper to order and pay for his food at the restaurant counter.
Goal	Geoff will order and purchase at the restaurant counter and eat his own meal.
Hypothesis for observed behavior	If Geoff's need for a helper is because he lacks opportunities to practice, then providing regular chances to order and pay for his food will enable him to be independent in this way.
Intervention plan	Schedule at least 3 trips to a restaurant with a counter per week during off-peak hours. Identify the parts of the process that he gets help with; provide direct instruction to Geoff about how to complete each part, and then let him try. Be prepared with physical prompts and verbal prompts if Geoff is not completing a step in the process. Practice steps in kitchen at home to get his meals; make a cue card for the wall that Geoff can reference. Make a video of Geoff doing the steps successfully that he can watch on his computer.
Measurement strategy	Coach will mark each skill as "YES" (independent), "verbal" or "physical" prompt. Coach and therapist will review Geoff's performance once a week and make adjustments as needed.
Criteria	(Note: Team does not care about the order Geoff learns the skills.) By 6 weeks, Geoff will order and purchase his own meal at the restaurant counter and eat independently 3 days in 1 week.

Table 7-18.

Geoff's Graph of Data Regarding Ordering, Purchasing, and Eating His Meal Independently

	WK1			WK2			WK3			WK4			WK5			WK6		
DATES:																		
Throws trash away and exits restaurant (5 minutes)	P	P	P	P	V	V	V	YES	YES	V	YES	YES	YES	V	YES	YES	V	YES
Eats food independently	P	P	P	P	P	V	V	P	P	V	V	V	YES	V	YES	V	YES	YES
Gets food, straw, napkin, utensils to table without spilling	P	V	V	V	YES	YES	YES	YES	YES	V	YES	YES	V	YES	YES	YES	YES	YES
Manipulates money, pays for food	P	P	V	YES	V	YES	YES	V	V	YES	V	YES	YES	YES	YES	YES	YES	YES
Places the order within 2 minutes	O	V	V	V	V	V	V	V	V	V	YES	V	YES	YES	YES	V	YES	YES
Selects his choices within 3 minutes	P	YES	YES	V	YES	V	V	YES	YES	V	V	YES	V	V	V	YES	YES	YES
	Meet 1 skill? *Yes*			Meet 2 skills? *Yes*			Meet 3 skills? *Yes*			Meet 4 skills? *Yes*			Meet 5 skills? *Yes*			Meet 6 skills? *Yes*		
	WK1			WK2			WK3			WK4			WK5			WK6		

P = physical prompting, V = verbal prompting, O = did not attempt, YES = completed independently.

order; people do not always learn life tasks sequentially. He made adequate progress each week, suggesting that the plan they had in place was effective for Geoff.

Planning Changes in Programs Including Discontinuing Services

In addition to monitoring progress, the team has a responsibility to compare the child's initial performance in relation to the established goals (e.g., on the IEP) during periodic reviews. If the child has not met the standards for performance in a particular classroom, we would continue services and make appropriate modifications in the program, intervention, or environment as the child entered the next year's classroom. If the child has met all the established goals and there is no further need requiring the expertise of occupational therapy, the child is discontinued from occupational therapy services, and the team records the decisions and factors. Occupational therapists recognize each child's functional abilities to participate separate from the presence of a temporary or long-term disabling condition.

Sometimes, parents are reluctant to discontinue services they see as supportive to their children. Parents feel anxious; they grow accustomed to having supports, and they worry that, without services, their child will flounder. One reason this happens is that teams fail to point out the good news to parents: that the child has made significant progress and therefore does not need the same supports any more. We reduce services when the team concludes that the child can function in a natural setting with peers without additional supports. This good news message needs to be the first information the family receives.

Once the team introduces the idea that the child does not need particular services, then they can design a follow-up or contingency plan with the family. In this process, the team solicits the parents' fears and concerns regarding their child's vulnerabilities if services are discontinued. The team can then set criteria for each fear and agree that if any of these criteria are met in the next period of time (e.g., the next school quarter), the professionals will immediately investigate and provide service support. If the quarter goes by and the child does not need additional supports, parents can see through the data that their child can indeed function independently of this support. When the family sees that the team is willing to serve their child, it is easier to recognize that it is the child's progress that leads to a reduction in services rather than the team's unwillingness to serve the child.

For example, parents might worry that their son will fall behind in his seatwork. The team can set criteria about seatwork:

Sam will complete at least 80% of his seatwork with at least 75% accuracy during each week. If during any week Sam falls below these criteria, the team will immediately meet to plan a strategy to support Sam's educational progress.

This provides two benefits. First, the parents feel that their son has a safety net. Second, when Sam continues to meet this criterion, it will become clearer to the parents that Sam is ready to be completely included in regular education.

Future Roles in Planning

Thus far, we have focused on children who have identified needs based on diagnoses, conditions, or impairments. This is how our systems are currently constructed. There is an increasing discontent with this structure for services; advocates for change emphasize the concept that everyone has individual differences that have the possibility of interfering with participation. From this point of view, it is artificial to require children to have a diagnosis or label of some sort to "qualify" for the expertise of team members like occupational therapists. The increasing attention to the RtI process is an early indicator that educators are interested in creating classrooms that support a wide range of learners, with a focus on strengths and success.

For example, researchers found higher sensory sensitivity (using the Sensory Profile) in a study of students who are gifted (Gere, Capps, Mitchell, & Grubbs, 2009). They referenced the gifted literature to link this sensitivity to two common features of giftedness. First, they proposed that increased sensitivity contributes to these children's challenges with social interactions. They suggested that the children noticed more aspects of social contexts and, therefore, could be unable to pick out salient aspects or could be overwhelmed by the flood of input. However, they also linked sensory sensitivity to these children's ability to problem-solve better than their peers, a skill that is highly desirable. In a response to this paper, Dunn (2009) commented that this frames the possible role of OT very differently. Children who are gifted cannot be considered children with disabilities, yet there are certainly supports that an OT could provide so a student who is gifted could improve social interactions if they were interested in doing so. Therefore, we will need to think more expansively about our contributions to children's ability to participate, rather than limit our thinking to disability-related supports. We discussed the strengths-based perspective in Chapter 1; review these materials to refresh your mind about the possibilities.

In the next decade, there will be an increasing recognition of the need to apply professional expertise to everyone, across all settings and activities. Occupational therapy can take a leadership role in serving children by looking broadly at the applications of our expertise. I predict this theme will be the central focus of the next edition of *Best Practices*!

References

Baranek, G. T. (2002). Efficacy of sensory and motor interventions for children with autism. *Journal of Autism and Developmental Disorders, 32*(5), 397-422.

Chapparo, C. (2010). *The impact of the sensory protocol on functional and behavioural performance of children with severe sensory defensiveness, behavioral disturbance and intellectual disability*. Paper presented at the World Federation of Occupational Therapy meeting, Santiago Chile.

Dunn, W. (1990). A comparison of service provision models in school-based occupational therapy services: A pilot study. *Occupational Therapy Journal of Research, 10*(5), 300-320.

Dunn, W. (2009). Invited commentary on sensory sensitivities in gifted children. *American Journal of Occupational Therapy, 63*(3), 296-300.

Dunn, W. (2000). *Best practice occupational therapy in community service with children and families*. Thorofare, NJ: SLACK Incorporated.

Fuchs, L. (1989). Evaluating solutions, monitoring progress and revising intervention plans. In M. R. Shinn (Ed.), *Curriculum-based measurement: Assessing special children*. New York, NY: Guilford Press.

Fuchs, L., & Shinn, M. (1989). Writing CBM IEP objectives. In M. R. Shinn (Ed.), *Curriculum-based measurement: Assessing special children*. New York, NY: Guilford Press.

Gere, D., Capps, S., Mitchell, W., & Grubbs, E. (2009). Sensory sensitivities of gifted children. *American Journal of Occupational Therapy, 63*(3), 288-295.

Giangreco, M., Cloniger, C., & Iverson, V. (1990). *C.O.A.C.H. microform: Cayuga-Onandaga assessment for children with handicaps: Version 6.0*. Burlington, VT: University of Vermont, Center for Developmental Disabilities.

Hopkins, H., & Smith, H. (1993). *Willard and Spackman's occupational therapy* (8th ed.) (pp. 387-390). Philadelphia, PA: Lippincott.

Lewis-Jackson, L. (1994). Third-party billing in public schools. *AOTA School System Special Interest Section Newsletter, 1*(1), 4-6.

Mailloux, Z., May-Benson, T., Summers, C., Miller, L., Brett-Green, B., Burke, J... Schoen, S. (2007). Goal Attainment Scaling as a measure of meaningful outcomes for children with sensory integration disorders. *American Journal of Occupational Therapy, 61*(2), 254-259.

Rodger, S. (2010). *Occupational performance coaching: Enabling occupational performance in families*. Paper presented at the World Federation of Occupational Therapy meeting, Santiago Chile.

Vandercook, T., York, J., & Forest, M. (1989). The McGill Action Planning System (MAPS): A strategy for building the vision. *Journal of the Association for Severe Handicaps, 14*(3), 205-215.

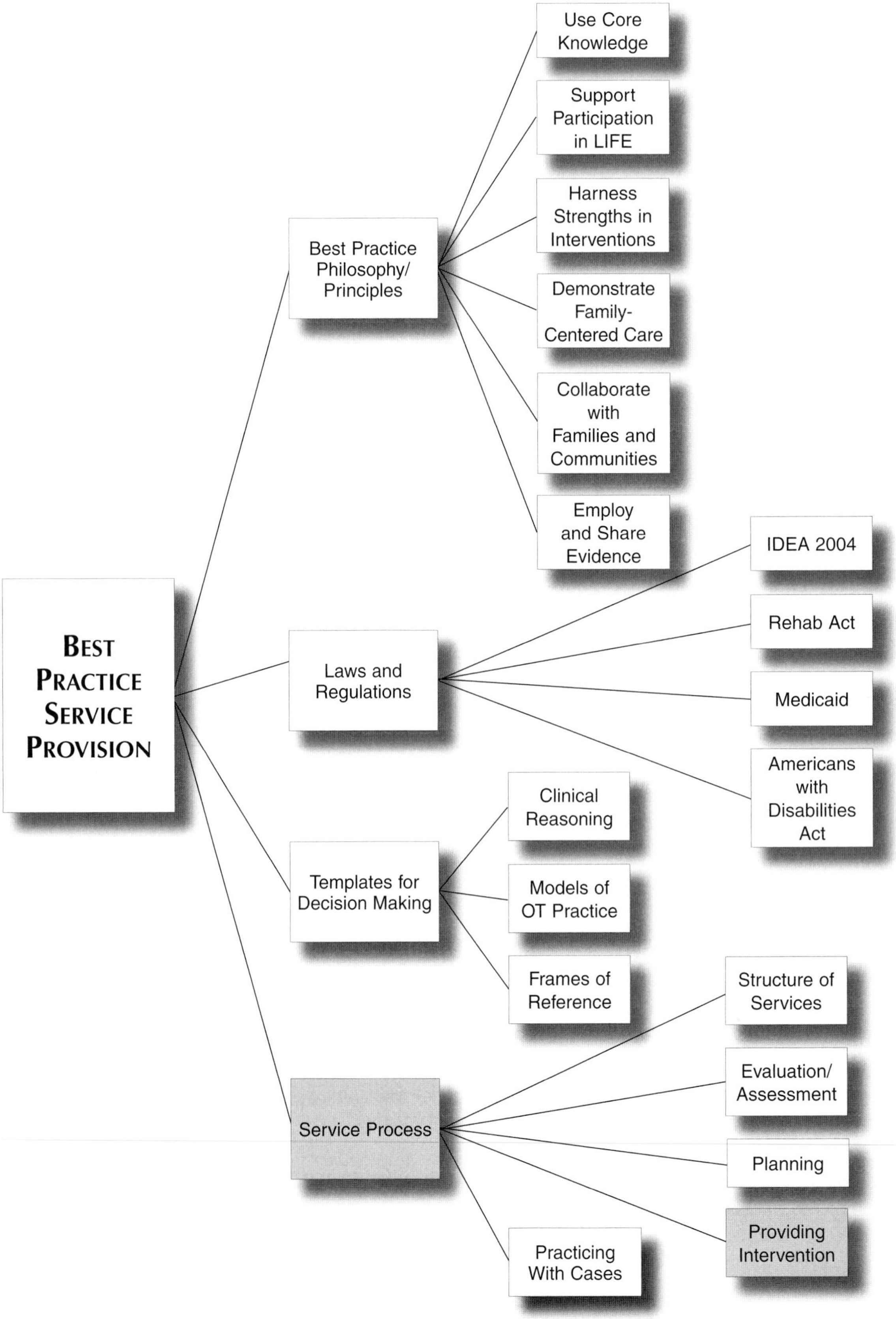
Best Practice Service Provision
Best Practice Philosophy/ Principles
Use Core Knowledge
Support Participation in LIFE
Harness Strengths in Interventions
Demonstrate Family-Centered Care
Collaborate with Families and Communities
Employ and Share Evidence
Laws and Regulations
IDEA 2004
Rehab Act
Medicaid
Americans with Disabilities Act
Templates for Decision Making
Clinical Reasoning
Models of OT Practice
Frames of Reference
Service Process
Structure of Services
Evaluation/ Assessment
Planning
Providing Intervention
Practicing With Cases

CHAPTER 8

Designing Best Practice Services for Children and Families

Best practice service provision is a fluid and complex activity because it requires ongoing decision-making. In this chapter, we will study ways to design and provide interventions that reflect the best practice philosophy (from Chapter 1), which are imbedded in everyday routines and situated in authentic contexts for children, their families, and others. We learned about planning in Chapter 7; now, we will learn how to craft interventions that support children to achieve desired outcomes. Table 8-1 summarizes the core concepts from prior chapters for your reference.

Services for children and families begin with an individualized plan that outlines the desired outcomes; within a family-centered care model, this means that we listen and respond to the family's and child's interests and desires about what they want and need the child to do as well as what the family needs to support their child's growth and development. Depending on the service system and the child's age, the team might design an IFSP, an IEP, an Individualized Habilitation Plan (IHP), or another similar service plan. Therapists design interventions based on referral concerns, RtI data, and assessment data (see Chapters 5 and 6), in collaboration with other team members, family, and the child, if possible. The process we describe in this chapter provides a way to link assessment with intervention planning towards the desired functional outcomes.

As we discussed in Chapter 7, many children receive services through more than one agency and provider. We must also take responsibility for integrating and coordinating these services with the family. Sometimes, there is a professional who provides case management with the family, while at other times, the family takes primary responsibility for coordinating services. In service coordination situations, therapists and other professionals must be vigilant in making sure that everyone understands the family's desired outcomes and how various agency services are contributing to these outcomes.

When professionals collaborate with each other and with families, they share responsibility for identifying the problem, creating possible solutions, trying the solutions, and then altering them as necessary for greater effectiveness. Occupational therapists understand behavior across the lifespan, recognize the impact of behaviors on participation, and understand the context of performance. These skills are easily translated into collaborative consultation. Other

Dunn W. *Best Practice Occupational Therapy for Children and Families in Community Settings, Second Edition* (pp. 157-179)
© 2011 SLACK Incorporated.

Table 8-1.

Summary of Core Concepts to Recall for Intervention Planning

Philosophy Principles	Clinical Reasoning	Practice Models	Assessment Procedures	Intervention Approaches
Professionals have a knowledge base that represents their profession and enables them to derive particular meaning from situations; individuals expect professionals to provide services that reflect the *expertise of the discipline.*	Scientific	Developmental	Records review	Establish/ Restore
Individuals have the right to *participate in daily life activities of their choosing;* communities have the responsibility to provide reasonable access to these activities.	Narrative	Sensory processing	Interviews	Adapt/Modify
Professionals who serve children and families have the responsibility to provide *family-centered care,* i.e., to honor the family's priorities and style in designing and implementing intervention plans.	Pragmatic	Biomechanical	Skilled Observations	Alter
Individuals have characteristics that support their participation; professionals have the responsibility to *focus on these strengths* as the foundation of service programs and satisfying outcomes.	Ethical	Motor control/ Motor learning	Activity analysis	Prevent
Professionals and families have the mutual and reciprocal right and responsibility to *involve each other in the organization and structure of services* within community-based systems.	Integrated	Coping	Response to intervention	Create
Individuals have the right to *consider options and choose interventions;* professionals have the responsibility to provide information regarding the effectiveness of the options we offer as potential solutions.		Behavioral	Criterion-based assessments	
		Cognitive	Standardized or formal assessments	

professionals contribute to the collaborative relationship in different ways. For example, classroom teachers focus on the products of learning, such as written work, verbal responses, staying on task to complete assignments, and attaining subject matter competencies. The combined perspectives of teachers and occupational therapists provide fertile ground for solving complex problems.

The Need to Provide Integrated Services

The core philosophical principles of best practice are the most apparent in intervention programs within community settings. Because we are present in the children's actual lives, we have opportunities to see the impact of contexts and expectations within activities; although we recognize that children's capacities play a part as well, we understand that person factors, environment, and occupations all contribute to children's ability to participate successfully. We also serve children alongside colleagues from other disciplines, which emphasizes both shared knowledge and unique perspectives from each discipline. In referring to "integrated services," we include coordinating all of these factors as we serve children and families. As community-based services have evolved, there has been an increasing emphasis on including children with disabilities in settings with their peers who do not have disabilities. Shifting to inclusion philosophies challenges our standard practices and requires different professional activities to support the success of this evolution.

Consider this scenario: Bobbie's family is concerned that he falls down a lot, which they notice in the community soccer league. Although you might identify weak equilibrium responses, the only reason this matters to the family is so Bobbie is safer to play soccer (and perhaps other daily life activities). If Bobbie wants to play soccer with neighborhood children, we would establish goals related to playing soccer, not improving equilibrium. In this paradigm of intervention, we link the person factor (equilibrium) to participation (soccer) as a way to integrate his community participation with our expertise. Better equilibrium by itself is irrelevant. We might be interested in equilibrium because we have studied about it and detect it in Bobbie's movement repertoire, but that is an interest and focus of ours; for the child and family, equilibrium only matters as it supports or interferes with activities of interest (in this story, soccer).

In the case study of James (see Chapter 9), we see that he is clumsy when moving about. The therapist constructed one of his goals to be, "in order to increase opportunities for play with peers, James will arrive at a new learning center at the same time as peers three of four times per week." You see that the goal is focused on having more time with peers; the team will certainly need to work on his movement skills so he can accomplish this goal. We could also write a goal about the nature and quality of James' participation with peers.

An important area for integrating services occurs when families have multiple agencies involved in their care. Coordinating between community settings like EI, preschool, or schools and agencies like hospital services is a common example for occupational therapy. Children with special health-care needs or who are followed by a medical team for care (e.g., children with cerebral palsy, Down syndrome) also attend their neighborhood programs. Many parents are concerned about feeding and eating, and this activity occurs frequently, so let's use this as an example. Table 8-2 illustrates the differences in emphasis between the medical team's occupational therapist and the EI team's occupational therapist, both who support the same family. Sometimes, they use the same strategies, but the emphasis is different.

Methods for Providing Intervention

Background

During the past 4 decades, many dramatic changes have occurred in our methods for providing intervention. Prior to this time, it was most likely that occupational therapists would serve children in hospitals, segregated schools, or in other institutions that provided care for children. It was very unlikely that occupational therapists would have the opportunity to serve children in their everyday contexts. Over this time, the culture of children's services has changed, and our profession has changed as well.

Table 8-2.

Comparing the Medical and Early Intervention Team Roles in Feeding

Factor for Family	Medical Team	Early Intervention Team
Our child will only eat pureed foods	**Observes the child eating easy and challenging foods (or being fed if appropriate)** OT conducts oral motor/feeding evaluation Recommends "swallow study"	**Observes the child eating easy and challenging foods (or being fed if appropriate)** Has family keep a food diary of what foods and liquids their child consumes Finds out context for eating and drinking Interviews family about family traditions surrounding eating Obtains coaching from team dietitian
Our child won't give up the bottle	**Interview family about why they think the child wants to keep the bottle** Review medical records to determine any contraindications Give family a recommended plan for weaning	**Interview family about why they think the child wants to keep the bottle** Coaches family re: what they have tried, how it worked, etc., to discover a plan Work side-by-side with family to wean the child from the bottle based on what the family figured out might work from the coaching process
Our child is not gaining weight	Obtain dietary log Get dietary log analysis from the dietitian Give parents a recommended list of foods/supplements	Obtain food diary Analyze food diary in consultation with dietitian With coaching from the dietitian, identify the characteristics of foods to consider (e.g., things with protein) Visit during meals to work with family to introduce foods with desirable characteristics that fit into the family preferences

Same strategies are marked in bold.

What was formerly routine practice is now considered dated; not only are our conceptual ideas better developed, but our methods and approaches are also evolving. Contemporary professionals must be nimble, keeping up with current evidence about both concepts and methodologies for providing the most effective interventions.

For example, in the last edition of this book, we discussed "direct service," "supervised therapy," and "consultation" as the methods for providing interventions (Dunn, 2000). At that time, having options other than direct service was still a little controversial; we had come to believe that spending time with children ourselves was the best method for providing our services. However, we were beginning to understand that children had needs during the whole day, and we had ideas about how to support them. So, we began talking more to teachers and parents about ways to adjust activities to make them more successful for our vulnerable children, thus expanding our repertoire for how to use our expertise.

Here we are with another decade of experience; most of us embrace the idea that we can have an impact on children's lives in more ways than in a one-to-one therapeutic interaction. So, are you not wondering what the controversy might be today as we embark on the next decade? I believe that our next evolution involves applying interdisciplinary research to our practices and embellishing these practices with our unique perspective.

For example, in Chapter 1, we introduced the Mission and Key Principles for Providing EI services in Natural Environments (www.nectac.org/topics/families/families.asp). This document was developed by an interdisciplinary expert panel and outlines the seven key principles for serving children and families through everyday learning opportunities. Each principle is built on evidence from the interdisciplinary literature and so provides all of us with guidance about how to frame our intervention practices. Principle 1 states that children learn best during everyday experiences in familiar environments. Every discipline can implement this principle within their practices, and each method will reflect the unique perspective of that discipline. An occupational therapist might suggest methods to make getting dressed easier for a young child who is sensitive to the textures of the clothing; a physical therapist might focus on making sure the young child has a stable base of support for getting socks or pants on. Both professionals are applying the interdisciplinary evidence (i.e., children learn best in everyday experiences) while using their own expertise.

This next step in the evolution of our intervention practices is a great place for occupational therapists serving children and families. Our core purpose is to support successful and satisfying lives; the interdisciplinary literature provides lots of support for our particular expertise. Let's consider what methods are appropriate for us to embrace now.

Contemporary Intervention Methods

A prevailing theme in service literature today is the concept of coaching. In general, the goal of coaching is to offer guidance that enables another person to solve a specified problem. Coaching in early childhood is seen as a particular type of help-giving practice that focuses on capacity building; coaches support people to use existing abilities and develop new skills (e.g., Dunst, Boyd, Trivette, & Hamby, 1996; Dunst & Trivette, 1996; Dunst, Trivette, & LaPointe, 1992; Rappaport, 1981). Through interactions with the "coachee" (i.e., the person being coached), coaches provide a systematic method for the person to understand, gain insights, and identify solutions to their own challenges. Coaches do not solve the problem or offer solutions or advice; they facilitate others to address their own challenges successfully.

In the education literature, authors say "instructional coaching" (Knight, 2007a, 2007b, 2009a). An instructional coach (IC) is a professional who teaches educators how to use proven teaching methods (Knight, 2009a). Instructional coaches meet with a teacher to find out (1) the best way to collaborate and (2) the teacher's concerns. Sometimes, the coach models instructional practices in the teachers' classrooms; other times, the coach observes the teacher and provides feedback. Knight (2005) outlines key principles of effective instructional coaching. The teacher and coach are equal partners in the process, and both partners have the choice about how they will communicate and address the teacher's concerns. In this partnership, they engage in conversations that facilitate reflection and adjustment as they try ideas; the coaching relationship occurs over time to allow this process to occur. Evidence suggests that teachers involved in a coaching relationship are significantly more likely to change their teacher practices (85%) when compared to teachers who have traditional in-service or workshop-style training (10%) (Knight, 2009a, 2009b; Showers, Murphy, & Joyce, 1996).

Service systems that support adults talk about "job coaches" (e.g., Virginia Board for People with Disabilities, 2007). Typically, job coaching services focus on finding the right match between a person and the employment opportunity and supporting people to learn and retain the jobs. Job coaches consider the person's interests and skills; they also investigate the employer's needs in the process of identifying the best possible placements. It is common for job coaches to remain involved in the early employment process to assist with problem-solving as unforeseen difficulties arise; staying involved increases retention. In early intervention, people have used the term *primary coaching* when there is a primary provider who works with the family to identify solutions for the family's needs with their young child (Rush & Shelden, 2010).

Life coaching (e.g., www.lifecoaching.com) involves supporting people to make the best decisions for their own life trajectory. Life coaches also explore a person's interests and talents and then, through a series of discussions, support people to discover solutions that will be the most satisfying for their lives. Executive coaches (e.g., American Management Association) is a hybrid version of coaching that involves supporting leaders to build their businesses and create more effective employee work patterns and a more positive, growthful work environment. Executive coaching has evolved from addressing problem employment situations to this more positive approach for making leadership more effective. Executive coaching is a more positive choice that is built on business and marketing literature about how to increase effectiveness. Related to executive coaching is peer coaching in which a pair of workers serve as coach to each other to improve their part of an organization (Douglas & McCauley, 1999). Coaching in business has grown in popularity as skilled workers have become scarcer, as a "value added" characteristic of a company.

Graham, Rodger, and Ziviani (2009, 2010) have applied coaching principles to occupational therapy intervention, calling it occupational performance coaching. In their work, they have been able to show that parents' perceptions about their own and their children's capacity improve significantly after occupational performance coaching to address daily life concerns. They also point out that the process of problem identification and identifying desired outcomes in everyday life seemed to be the most powerful ingredients to contribute to changes for the families. When parents learned to consider options to improve their children's performance, such as changing the activity demands or changing the environmental factors, they felt like they could be more effective parents.

So what do all these applications of coaching have in common? They are all based on a reciprocal communication relationship between the person serving as a coach and the person being coached. In each case, the "coachee" identifies the issue rather than an expert approach in which the professional would define the problems. The communication is focused on solving the problem, which includes making a situation better, not just fixing something. Most importantly, in a coaching relationship, solutions grow out of the coachee's insights (as they are facilitated by the coach's questions and guidance). Because the solutions grow out of insights, they are situated within the authentic environments and activities in which the solutions are needed. These core components of coaching comprise a contemporary method for providing intervention; OT researchers have provided early evidence that coaching methods apply successfully to OT interventions (Graham et al., 2009, 2010).

CORE COMPONENTS OF CONTEMPORARY METHODS OF INTERVENTION

1. The relationship is based on reciprocal communication
2. Person we are serving identifies the issues
3. Communication is focused on solving the problem/issue
4. Solutions grow out of the other person's insights
5. Solutions are situated within authentic environments and activities

Example of a Contemporary Method of OT Intervention

Let's look at an early intervention situation. Will is a baby whose child-care provider is frustrated about diapering. The parents have given permission for the OT to provide supports both in their home and at the child care. Because the person we are coaching must be an active participant in the relationship, the therapist listens to what the child-care provider needs and frames the discussion to address this need. So, in this situation, if the therapist took a more traditional approach and immediately offered "expert" solutions, the child-care provider may see all the therapist's suggestions as interference that lengthen the time to get diapering completed (i.e., doing a "therapy" session with Will). If the therapist can explore with the child-care provider what she sees as the barriers, then the child-care provider will be more likely to implement the therapeutic intervention on the child's behalf. The therapist knows how positioning and handling strategies can make it easier to get the diapers off and on (due to Will's spasticity) and also understands the coaching evidence, which emphasizes the importance of having a reciprocal relationship with the child-care provider to solve her dilemma. The therapist listens for opportunities to guide the discussion toward insight and discovery of a workable solution. Let's look at a possible dialogue (see Table 8-4 later) between the child-care provider and the therapist in this situation, using the coaching approach that we outlined in Chapter 5.

In this coaching intervention, you see that the therapist guides the child-care provider toward a solution that fits in with the current routines. The therapist could have just picked Will up and demonstrated a handling strategy to get Will's legs to relax, but the therapist might have made incorrect assumptions about the situation. She might have presumed the child-care provider could not identify any times when Will was relaxed or that the child-care provider would be willing to do *anything* suggested. By taking the time to find out what the child-care provider's perspective and awareness was, the therapist was

Table 8-3.

Example of Analysis of Reflective Questioning for a Conversation Between the OT Coach and a Child Care Provider

Child-Care Provider Comments	OT's Guidance (Coaching the Child-Care Provider)	Analysis of Coaching: Reflective Questioning Strategy of Interacting
(start here) "Diapering is a real problem!"	"How are you doing the diapering?"	To promote awareness of the parts of the task
"Like I have always done diapering with my kids.... I lay the baby down on his back, and usually I can pull the diaper right off. But with Will, his legs stay together, and I cannot get the diaper out from between his legs."	"So, with other children, their legs separate, but with Will, his legs stay together.... Do you have ideas about what might make it work better?"	Pointing out that the child-care provider is analyzing: making comparisons Asking child-care provider to consider options/alternatives
"Well, I tried prying his legs open, but this made him and me upset. So, the other day, I tried playing with him for a little while after I laid him down. His legs just got tighter!"	"That was a good idea to try.... I wonder if you can think of a time when Will's legs were apart?"	Inviting child care provider to make comparisons (analysis)
"Hmmm.... You know what? When I hold Will up over my shoulder, or when I kind of cradle him like this (demonstrates) so his body is in a ball, his legs do go apart!"	"So, can you think of some ways we could use those positions to change his diapers?"	Working on a plan (action)
"It would be weird to try to change his diaper over my shoulder; I wouldn't feel safe doing that. "	"Good point. What about when his body is in a ball? Are there ways we could get that shape to work for diapering?"	Trying to generate alternatives so we can move to an action plan
"You know what? He gets in that shape in the infant seat. I could put a towel in there and change his diaper that way!"	"Are you willing to try this next time and take note of how it works for you and Will? It seems to be a good match, but we can think some more if it doesn't work like you need it to. Let's check in about this by phone in a couple of days."	Getting a commitment to an action plan Providing an opening for considering alternatives next time
"Thanks so much. This has been helpful. I have so much to do all day; I cannot be spending all my time consoling Will after he gets upset from diaper changes."		

able to identify the precise way that a therapeutic intervention (getting more relaxation of spasticity) could be imbedded into the child-care provider's and Will's routine (Table 8-3).

Let's look for indications of the core components of contemporary intervention methods in this scenario. Use Table 8-4 to record the indicators from this scenario.

The People in the Context Matter, Too!

Context also includes the people supporting the child. For example, when working with a first-year classroom teacher, the therapist might try out some strategies to identify the best options and then support the teacher to learn the best ways to facilitate the child's performance. With a very experienced

Table 8-4.

Analyzing an Intervention Scenario for Presence of Contemporary Intervention Components

Core Components of Contemporary Methods of Intervention	Will and Child-Care Provider Need Better Diapering Strategies
1. Reciprocal communication relationship	
2. Person we are serving identifies the issues	
3. Communication is focused on solving the problem/issue	
4. Solutions grow out of the other person's insights	
5. Solutions are situated within authentic environments and activities	

special education teacher, the coaching process is more reciprocal from the start because this teacher understands what factors might be relevant for this student in this classroom environment.

Similarly with families, there will be some members who enjoy experimenting, and so the therapist will ask the family member to try several things and give feedback about the best strategy at their next meeting time. Other family members will want the strategy that "works," thus dictating that the therapist will need to be more involved in the discovery process with the child and parent.

Intervention to Affect System Change

We can also use the coaching method to focus on improvements of the system within which services are provided. Another name for this type of work is "population-based services" (see AOTA, 1999; NBCOT, 1997). Participation in a system-wide curriculum committee and serving as a speaker in a preschool Parents' Information Night are examples of system-level intervention—where the objective is to improve how the system works so that all children will benefit. In Chapter 9, we have a case about "Service to the Westwood School," which provides an example of population-based service to a charter school. In each case, the therapist is using occupational therapy expertise to improve a situation of concern to others.

What Happens to More Traditional Intervention Methods?

This discussion might be uncomfortable because we have not discussed more traditional intervention methods that were discussed in the previous edition (e.g., direct services). With the knowledge and evidence available for this new edition, it seems it is time to restructure our thinking about how we provide interventions. In the past, direct services have been the first consideration and sometimes our primary method for providing intervention. It has become more difficult to select traditional direct service methods because they do not meet the standards of best practice principles. For example, traditional direct service methods segregate children from their authentic routines and settings and, therefore, do not provide natural opportunities to practice. Therapists who have used direct service methods might argue that this one-to-one interaction gives them a chance to really understand the child's movements, reactions, etc. They might also believe that they are better at stimulating or facilitating the child's responses. No one can argue that occupational therapists are very skilled at creating just the right cues and supports to engage children successfully. However, if we are truly dedicated to improving children's lives, we recognize that isolated direct services do not afford adequate practice, are less likely to generalize, and fail to build the family's or teacher's capacity on that child's behalf.

Using best practice principles as a guide, direct service options can only be considered in narrow circumstances, must be a brief part of the overall method, and must be situated within intervention methods that are more contextually relevant. This is certainly true for therapists working in community settings like EI programs, preschools, public schools, or transition-to-work programs, but it is also true for therapists working in other settings such as a children's hospital or a private practice. Families get to set priorities; we have a responsibility to know their life routines and schedules so we can be relevant to their needs. When therapists commit themselves to a best practice philosophy, they expand the possibilities no matter where they work.

Last year, some pediatric therapists in our community worked together to move closer to best practice in each of their settings. One particularly challenging situation was a therapist working in a children's hospital. They came up with a great idea to move this practice closer to authentic settings and routines: they suggested that the therapist meet parents in the parking lot to support them as they got their children out of the car seat and into the building. Parents frequently apologized for being a little late because of how much time and hassle this transition was; by joining with the parents in this authentic routine, the therapist accomplishes several things. She communicates her emphasis on what the parents need; she indicates she is listening to them; she changes the "late" time to intervention time; she builds rapport while also building the parents' capacity to understand how to make this transition efficient. These parents will understand that occupational therapy is concerned with everyday life. This one change invites more discussion about family routines; families might bring videos to analyze and problem-solve together. Let's look at a few more examples.

Sometimes, our intervention strategies require us to be more closely involved because of safety or training needs. A school might have a new teacher's aide without experience with children who have moderate physical involvement; a work supervisor might be hiring someone who needs particular accommodations that have not been provided before; there might be unsafe ways to feed someone. We might wonder whether a contemporary approach is still appropriate when we need to teach a procedure or apply a safety procedure. It is certainly appropriate to provide procedural, safety, or precautionary information; the person we are collaborating with in these cases would not have a repertoire that would include new safety or procedural information. In these situations, we can take a cue from classroom teachers. When a child needs to learn a brand new skill, the teacher provides direct instruction briefly and then immediately situates the child back into the authentic learning environment for practice. Teachers know that children remember better when they practice in situations that will require them to use that skill again.

For occupational therapy intervention, we might be concerned about the strategies and precautions for feeding a child who cannot eat independently. We do not want the child to be at risk because of failing to set precautionary measures in place. If the aide has had experience with the child, we could employ coaching principles to discuss the challenging moments during lunch and when things go smoothly. Sitting with the aide at lunch time, we can employ coaching methods by providing commentary about why particular strategies are helping or interfering with feeding so that the ideas are situated in the context of the authentic routine. If the aide is new to this duty, we might model a strategy for one spoonful of food and then have the aide model that same strategy. We can build a repertoire of safe methods in this way. Even when care needs to be taken, we rely on the evidence, which suggests that imbedding the strategies in the everyday learning opportunities is the best method for generalization.

An adolescent who needs to practice social engagement skills needs cues and supports throughout the school day; if the occupational therapist only worked on these skills using a direct service model, there would be little likelihood that the skills would generalize to the needed settings for performance. By using a coaching method, a therapist can design a rich context for supporting the child's skill development. We can coach the student, willing peers, and other teachers so they provide appropriate cues, supports, and feedback for the interactions they have with the student. We illustrate the occupational therapist collaborating in this way in the cases of Derek and Cameron in Chapter 9.

Approaches to Intervention

The Ecology of Human Performance (EHP) conceptual framework (see Chapter 4) provides a comprehensive view of intervention approaches (Dunn, Brown, & McGuigan, 1994) by describing whether the intervention is focused on person, task, and/or context factors. When therapists consider several approaches to intervention planning, it is much easier to identify the best-matched interventions for the child, the family, other service providers, and the life environments. The EHP outlines five approaches to intervention: establish/restore, adapt/modify, alter, prevent, and create interventions.

Establish/Restore Interventions

The "establish/restore" intervention addresses person factor skills and barriers to performance; interventions are directed toward improving the person's repertoire of sensory perceptual, motor and praxis, emotional regulation, cognitive, communication, and social skills. For example, if a child has low endurance that is interfering with playing with friends on the playground and in intramural sports, the occupational therapist might consult with family and the school team to construct some endurance-building activities into the child's weekly routines. The parents might sign the child up for gymnastics, karate, or swimming. The physical educator might work with the child to design a "personal fitness" program. The classroom teacher might include this child in cleaning the chalkboards and transporting books to the library. These activities address the "person variable" of low endurance that is interfering with play and socialization. When using this approach, the therapist is using occupational therapy knowledge and expertise to find ways to improve the child's skills to support performance.

Adapt/Modify Interventions

The "adapt/modify" intervention addresses the context and task characteristics that might be creating barriers to performance; the therapist changes aspects of the context and environment or the activity demands to make participation more possible. For example, if a child is having difficulty copying from the board, the therapist might provide the child with a slant board (i.e., a writing surface that changes the angle of work) to make the perceptual task of copying easier for the child. This change in the way the child performs the task does not make the child's perceptual skills better, but rather supports the child to complete the task in spite of perceptual challenges. For Cameron (see Chapter 9), the team designed adaptations to make the school more accessible.

Alter Interventions

The "alter" intervention takes advantage of the natural features of contexts, environments, and activities; therapists select the best natural environment for the person without requiring the person to develop new skills and without requiring the context to be changed. For example, if a child has difficulty completing seatwork in the busy classroom, the occupational therapist might suggest that the child go to the library for work periods. The library has qualities that make it better for the child to work; the therapist has not improved the child's skills or asked the librarian to change the library. The therapist is taking advantage of the characteristics that are more suited to this child's current performance to advance his educational endeavors.

Prevent Interventions

The "prevent" intervention acknowledges the performance difficulties that may occur in the future and sets a course to keep negative performance outcomes from occurring. For example, a child who has cerebral palsy could be at risk for developing pressure sores, which would interfere with health and participation in the preschool program. The therapist would not wait for a pressure sore to develop, but would act on this knowledge about the risk. The therapist might develop a positioning program with the staff so that the child gets moved around throughout the day to prevent skin breakdowns. When we can anticipate a negative outcome, prevention enables us to use our expertise to re-design daily life to support a more positive outcome. It is not a prevention intervention if the problem already exists for the child; prevention is reserved for addressing potential problems and, by doing so, keeping them from happening in the first place.

Table 8-5.

Seven Core Principles of Universal Design

Universal Design Principle	Definition
Equitable use	The design is useful and marketable to people with diverse abilities.
Flexibility in use	The design accommodates a wide range of individual preferences and abilities.
Simple and intuitive use	Use of the design is easy to understand, regardless of the user's experience, knowledge, language skills, or current concentration level.
Perceptible information	The design communicates necessary information effectively to the user, regardless of ambient conditions or the user's sensory abilities.
Tolerance for error	The design minimizes hazards and the adverse consequences of accidental or unintended actions.
Low physical effort	The design can be used efficiently and comfortably and with a minimum of fatigue.
Size and space for approach and use	Appropriate size and space are provided for approach, reach, manipulation, and use regardless of user's body size, posture, or mobility.

Create Interventions

Finally, the "create" intervention uses the expertise of occupational therapy in a way that promotes the availability of enriched contexts for everyone, without a specific focus on a disability or a person with a performance problem. Occupational therapy expertise is useful in designing universally accessible environments, such as playgrounds, homes, and community centers. Making recommendations that are in everyone's best interest taps our discipline's expertise to develop user-friendly communities. When spaces and activities are more transparent to individual differences, those who do have a limitation will have opportunities to participate with everyone else. Occupational therapists can serve on curriculum committees, community development boards, housing panels, and charter school boards to infuse occupational therapy expertise into the daily routines of our communities. Chapter 9 illustrates an occupational therapist's involvement in the Westwood Charter School.

One way to conceptualize the create intervention is through the Universal Design Principles (Connell et al., 1997). They define universal design as the "design of products and environments to be usable by all people, to the greatest extent possible, without the need for adaptation or specialized design." Please visit their Web site for additional information: www.design.ncsu.edu/cud. They offer 7 core principles of universal design (Table 8-5).

These are great principles to keep at your fingertips when you are designing interventions of all types, to get as close to a universal design as possible. The more our interventions fit into everyday life and environments, the more everyone will be included.

Factors in Selecting an Intervention Approach

We select service approaches in collaboration with families, team members, and, when possible, the child. Best practice prescribes that occupational therapists design interventions using several different approaches and present them to the families, teachers, etc., so they can decide what might be the best match for them. This requires negotiation and a shared understanding of what the intervention will look like and how it will fit into the daily routine.

This strategy of intervention planning requires therapists to have very creative and flexible thinking about performance problems, so that a variety of ideas emerge from planning. By only designing one approach, you limit the possibilities for the child and take the risk that the intervention will not be used, thereby diminishing any possible therapeutic benefit that might have been possible.

In Chapter 9, we provide examples of how to design a multifaceted intervention approach with several children. Search through the cases to find examples of each intervention approach being applied within a child's life. Let's look at some brief examples here to get you started.

For a child who is extremely hypersensitive to movement, the high level of activity and randomness of a preschool room may be overwhelming for the child. The occupational therapist would collaborate with the teacher to identify ways to reduce the impact of the hypersensitivity (an adapt/modify approach) so the child can interact with peers, pay attention to teacher instruction, and complete learning activities. They might move his seat to a less active corner, move furniture to create a "safe spot" from the high activity, and create work zones that are more or less sedate so the teacher could direct the child to a more manageable area during choice times. The therapist and teacher would also collaborate to collect data on the child's ability to participate throughout the preschool day. The case study of Peter (see Chapter 9) describes a situation similar to this one.

A student is having difficulty staying in the desk during work time (i.e., the student falls out of his chair). The therapist can use a seatwork period to provide interventions that support the student to work on seatwork. The therapist might encourage weight shift for improved balance in the chair by placing the work items on the counter next to the child's desk, requiring a little longer reach (an *establish/restore* approach). Alternatively, the therapist might suggest a new desk placement or a different chair that provides more support for the student during work time (an *adapt/modify* approach). Imbedding intervention within the setting of interest to being a successful student also allows teachers and aides to see what the therapist does to support the child and creates more opportunities for the student to practice the needed skill (i.e., staying in the desk while working) while simultaneously supporting participation (i.e., completing work).

There are some additional cases in Dunn (2007) that follow the Ecology of Human Performance model through three children's stories using worksheets and explanations of the situations. These will be helpful if you need additional examples of how to apply these approaches to intervention.

PRACTICE WITH MODELS AND APPROACHES TO INTERVENTION

The case studies in Chapter 9 summarize the OT process with infants, toddlers, children, and adolescents. Review the case studies, and mark the places you see evidence of the therapists employing the intervention methods and approaches you have just studied here. Compare your assessment with others to see if you are identifying the same examples. Discuss with each other when you have differences in your findings so you understand more perspectives. Then, identify places in which the therapists might have used a different approach or method, and discuss this with others.

ARTIE'S PARENTS WANT HIM TO PARTICIPATE WITH THE FAMILY AT MEALS

He is 4 years old and attends the neighborhood preschool.

Intervention Approaches	Example of Intervention Strategy Options With Each Intervention Approach
Establish/restore	
Alter	
Modify/adapt	
Prevent	
Create	

Using Evidence to Support Interventions

Another principle of best practice is that we base our plans on evidence. Please refer to other sources for details about evidence-based practices (e.g., Dunn, 2008; Law & MacDermid, 2008). As we have stated, we build our interventions based on interdisciplinary evidence, which not only guides the strategies we might select, but also informs us about the methods and approaches that are most likely to be effective.

There are many sources for evidence; some are more legitimate than others. In professional practice, we count on evidence that has been peer-reviewed, which means that people not involved in the studies themselves have indicated that the work meets certain standards. We cannot count on materials that claim certain outcomes but that have not been reviewed by uninterested parties. For example, Web sites that are dedicated to certain interventions might make a lot of claims about their procedures. However, when investigating, we might see only materials developed by those promoting the intervention, or the "evidence" section includes only self-written papers or testimonials. Interventions with only these endorsements do not meet the standards expected for professional evidence.

One of the most interesting developments in the past decade is the availability of information on the internet. It is very common for families to look up things about their children's conditions and talk to other families about what they have found. Families want to do everything in their power to give their children the best benefits possible. Because we provide family-centered care, we support families in this discovery process, rather than judge them. We also provide guidance and other balanced information so families can make truly informed decisions. It is challenging to discern which materials are legitimate and which are not.

For example, a family has identified a "new" intervention that you cannot find any legitimate evidence about. Using a coaching method, you might ask the parents what outcomes they would expect from using this intervention. In this process, you can help them operationalize how they will decide if the intervention is meeting their needs. You also give them feedback about what you found, giving them any materials you might have collected so their decision is informed by all available evidence (including telling them you found nothing in "peer reviewed" sources, if appropriate). In the coaching process, you can help them make decisions about financial and time investments as well. If they decide to go ahead with this choice, help them create goals and a timeline for evaluating the intervention's impact on their child.

Here is a strategy we use in Kansas to help novice professionals and parents be informed consumers about interventions that come along. The second part of the box summarizes criteria from the literature about what might make an intervention controversial (i.e., not tested). The source articles provide more detail about this discussion.

The cases in Chapter 9 provide some examples of evidence these therapists used to support their intervention ideas (look for the comment bubbles to the outside of the text).

DECIDING ABOUT THE LEGITIMACY/ PARAMETERS OF AN INTERVENTION

1. Identify key words that define the intervention
2. Conduct an internet search using these key terms
3. Conduct a search of professional literature (e.g., you can use Google Scholar, which accesses professional literature)
4. Compare what you find with each search

If only internet search finds things but not the professional search, then we have to be cautious about claims the intervention makes because they are not substantiated.

DETERMINING WHETHER INTERVENTION PRACTICES MIGHT BE CONTROVERSIAL*

The intervention claims to help or *cure* a wide range of diagnoses.

They claim *dramatic* results.

Testimonials are used as evidence.

Papers written by the designers that are not in outside journals.

People have to pay for special training to learn the procedure.

Equipment is expensive and only available from designer.

The intervention requires a lot of money/time from the family.

The intervention builds on oversimplified ideas from the literature.

They do not discuss possible side effects/impact.

**Adapted from McWilliam (1999) and Nickel (1996).*

Generating Specific Strategies for Use in Interventions

We can do all the planning in the world, and at some point we have to come up with actual strategies for intervention. Our repertoire of strategies emerges from coursework, evidence, and experience. There are some techniques to help you practice generating ideas.

Look for Everyday Learning Opportunities

Becoming more familiar with everyday routines and schedules provides a rich source of ideas. Think about your own schedule every day. When are you using particular skills, like memory, balance, eye contact? Situating your knowledge about person, context, and task factors within a daily life routine provides a framework for generating strategies. Activity configurations provide the scaffolding for seeing the possibilities.

Consider Madeline; she is a young professional who has just broken up with her long-term boyfriend. She is not sleeping well and complains that her morning routine is completely a mess. She is forgetful, distractible, and has been missing parts of this well-established routine, getting to work "not put together." She helped us fill out her morning schedule, focusing on getting dressed (Table 8-6), although she reminded us that it is taking her longer these days.

You will see on the right side of the table (shaded), we have begun filling out some of our analysis of Madeline's situation. Because Madeline indicates that she is distressed and depleted, we hypothesize that it is not her basic abilities (e.g., memory, motor skills, sequencing) that are interfering, but rather her current diminished capacity. With this hypothesis, we generated ideas about how to *modify/adapt* her morning routine to support her desired outcome of being "put together" when she gets to work.

Activity Configuration: Getting Dressed to be "Put Together" for Work

What strategies would you generate if Madeline had just returned home from head injury rehabilitation? What if she had arthritis? In each case, although the routine might stay the same, we might be more concerned about other factors as we generate a hypothesis and then possible strategies to support her desired outcome.

Obtain some other daily routines, and practice this process with various hypotheses. The more you practice, the easier it will get to generate ideas. For example, find all the times a parent might give a child the opportunity to balance (e.g., when getting pants on, going up steps, reaching for a toy out of reach) or remember (e.g., "What comes next when we are making your cereal?," "Where do we keep your socks?," "Go get your banana"). When we make the opportunities explicit, the family begins to notice the opportunities and then can capitalize on them as they occur in their lives.

Practice Generating Ideas

There are other ways to generate ideas as well. Brainstorm with your peers, and share your ideas so you can think on your feet when you are listening to a family's story. An artful part of occupational therapy intervention is being able to see the therapeutic possibilities in the everyday routines, objects, and settings.

There are some ideas in Table 8-7 to get you started. We are taking an *"establish/restore"* approach in these examples, because we want these children to develop needed skills. These examples illustrate how to imbed skill learning into daily routines.

We can also generate ideas this way using a *"modify/adapt"* approach. Think of all the ways you could adapt a student's classroom routines to keep his or her difficulty with auditory memory from interfering with completing his or her work during the day. We have some ideas in Table 8-8; you come up with some, too.

Now consider these examples in Table 8-9. In the first column is a list of variables that are interfering with participation. Think of ways to change activities and routines in everyday life that (1) establish the skill within daily routines, (2) adapt to minimize the need for using this skill, and (3) are alternative options to build on strengths. We completed the first one in Table 8-9; complete the others with partners. You can practice with any aspect of the OT Practice Framework from AOTA (2008) to increase your mental flexibility.

Table 8-6.

Madeline's "Getting Dressed" Routine With an Analysis

Time	Activity	Components	Way to Change Something (Modify/ Adapt) Based on Hypothesis
7:00 a.m.	Check weather for day	Scanning to find the remote Manipulating the buttons for channel, volume Attending to the information Making an association between the information and appropriate clothing options	Set the TV so the weather channel is the "turn on" station automatically Leave TV on with volume down so she can refer back to the weather if she forgets
7:05 a.m.	Select basic clothing (underwear, pants, top)	Remembering where items are stored Manipulating the drawers, hangers Scanning to find desired items Matching the pieces for a "put together" look	Consider putting a week's worth of outfits together on the weekend when there is more time Take pictures of a "put together" outfit for future reference Lay out the outfit on the bed
7:10 a.m.	Select accessories (shoes, jewelry, jacket)	Keeping basic clothing in mind Manipulating drawers, shelves Scanning to find desired items Matching the pieces for a "put together" look	Consider having a couple of standard sets of accessories during this challenging period to reduce the thinking required
7:20 a.m.	Complete personal hygiene (bathe, brush teeth, deodorant)	Remembering to complete all the parts Locating products, devices Manipulating the devices	Post a card on the wall reminding about parts that are getting lost (e.g., Did you put on your deodorant? In a strategic place) Make a basket of items needed so they are all in one place
7:35 a.m.	Additional personal hygiene (hair, make-up)	Remembering to complete all the parts Locating products, devices Manipulating the devices	Same options as above
7:45 a.m.	Put outfit on	Coordination required to get each item on Sequencing items properly Remembering all the parts	With items laid out on bed, having them right there will be a reminder
7:50 a.m.	Go to breakfast		

Table 8-7.

Imbedding Skill Learning Into Daily Routines

Thomas needs to learn the concept of "cause and effect" for playing with his toys.

10 things in a home that generate opportunities for learning "cause and effect"	*You come up with 10 more!*
1. Pushing the buttons on a remote controller	1.
2. Manipulating light switches	2.
3. Pushing the "open" button on the microwave	3.
4. Turning the water faucet on/off	4.
5. Pushing something off the edge of the table	5.
6. Holding food out on a flat hand (if you have a dog)	6.
7. Waving (the adult waves back!)	7.
8. Lifting the lid to find one's toy in the box	8.
9. Flushing the toilet	9.
10. Pulling on the drawer pulls/pushing on the drawers	10.

Sarah needs to grasp so she can hold her cup.

10 things in a home that provide opportunities for practicing grasping	*You come up with 10 more!*
1. Carrots	1.
2. Electric toothbrush	2.
3. Lotion bottle	3.
4. Markers	4.
5. Glue	5.
6. Garden hose	6.
7. Video game remote	7.
8. Railing by steps	8.
9. Wooden spoon	9.
10. Hair brush	10.

Table 8-8.

Ways to Adapt the Classroom Settings and Routines so Horatio's Auditory Memory Challenges Do Not Interfere With Keeping Up With His Work

Horatio needs to complete his school work every day in class.

Teacher writes assignments on the chalkboard so Horatio can refer to the list during the day	
Teacher uses Horatio's books to point out what to do and then hands him the book so he knows right where to start	
Teacher sets up work groups so Horatio has others he can ask about what to do	
Horatio has tasks in work groups that do not require auditory memory (e.g., taking a list of resource needs to the librarian, drawing the pictures for the project)	
Horatio learns to write down the instructions with a peer's guidance	
Horatio audiotapes the teacher's instructions so he can play them back when needed	
Parents get Horatio a "Livescribe" pen for class (this pen audio records while you write, so you can review notes with the instructions)	

Categorize the Evidence

It is impossible to read all the evidence available, so it is important to take advantage of collective work to review and summarize the evidence. There are some Web sites dedicated to summary reviews of topics particularly relevant to children's needs (www.canchild.ca and www.researchtopractice.info). Visit these sites, and obtain information relevant to your work. You can also gather smaller reviews from your peers; by each selecting a topic, you can accumulate a number of current reviews of relevant literature to support your practices.

Designing Intervention With the Occupational Therapy Process Template

With Becky Nicholson, MEd, OTR and Jane A. Cox, MS, OTR/L

We have found that novice learners need to see a number of ways to work their way through intervention planning. Typically, one way seems more synchronous than another for each novice. However, not all novices find a single method to be the best option. So, with this in mind, we have organized different

Table 8-9.

Changing Activities and Routines in Everyday Life

Factor That Seems to be Interfering With Participation	Ways to Provide Establish Strategies in Everyday Routines	Ways to Adapt Daily Routines to Minimize the Impact on Participation	Ways to Alter the Routines/Settings so This Factor Does Not Interfere Any More
Need for vestibular and proprioceptive input	Swing with dad in the back yard and at park Play horsey Use jungle gym at recess	Place books on floor next to desk so he has to bend over to get them during assignments	Select different recreational activities (e.g., karate vs. piano lessons) (he is likely to misbehave during piano lessons because of need for movement)
Need for firm touch			
Difficulty with bilateral integration			
Problems with sequencing			
Poor equilibrium			

cases in this book using different formats. To illustrate the occupational therapy process as an organizational structure, Table 8-10 illustrates a case study of a preschooler named T.J. This is the same case we introduced in Chapter 3 when discussing clinical reasoning concepts; we have reformatted the case into the OT process to illustrate the intervention process and to show you how information can be presented in different formats to meet different communication needs. Observe how this therapist worked through this case to design some interventions for T.J.

Program Evaluation Components of the Intervention Plan

Occupational therapists include a method for evaluating the child's progress in the intervention plan and as part of the documentation. Best practice dictates that these evaluation features must be easy to measure, measured in the natural context, and directly about desired participation. By designing evaluation criteria about performance, therapists ensure that they address the daily life and not isolated skills. Additionally, when the evaluation criteria are imbedded in the natural environment, we can see the potentially positive effects of all the service approaches, not just those directed at restorative interventions (i.e., person variable focused). Chapter 7 provides detailed information on methods for charting and evaluating a child's progress as part of comprehensive documentation.

Summary

Best practice intervention is a complex process. When therapists are vigilant about listening, observing, and considering options, children and their

Table 8-10.

T.J.: A Preschooler Who Wants to Play With Peers, and Who Is Experiencing Anxiety

Pre-assessment Hypothesis. At this point in the clinical reasoning process:	
Choose one theory that is guiding your reasoning? Refer to conceptual frameworks from Chapter 4. Provide a rationale.	*Model of Human Occupation*—I chose this model because of its focus on habituation in addition to performance capacities and volition. Because T.J. displays delays in all motor abilities and has anxiety about participation, we need to consider how we can get some routines developed to support his participation. By having routines, he will be able to anticipate what is coming next, thus reducing his anxiety reactions.
What practice model(s) or frame(s) of reference would you consider at this point to guide your further reasoning? Refer to chapter 4. Provide a rationale.	*Sensory Processing*—Identify opportunities to adjust activity demands and contextual features to support T.J. to continue to participate. *Biomechanical*—Identify current and desired movement patterns, and make a plan to bridge the differences for development of coordination and motor skills. *Developmental*—Parents and teacher want T.J. to participate in age-appropriate activities. We need to keep track of how to support his development.
What additional information do you need to competently move forward?	It would be useful to know what T.J.'s curriculum is and how the daily routine occurs so we can identify opportunities within his day.

Assessment Plan		
Therapy Intake Form	Informal	Developmental, sensory, and social history. Parent's main concerns
Record Review	Informal	Gather background information; review previous assessment results for comparison, determine need for further formal evaluations; review medical history; review previous intervention plans, previous goals, and progress; developmental progression
Skilled Observation	Informal	Gather information regarding social interactions, motor and communication skills, level of functional independence, reaction to sensory stimuli in school routines
Interview	Informal	Behavior at home and school, social interactions, priorities of the family
Miller Assessment for Preschoolers and Peabody Developmental Motor Scales	Norm-Referenced	Compare motor performance to same-aged peers; determine level of motor skills Obtain a score that indicates whether T.J. is performing within the expected range based on a bell curve
Sensory Profile and Sensory Profile School Companion	Other Not a traditional criterion-referenced or norm-referenced test	Scores provide a profile of T.J.'s unique sensory processing patterns. Provides information regarding T.J.'s sensory patterns so we can determine how they might be met within daily routines. By having parent and teacher perspectives, we obtain general (parent) and situation-specific (teacher-school companion) information about T.J.'s reactions.

(continued)

Table 8-10. (continued)

T.J.: A Preschooler Who Wants to Play With Peers, and Who Is Experiencing Anxiety

Findings and Interpretations	
Describe assessment results and provide your interpretation of the findings. Include a summary of the factors you believe support and hinder performance.	*Therapy intake form and record review*—Motor development overall delayed: stood at 15 months, walked at 16.5. Difficulty learning new tasks, clumsy, and easily frustrated. Sensory history includes fidgety, becomes irritable in response to noises or touch, difficulty paying attention or maintaining eye contact, seems to ignore people. Good eating. Tends to prefer the company of adults.
	Observations—T.J. often bumps into things and slouches in his chair. He is compliant but does not get excited about too many activities. He will tolerate messy activities for a short time but asks to wash his hands often. Looks up anxiously when hearing an unexpected or loud sound. Awkward movements when throwing, catching.
	Interview—Mom would like for T.J. to have body awareness to function at home and school and increase his social interactions. She is also concerned about his apparent anxiety. T.J. is generally happy but whines when requested to engage in activities he does not like. Does feel pain, but falls often. Teacher says that T.J. is a generally happy child who struggles to keep up with peers during play. Occasionally, he seems worried about new activities, and he is clumsy when compared to the other children, especially the other boys.
	Miller Assessment—T.J. falls into the below-average category (functioning in the 0% to 5% range) in four of five areas (sensory, coordination, non-verbal, and complex tasks). His verbal skills are adequate, but fall into the "caution" range. This indicates that T.J. will most likely have difficulty in the classroom and may need some support to function effectively in a classroom setting.
	Peabody Developmental Scale—T.J. fell into the below-average category in all five areas (looking at balance, movement, ball skills, grasping, and visual motor integration). This is likely to affect his play with typically developing peers, as well as his self-esteem. He does display some nice stationary skills, which could be used as a starting point to build confidence and increase his skill level.
	Sensory Profile—T.J. is just like his peers in his ability to notice sensory input (registration) and in his interest in sensory experiences overall (seeking). He is more sensitive than other children related to sounds and touch, which may account for his reactions in play, social interactions, and group situations. He also seems to have less endurance than other children, which might account for his motor challenges when interacting with peers.
	Sensory Profile School Companion—T.J.'s responses at school are very similar to those reported by the parents. He is just like peers in his noticing and interest in sensory input, but he is more sensitive to touch and sound.
Include a summary of the factors you believe support and hinder performance.	*Supports* T.J. is just as interested in experiences as other children; he also notices most inputs the way that other children do. He seems generally happy. Parents are involved with his development. Teachers enjoy T.J. in their classroom. The school has equipment and activities that are suited to T.J.'s needs. *Interferes* T.J. is more sensitive to touch and sound, making some situations at school more challenging for him. His motor development, coordination, and endurance seem to be interfering with peer play schemas. T.J. has anxious reactions that keep him from participating.

(continued)

Table 8-10. (continued)

T.J.: A Preschooler Who Wants to Play With Peers, and Who Is Experiencing Anxiety

Intervention Plan	
What practice models/frames of reference did you keep/discard when choosing interventions? Rationale?	Because the mom requested a sensory diet and because he had so many areas of differences on the sensory profile, I used the sensory processing model to plan interventions. Also, I used the biomechanical model to increase his motor skills to enable him to engage in the same types of activities as his same-aged peers.
Targeted outcomes (long-term functional goal)	T.J. will play with peers throughout a free-play situation. T.J. will participate successfully in a group activity within the classroom.
Short-term goals that reflect the targeted outcome	T.J. will kick a ball with a peer for 3 minutes. T.J. will hold the weather chart for the other children to see during the morning greeting.
Specific objectives designed to achieve goals	T.J. will kick the ball twice with support from an adult. T.J. will stay in his designated spot for the morning greeting (others cannot bump into him) to establish this routine of participation.
Intervention approaches selected and rationale for selection (OT Practice Framework—Establish/restore, modify, maintain, prevent, create/promote)	*Establish* motor and social skills through structured interactions. *Modify* environment to allow T.J. to be successful (e.g., make sure that routines stay in a predictable pattern). *Create* a daily routine so that T.J. is aware of what activities he will be doing next; this will decrease his anxiety.
Specific intervention methods used under each intervention approach selected. (provide examples here)	*Establish:* Identify times and activities in the curriculum when the class is working on motor skills and interactions with others. Emphasize balance and coordination components of the activities for T.J. Prompt interactions with peers during play. *Modify:* Select a set place for T.J. to stand during the morning greeting time. Introduce an adapted kicking strategy that T.J. can do so he can play with peers. *Create:* Work with the team to organize and post the routine for the day. Have the teacher move a star to each activity as they transition so everyone (including T.J.) can see what is coming next.

(continued)

Table 8-10. (continued)

T.J.: A Preschooler Who Wants to Play With Peers, and Who Is Experiencing Anxiety

Summary of the Intervention Process

OT meets with the team weekly to review T.J.'s participation and evaluate the effectiveness of strategies used the prior week. The team employs activities for all the children into the curriculum that were particularly helpful for T.J. (e.g., obstacle courses incorporating balance, ball skills, gross motor activities, and hand-eye coordination, playing in several different textures, such as sand, flour and water, play-dough, etc. (as T.J. can manage this, we will take cues from him], fine motor activities like cutting and coloring to make cards, pictures, and other age-appropriate craft projects).

The teacher establishes a place where children can get away from the group when they need to "regroup." Although all children can use this, the teacher watches for times when T.J. might need it to keep him on an even keel in class.

Additionally, the OT supported T.J. to interact with others by prompting the use of appropriate social responses during the school routines.

Outcome Summary

Comparison of targeted/desired outcomes and true outcomes achieved.

T.J. is joining in during messy activities (e.g., during art time) and seems interested in "sharing" materials with peers. He is also interacting with peers during outdoor play, running and watching other children, fetching the ball, and sometimes attempts to kick it or throw it to others.

His mom reported that he is showing less anxiety during social situations with family. He is now able to kick, throw, and catch a ball at home, but not at a distance of more than 2 feet. They made a card for grandmother, and he used the scissors, although mom still had to cue him to orient the scissors and the paper.

Future Client Recommendations and Rationale

T.J. should continue to receive support from the OT as he works on his interactions and play. It is particularly important to begin making a transition plan for his move to public school. The team will need to collaborate to make recommendations and meet with the public school team members to make a smooth transition. The OT will encourage the school-based therapist to visit the preschool and get to know T.J.

support groups (i.e., families and teachers) receive the very best of occupational therapy wisdom. Using systematic steps to establish the process ensures that therapists will consider all factors when planning the best possible services for children, families, and other providers.

References

American Management Association. *Coaching: A strategic tool for effective leadership*. www.amanet.org/training/seminars/Coaching-A-Strategic-Tool-for-Effective-Leadership.aspx. Accessed June 2010.

American Occupational Therapy Association. (1999). *Occupational therapy practice guidelines*. Rockville, MD: Author.

American Occupational Therapy Association. (2008). *The occupational therapy practice framework*. Rockville, MD: Author.

Connell, B., Jones, M., Mace, R., Mueller, J., Mullick, A., Ostorff, E... Vanderheiden, G. (1997). *The principles of universal design*. Raleigh, NC: NC State University, The Center for Universal Design.

Douglas, C. A., & McCauley, C. D. (1999). Formal development relationships: A survey of organizational practices. *Human Resource Development Quarterly, 10*, 203-220.

Dunn, W. (2000). *Best practice occupational therapy in community service with children and families*. Thorofare, NJ: SLACK Incorporated.

Dunn, W. (2007). Ecology of human performance model. In S. Dunbar (Ed.), *Occupational therapy models for intervention with children and families* (pp. 127-156). Thorofare, NJ: SLACK Incorporated.

Dunn, W. (2008). *Bringing evidence into everyday practice: practical strategies for healthcare professionals*. Thorofare, NJ: SLACK Incorporated.

Dunn, W., Brown, C., & McGuigan, A. (1994). The ecology of human performance: A framework for thought and action. *American Journal of Occupational Therapy, 48*(7), 595-607.

Dunst, C., & Trivette, C. (1996). Empowerment, effective help giving practices and family centered care. *Pediatric Nursing, 22*(4), 334-337.

Dunst, C., Boyd, K., Trivette, C. & Hamby, D. (1996). Family-oriented program models, help giving practices, and parental control appraisals. *Exceptional Children, 62*(3), 237-248.

Dunst, C., Trivette, C., & LaPointe, N. (1992). Toward clarification of the meaning and key elements of empowerment. *Family Science Review, 5*(1/2), 111-130.

Graham, F., Rodger, S., & Ziviani, J. (2009). Coaching parents to enable children's participation: An approach for working with parents and their children. *Australian Occupational Therapy Journal, 56*, 16-23.

Graham, F., Rodger, S., & Ziviani, J. (2010). Enabling occupational performance of children through coaching parents: Three case reports. *Physical & Occupational Therapy in Pediatrics, 30*, 4-15.

Knight, J. (2005). A primer on instructional coaches. *Principal Leadership, 5*, 9.

Knight, J. (2007a). *5 key points to building a coaching program. National Staff Development Council, 28*(1), 26-31.

Knight, J. (2007b). *Instructional coaching: A partnership approach to improving instruction*. Thousand Oaks, CA: Corwin Press.

Knight, J. (2009a). Coaching: The key to translating research into practices lies in continuous, job-embedded learning with ongoing support. *National Staff Development Council, 30*(1), 18-22.

Knight, J. (Ed.) (2009b). *Coaching approaches and perspectives*. Thousand Oaks, CA: Corwin Press.

Law, M., & MacDermid, J. (2008). *Evidence based rehabilitation: A guide to practice*. Thorofare, NJ: SLACK Incorporated.

McWilliam, R. (1999). Controversial practices: The need for a reacculturation of early intervention fields. *Topics in Early Childhood special Education, 19*(3), 177-188.

NBCOT. (1997). *A national study of occupational therapy practice final report*. New York, NY: Professional Examination Services.

Nickel, R. (1996). Controversial therapies for young children with developmental disabilities. *Infants and Young Children, 8*(4), 29-40.

Rappaport, J. (1981). In praise of paradox: a social policy of empowerment over prevention. *American Journal of Community Psychology, 9*, 1-26.

Rush, D., & Shelden, M. (2010). *Early childhood coaching handbook*. Baltimore, MD: Paul H. Brookes Publishing.

Showers, B., Murphy, C., & Joyce, B. (1996). The river city program: Staff development becomes school improvement. In B. Joyce & E. Calhoun (Eds.), *Learning experiences in school renewal*. Eugene, OR: The ERIC Clearinghouse on Educational Management.

Virginia Board for People with Disabilities (2007). *Job coaching services and benefits to businesses and people with disabilities*. Retrieved from: www.worksupport.com/documents/va_board_factsheet1.pdf.

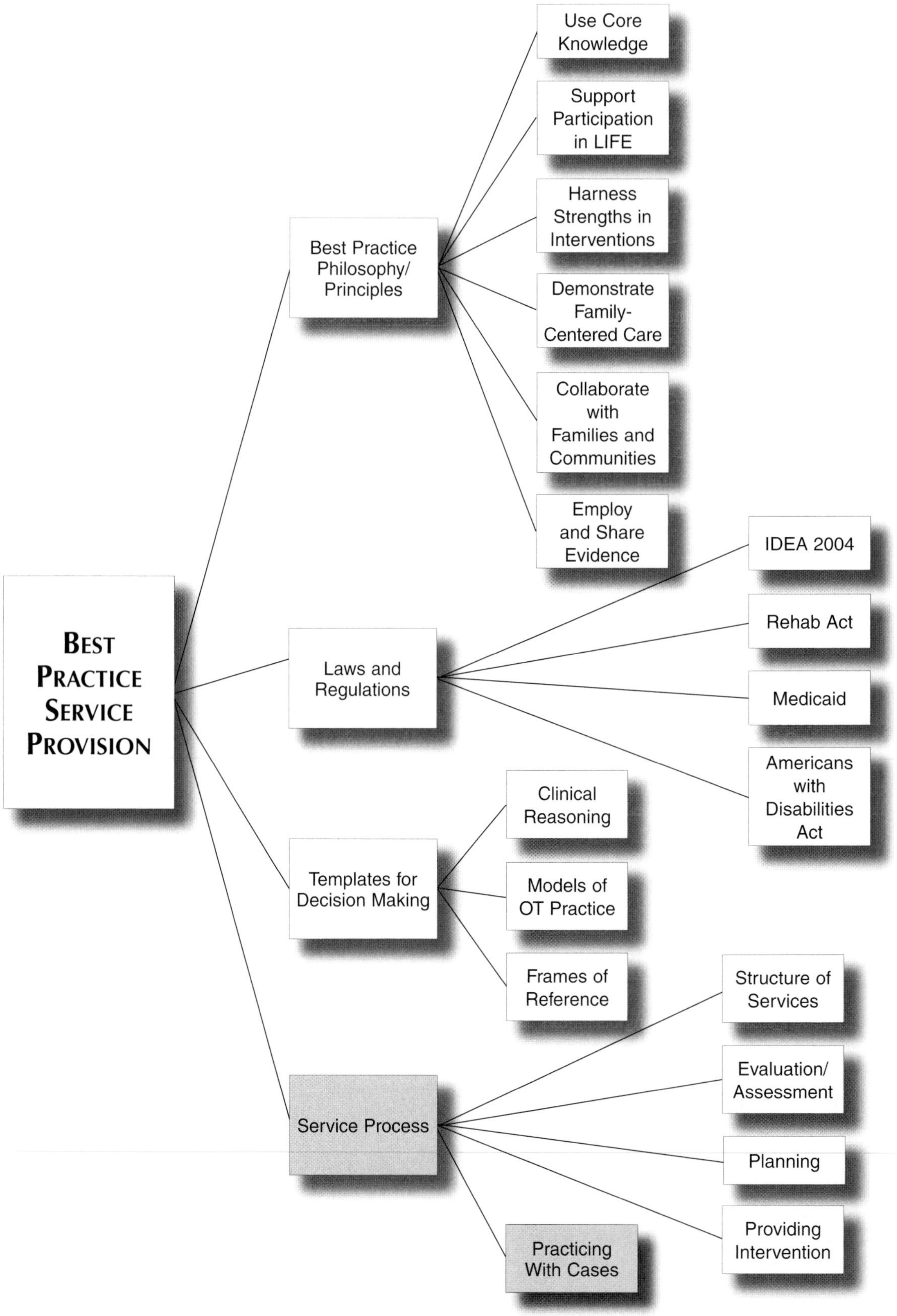
Best Practice Service Provision
Best Practice Philosophy/ Principles
Use Core Knowledge
Support Participation in LIFE
Harness Strengths in Interventions
Demonstrate Family-Centered Care
Collaborate with Families and Communities
Employ and Share Evidence
Laws and Regulations
IDEA 2004
Rehab Act
Medicaid
Americans with Disabilities Act
Templates for Decision Making
Clinical Reasoning
Models of OT Practice
Frames of Reference
Service Process
Structure of Services
Evaluation/ Assessment
Planning
Providing Intervention
Practicing With Cases

9 CHAPTER

Case Studies Applying Best Practices in Community Programs

We have proposed many strategies for thinking, organizing, and documenting your work on behalf of children and families in this book. These ideas about how to implement best practice are merely conceptual and theoretical if we cannot also show you how it will look in actual practice. The purpose of this chapter is to illustrate best practices as they occur with children, families, and other service providers in actual community settings and situations.

In the teaching/learning process, we can fall prey to using "perfect" examples. This strategy has a useful function because it allows teacher and learner to focus on the idea, or point of the story, as the salient place for attention. However, after we study concepts, we must be able to use them with the flexibility and generalization required by human beings as they live their lives, which is never (nor would it be desirable to be) perfect. The nuances that make our decision-making complicated are also what make the practice of occupational therapy an interesting and intimate endeavor. We are always vigilant in practice to notice what might support or hinder a positive outcome; it does not matter how theoretically brilliant our recommendations are if families, teachers, and children don't use them because some contextual feature prohibits implementation. The artful dance of practice lies in a therapist's ability to stay relevant to the child's and family's lives. So, these stories are not perfect; they hold the comfort of reality and the possibility of learning how to navigate in the complex lives of the children we serve.

Chapter Organization and Structure

We have organized the chapter to facilitate your learning and practice. We present eight children of all ages with a variety of backgrounds and participation strengths and needs; we also present a consultative case study with a charter school to illustrate population-based practices. Table 9-1 summarizes the cases for quick reference. We have tried to emphasize different situations with the different children so you will have examples of all aspects of practice (e.g., initial referrals, changing services, dismissing services, differing presenting performance challenges, various levels of resources in families, and school personnel). We have also only completed one target goal

Dunn W. *Best Practice Occupational Therapy for Children and Families in Community Settings, Second Edition* (pp. 181-234)
© 2011 SLACK Incorporated.

Table 9-1.

Overview of the Cases in Chapter 9

Case No.	Contributors	Child's name	Age	Participation focus of case study
1	Dunn, Pope	David	2 mo.	Daily routines are interrupted by irritability
2	Dunn, Cox	Ted	32 mo.	Transitioning from EI to preschool services
3	Dunn, Cox	James	3 yrs.	Eating and talking and playing
4	Dunn, Nicholson	Peter	6 yrs.	Manage self in classroom; Play appropriately with peers
5	Dunn, Nicholson	Derek	10 yrs.	Being included with peers at school
6	Dunn, Nicholson	Cameron	12 yrs.	Transition to middle school
7	Dunn, Nicholson	Sarah	16 yrs.	Reintegration into school after head injury rehabilitation
8	Dunn, Cox	Tammy	19 yrs.	Transition to work life
9	Dunn	Westwood Charter School		Improve student, teacher, and school success

for each child as an illustration of the direction of the therapist's and team's thinking; these are not complete plans for the children. We encourage you to "complete" the child's record by creating other goals and documentation plans as rehearsal for applying the concepts within your own service.

You will notice that we have altered the margins in this chapter. We have done this to enable you to make notes in the margin. You will see that we made notes on some parts of each case to provide you with background information, further explanation of a key point, or to provide a reference or Web site source for you. We encourage you to make the same type of notes on other children and then compare them with colleagues; the discussions you have will be an important part of your learning. Table 9-1 summarizes the main concepts from other chapters; use this table to make additional notes on the cases for yourself. The outside column is for identifying the processes at work in the stories (i.e., what clinical reasoning, what practice models, what philosophies, etc., are at work in the story). We hope all of these formatting cues help you to practice your own strategies for clinical reasoning.

You might remember that we provided a picture reminder of each of the core principles of the best practice philosophy in Chapter 1. You can print stickers of these pictures with a key word on them and use them to mark examples of the best practice principles in your cases as well. Figure 9-1 illustrates how these stickers will look; they are 1-inch circular stickers. You can download the templates from www.efacultylounge.com and print them onto sticker sheets. Then, you can stick them onto the appropriate places on the case studies so you never forget the core principles of best practice... sounds like fun, doesn't it?

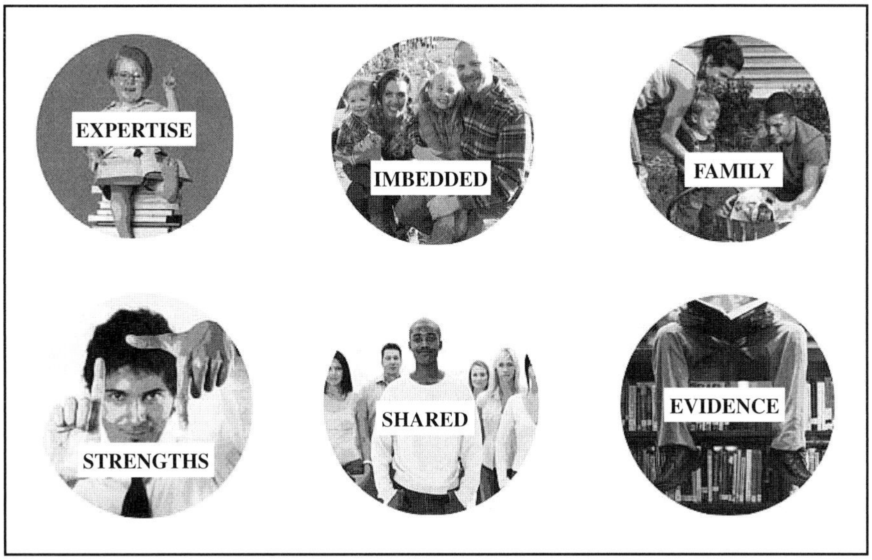

Figure 9-1. Illustration of the best practice principles stickers.

We want you to see the principles as they look in actual practice (e.g., as a therapist is talking with the mother or planning with the teacher). We also have shaded boxes with examples and tips in them; sometimes, we provide an excerpt from a report or a conversation to bring the factual material into narrative relief. We also want you to hear how a therapist thinks through the case; you will see our explanations about how we are interpreting our findings as we go through each case as well. Many times, novices watch experts and marvel at the expert's skills, but remain unclear how the expert got to the solution or the options. We want to illustrate how we have traversed the territory from the referral/performance problem to our suggestions and recommendations about how to proceed toward a more satisfying outcome. We are trying to show you our metacognitive processes (i.e., how experienced therapists are thinking through the problems of the case).

Have fun getting to know our therapeutic processes!

David

Winnie Dunn, PhD, OTR, FAOTA and Ellen Pope, MEd, OTR

Evaluation

Occupational Profile

David was referred to the local Part C early intervention program by the neonatal intensive care unit (NICU) social worker. This program serves infants and toddlers with disabilities and developmental delays. David was born prematurely and is screaming several hours a day, is inconsolable most of the time, and is unable to enjoy or complete feedings. Changes in formula have not helped. Subsequent laboratory tests and x-rays suggested no physical reason for David's irritability. David's mother is stressed due to these difficulties.

This information is part of our Scientific Reasoning: it helps us think about David's situation and what might be possible to do, or what might be a precaution we would have to take as we plan with this family.

History

David is a premature infant born at 28 weeks gestation weighing 2 pounds, 10 ounces. In the first 5 days of life, he suffered initial prolonged hypoxia followed by several short periods of hypoxia. No seizures, infections, or intraventricular bleeds occurred during his intensive care stay. He is being dismissed from a neonatal intensive care unit (NICU) to his mother's care after spending the first 2 months of his life in the hospital. David's mother is a single teenage mother who lives with her mother. She is trying to work on completing her general equivalency diploma (GED). David's father lives with his parents in a town 20 miles away from where David's mother lives and visits infrequently. He is trying to complete high school graduation requirements.

Prior to discharge, the NICU social worker made a referral to the local Part C early intervention program and to the county health department. A discharge planning meeting was scheduled 1 day prior to discharge with a representative of the early intervention program in attendance as well as the county health department nurse.

The nurse from the county health department immediately began making weekly home visits to the mother's home to aid in the transition from the hospital and to monitor the use of the apnea monitor, feeding issues, and general care. Although the mother was concerned about David's crying and feeding issues, she was not extremely receptive to having the local early intervention program evaluate David, but the nurse home visitor was able to convince this mother that it would be a good idea to get additional help for her and her son.

Analysis of Occupational Performance

The local early intervention program (Part C) contacted the mother to schedule an initial evaluation at her home. Two professionals from different disciplines on the local Part C team were assigned to complete the comprehensive evaluation. These two professionals were determined based on the referring concerns and geographic area where the client lives. In addition to the occupational therapist and speech and language pathologist, the Part C team is made up of a physical therapist, an early childhood special education teacher, a social worker, a dietician, and a psychologist. This team meets weekly to coach one another to support families. The occupational therapist and the speech pathologist were the two professionals assigned to complete the evaluation. The occupational therapist took the lead and served as the interim family service coordinator. The evaluation was scheduled during a feeding time and was also coordinated with the father and with the nurse from the county health department. Prior to the first visit with David and his mother, the speech pathologist and occupational therapist reviewed the records and discharge summary from the NICU.

Upon arrival at the mother's home, required paperwork was signed by mom to give permission to evaluate David and to obtain and share information with all parties involved including the hospital where David was born, the county health department, the primary care physician, and David's grandmother, because David and his mother are living in her home and she is a resource for David's mother. The occupational therapist also explained to the mother what the evaluation process would be as well as an overview of the early intervention program itself.

> You will notice that the team is implementing Key Principle #4 from the Mission and Key Principles for Providing Early Intervention Services in Natural Environments.
>
> *Principle #4.* The early intervention process, from initial contacts through transition must be dynamic and individualized to reflect the child's and family members' preferences, learning styles, and cultural beliefs.

As part of the comprehensive evaluation, an asset-based context (ABC) matrix (Wilson & Mott, 2006) was completed. This is an interview conducted with the mother about her daily routines and activities with David, including routines that are going well and routines that are challenging. In addition, observing and interacting with David and asking David's mother additional questions completed the Hawaii Early Learning Profile (HELP) (Parks, 1992), a curriculum-based assessment. These two assessments are completed routinely with families and their infants/toddlers entering the early intervention program.

Quality interviewing skills need to be employed. "Can you describe a typical feeding?" and "What calms your baby when he is upset?" are examples of open-ended questions used to gain more information. The OT observed the mother feeding David. Observations were made, such as changes in state (ranging from calm to irritable), changes in emotional responses (ranging from joy to fright), and changes in postural responses (ranging from decreased to increased tone; flexion to extension; approach to avoidance). In addition, what techniques David and his mother use to calm or excite were also observed.

The occupational therapist also decided to complete an Infant Toddler Sensory Profile (ITSP) (Dunn & Daniels, 2001) due to the referring concerns of inconsolability and fussiness, as she wanted to further explore some of David's sensitivities and preferences.

Sometimes, an Interest Checklist is used to determine the interest of the infant or the interests of the caregiver, but it was not used at this initial visit (Swanson, Raab, Roper, & Dunst, 2006).

During the initial eligibility phase of entering a Part C program, the primary provider completes the Early Child Outcomes (ECO) Summary Form.

In 2005, the Office of Special Education Programs (OSEP) began requiring State Early Intervention and Preschool Special Education programs to report on child and family outcomes.

Each infant entering and exiting a Part C program is rated on the following outcomes:

1. *Positive social-emotional skills (including social relationships)*
2. *Acquisition and use of knowledge and skills (including early language/communication [and early literacy])*
3. *Use of appropriate behaviors to meet their needs*

The following family outcomes are also assessed:

1. *Know their rights*
2. *Effectively communicate their children's needs*
3. *Help their children develop and learn*

Findings and Interpretations

The evaluation data gained on David was both formal and informal and from multiple sources (i.e., record review, observation, interview, and standardized assessment).

When David began to fuss during the visit, his mother began to breastfeed him. The therapist made these observations:

> *He initially settled and began sucking, but after a few sucks, he began to squirm and then arch his back and begin to cry. He became more irritable as his mother tried to reinitiate the breast feeding. His mother describes his quickly escalating crying as "panic screaming." David does quiet, although he remains partially stiff, when held vertically over the mother's shoulder while being bounced and walked. David's mother reports that this is a typical feeding and that a feeding often takes 45 to 60 minutes.*

A more formal evaluation of an infant such as David would not yield the quality and quantity of information gained from a more informal interview and observation of David and his family.

The more informal approach is also less invasive for families who are already in a vulnerable and scary position and typically dealing with multiple members of the medical community.

The therapist also talked with mom and grandmother. The mother and grandmother disagree about whether or not David calms to or enjoys minor roughhousing in the form of firm patting on the back or buttocks, knee bouncing in a supported sitting position, or linear (heel to head) rocking prone over knees. David's grandmother feels that David enjoys these kinds of play. The grandmother also feels David maintains a more organized state following these kinds of play. David's mother feels that he has a delayed reaction to these sessions, becoming even more irritable and less consolable an hour or so later.

Excerpts of the report about the other assessments are included in Figure 9-2.

The assessment process is ongoing, and for a very young infant, the early interventionists will probably just be able to gain some preliminary information. Often, the therapists or teachers may need to make repeat visits to the family's home to gain more complete information due to the infant's sleep-wake patterns or any medical difficulties the infant may have at the time of the initial evaluation as many of this information changes rapidly with such a young infant.

David was eligible for Part C Infant Toddler Services based on his risk factors as well as his current challenges. Note that David is eligible for all of the needed Part C services in order to meet his outcomes and that it is not appropriate, for example, to write that he is eligible for occupational therapy or speech and language pathology services. Services will be determined after the family writes outcomes.

Intervention (Developing the Plan)

Following the eligibility evaluation, the team met with the mother and grandmother. The team consisted of the county health nurse, the speech pathologist, the occupational therapist, and the primary care physician. The father was invited to the Individual Family Service Planning (IFSP) meeting at the mother's home. A letter was sent and a phone call was made to the father's home with no response.

Research reflects that fathers often feel left out of the services and service systems of professionals (Turbiville, Umbarger, & Guthrie, 2000). David's mother and father did not have a good relationship before David was born and David's father chose not to spend time with David in the hospital. Because he is the biological father, it is the responsibility of the infant toddler program to notify him of meetings and send paperwork to him about David even if he does not respond. The team felt it was important to reach out to David's father by not only notifying him of the meeting but to also phone him to explain the process and the program. By doing this, even if David's father chooses not to participate at this time, he may choose to be more involved in the future.

The team met at the mother's home and proceeded to develop the IFSP. This is the plan that will be followed in order to meet David's needs as well as the family's needs related to David's development. The occupational therapist, who serves in a dual role as an OT and as the family service coordinator, leads the meeting. Evaluation information was again reviewed with the mother, including David's strengths as well as David's mother's priorities and resources. Because the feelings of incompetence as a parent are so strong in families that include a child with sensory sensitivities, it is especially important for the therapist to note when any family member has initiated or has responded in a way that enhances interaction (i.e., "When you hold him over your shoulder like that and bounce, he seems much happier and is able to look over and give Grandma a smile"). It is extremely important to have conversations with the family about what is working, what they already know, and what they have tried, throughout the process of intake and evaluation.

The first priority for David's mother was for him to be able to sleep for longer periods of time during the nighttime so that he could be more alert and interactive during daytime hours. This outcome was also important for

Report Excerpt: Findings from Specific Assessments

Infant Toddler Sensory Profile:

The results indicate that David's biobehavioral state is often very highly aroused, and he is vulnerable to frequent episodes of sensory overload. Sudden touch or movement, position changes, or any noise seem to result in startle responses and intense crying. He is extremely difficult to calm and has few strategies to calm himself (e.g., he does not suck on his fingers, hand, or a pacifier). During the observation, he made several attempts to get his hands to his mouth but each attempt resulted in a total extension pattern, which reflexively moves his hands away from rather than towards his face and mouth. Once calm, the mother knows of no specific clues as to how to maintain that calm or what might 'set him off" the next time.

ABC Matrix:

The Asset-Based Context Matrix (Wilson & Mott, 2006) was used to identify activity settings, child and family assets, and opportunities and possibilities for participation for David and his mother. The OT asked David's mother a series of questions about what routines and activities she does with David most days and activities or people that David enjoys or is interested in. Additional information was obtained from David's mother about David's and the family's strengths and skills. Mom reports that David typically wakes up about 6:00 a.m. at which time she immediately breastfeeds him in bed with her. This feeding typically takes about 45 minutes, after which time David is awake and alert for the day. Mom describes this as David's best time of the day. David's mom moves David to his infant seat in the in front of the television in her bedroom so she can get dressed and ready for the day. She states that David seems to like the bright, moving images on the television. David objects strenuously when placed on his stomach and prefers being held and carried with his head in a vertical position. He goes to sleep only when walked and bounced in a vertical position, but usually wakes and cries immediately when placed in any other position (prone, supine, or sidelying) in his crib. He sleeps for 2 or 3 hours when held close to his mother's or grandmother's chest.

HELP:

On the HELP in the cognitive domain, David responds to sounds and voices and shows an active interest in a person or object. In the language domain, David cries when he is hungry or uncomfortable, makes sucking sounds, and is beginning to vary the pitch, length, and volume to indicate his needs. In the gross motor domain, David turns his head to both sides in supine, holds his head up to 45° in prone, and lifts his head when he is held at shoulder. In fine motor, David moves his arms symmetrically, regards a colorful object for a few seconds, and follows a moving person with his eyes when in supine. In the social domain, David smiles reflexively, establishes eye contact, and draws attention to self when in distress. In the self-help domain, David opens and closes his mouth in response to food stimulus. He does not yet have coordinated sucking, swallowing, and breathing. The OT observed the following when David's mother tried to feed him: When David began to fuss, his mother began to breastfeed him. He initially settled and began sucking, but after a few sucks, he began to squirm and then arch his back and cry. He became more irritable as his mother tried to reinitiate the breastfeeding. His mother describes his quickly escalating crying as "panic screaming." David does quiet, although he remains partially stiff, when held vertically over the mother's shoulder while being bounced and walked. David's mother reports that this is a typical feeding and that a feeding often takes 45 to 60 minutes. The mother and grandmother disagree about whether or not David calms to or enjoys minor roughhousing in the form of firm patting on the back or buttocks, knee bouncing in a supported sitting position, or linear (heel to head) rocking prone over knees. David's grandmother feels that David enjoys these kinds of play. The grandmother also feels David maintains a more organized state following these kinds of play. David's mother feels that he has a delayed reaction to these sessions, becoming even more irritable and less consolable an hour or so later.

ECO:

The following ratings were based on a scale developed by the Early Childhood Outcomes (ECO) Center:

1. Positive Social-Emotional Skills: Rating of 3 (emerging) on a 7-point scale
2. Acquiring and Using Knowledge and Skills: Rating of 6 (between somewhat and completely) on a 7-point scale
3. Taking Appropriate Action to Meet Needs: Rating of 3 (emerging) on a 7-point scale.

Figure 9-2. Excerpts from reports on David.

David's mother who would like to have more continuous sleep at night as well. By getting more sleep, the mother would have more personal resources to care for David as well as for her education. The second outcome focused on reducing the stress that was generated during mealtime so that David could eat successfully in less time. In addition, an outcome was written that focused on David's mother as she expressed interest in searching for a child-care setting where David could go several days a week while she finishes her GED and looks for a job.

These questions provide scaffolding for families to give us specific information about what the outcome will look like in THEIR lives.

The outcomes written for the IFSP include the following:

- Outcome #1: I would like David to remain quiet and calm during feeding and when we play.

  How will we know we are making progress? What will be observed? Where/with whom?

  When David is able to feed within a 30-minute time period without crying and when he is able to be awake and alert for short periods during the day without crying.

- Outcome #2: I would like for David to sleep through the night, waking up only one time for a feeding.

  How will we know we are making progress? What will be observed? Where/with whom?

  When David goes to sleep by 10:00 p.m., wakes up one time for a bottle and, doesn't wake up again until at least 6:00 a.m. for a week as reported by David's mom.

- Outcome #3: I would like to find child care for David so I can finish my GED and find a job.

  How will we know when we meet the outcome?

  When David is enrolled in a quality child-care program 2 days a week and Mom finishes her GED.

What we know from families who have been enrolled in early intervention programs is that the more individual services (OT, PT, SLP, ECSE, Social Work etc.) involved directly with the family, the greater the negative impact on family functioning (Dunst, Brookfield, & Epstein, 1998).

After the team wrote the outcomes, they discussed what services would support David to achieve those outcomes. Although both the occupational therapist and the speech and language pathologist have expertise in feeding, the team decided that the occupational therapist would be the primary implementer for David's family with the speech pathologist providing support to the OT and the family through joint visits and the entire team supporting the OT and SLP through regular team meetings.

The team also agreed that the county health nurse would continue to monitor David's equipment while the occupational therapist would focus on decreasing the impact of sensory sensitivity on David's ability to interact with family in a calm way. The OT also helped mom find a quieter and more supported (i.e., positioning in his chair) method for feeding David. Because David's mother needed help right away to make the changes that she wanted, she chose to have the occupational therapist come twice a week for the first 2 weeks. During this time, they developed strategies for David to be calm so he could successfully feed, sleep, and play. David's mother chose the times of the day that are most challenging for her and David for the OT to conduct the home visits.

Note: Developing services that support the family and child in meeting outcomes is often a "best educated guess" about what will be needed. Many Part C programs are now listing

Possible Script to Explain Evidence for David's Mom

"One of our colleagues has suggested that we look at children's responses to sensory experiences by considering how fast they respond to particular events. Her research has shown that when children respond quickly to sensory input, it makes some daily life experiences more challenging (see Dunn, 1997; Dunn & Brown, 1997). In David's case, he is responding very quickly to touch, movement, and sound; that is probably why he gets overloaded and irritable so quickly. Dr. Dunn suggests that we select strategies that are less likely to overload the child. For example, we know that certain kinds of movement and touch are calming (Kandel, Schwartz, & Jessel, 2000), and so I am suggesting activities that have these features in them for you to try with David."

Figure 9-3. Possible script for David's mother.

the services on the service page in a much more flexible manner to be more responsive to families and to provide supports during times the family needs them most. Therefore, instead of listing one-time-a-week services for 60 minutes, which has been the traditional way of providing services, programs are now writing 14 sessions of OT for the first 3 months. This allows the OT to provide more intense services at the beginning (2x weekly) and then allowing time for the family to implement and practice strategies that were developed in collaboration with the OT, SLP, and nurse. Subsequently, the family may not feel a need to see the OT every week when things are going smoothly, but the family then may need more support when new issues arise for David or for his family.

Intervention Implementation

David needed to develop a larger repertoire of self-regulatory strategies so that he could engage the environment more frequently in a goal-directed way. The therapist decided to design an intervention approach that incorporated the sensory qualities and physical properties of objects and tasks and the inherent characteristics of the environment (Dunn, 2009). One must remember that sensory experiences and reactions are difficult to conceptualize because therapists observe only reactions to stimuli, which are motoric in nature and demonstrate the intimate relationship between input and response (Dunn, 1990).

In David's case, the OT wanted to support David's sensory processing needs so he could establish and maintain an organized state for participation. Because David responds positively to Grandma's vertical bouncing, we consider that a strength related to keeping him in calm state. Therefore, we can think of other similar activities that could form the basis for the intervention strategies. A strengths approach dictates that we focus on activities that David can handle, while minimizing the impact of more challenging sensory processing areas. For example, David is fussier in noisy environments, so we will also work on creating quiet contexts for play, feeding, and interacting with family.

We also employ principles of best practice; using evidence in our practices also means we must give mom information from evidence about what supports our suggestions. Figure 9-3 shows a possible script we might use with David's mom.

In addition, focusing on David's and David's mother's interests (Raab, Swanson, Roper, & Dunst, 2006) as well as David's mother's responsiveness (Mahoney, 2009) to David will be key in designing successful strategies.

Researchers in therapy procedures have demonstrated that children like David have an easier time interacting with other people and accepting food items when we make sure that David's nervous system can stay calm and does not have to work to keep his body organized (Crott, Giesel, & Hoffman, 1998; Royeen & Lane, 1991; Vergara, 1993).

Outcome

I would like for David to remain quiet and calm during feedings and play.

When working in early intervention, the target person is the mother, father, or primary caregiver for the child; therefore, the OT will be working primarily with the mother and grandmother.

> You'll notice that this team is implementing Key Principle #3: The primary role of a service provider in early intervention is to work with and support family members and caregivers in children's lives.

The mother has already identified 3 activity settings that she has found to be challenging with David: eating, playing, and sleeping. The focus of intervention will be on these activity settings. On the first home visit, the OT will first observe David during a playtime with his mother and then during a feeding time. Rush and Shelden (2008) developed a Framework for Reflective Questioning that provides awareness, analysis, alternatives, and action questions. These questions help the practitioner discover what the family knows about their child's condition/issue and what the family has already tried to address the issue. In addition, other questions assist the family in reflecting upon what they have done, discovering alternatives, and making plans to address the issue(s). The occupational therapist uses these questions with David's mother so that they can develop strategies together to address David's sleeping and feeding challenges (Figure 9-4).

The touch pressure and proprioceptors send input from the muscles and joints into the brain through the dorsal columns. These neurons send very specific information to the brain for mapping the body and for creating body awareness (Dunn, 1998). These neurons do not activate the reticular formation with collateral fibers, so this type of input does not generate additional arousal (which would be bad for David).

The occupational therapist explains to David's mother that dispersed pressure across the body is more calming than distinct, isolated touch. They discuss the idea of using the quilt, which is heavier than a typical infant blanket, or the stuffed animal across David's body when he is being held and transitioning to laying down. This small amount of dispersed weight may provide the necessary calming so that David can be moved from a vertical to a supine position. Wrapping David tightly in a blanket or in stretchy, tight onesie pajamas may also have the same effect. They also discuss that, for safety reasons, the stuffed animal should not remain in the crib while David is sleeping (Figure 9-5).

Then, the occupational therapist and David's mother try some additional strategies that may calm David. The occupational therapist explains to David's mother how rhythmic input can be more calming to David so that when she holds him in his preferred vertical position, the bouncing that she provides should be very even and rhythmical. This should calm him faster so that he can engage with his surroundings without being held. The OT also explains to David's mom that when David is calm in this position, this might be an opportunity to give him a toy to hold. For David, having something in his hands gives him additional touch input and clears the way for him to play with toys as he grows.

During this discussion, David begins to fuss so Mom picks him up, and with coaching from the OT, she tries the different strategies that they have discussed.

At the end of the home visit, the OT reviews all of the ideas that they have either discussed or tried, and David's mother decides which of these she wants to try over the next several days before the OT comes back for a

The conversation goes like this:

OT: "What have you tried to get David to calm or quiet?" *(awareness)*
Mom: "Sometimes, when I hold him in this position at my shoulder and pat him on his bottom, he calms down. My mom showed me how this worked for her."
OT: "It sounds like you have at least one good strategy to calm him, which is great. Tell me about other times when he is calm." *(awareness)*
Mom: "He seems to be calmer when I put him in his infant seat and turn the TV on without the volume. He really seems to like the bright, moving pictures on the TV. But, when he is in his infant seat, I notice that he seems to like to have something on top of him, like one of his big stuffed animals or a quilt that my mother made him."
OT: "What do you think would happen if you used the blanket when he is trying to get to sleep?" *(analysis)*
Mom: "I don't know. He might fall asleep quicker. I had not really thought about it."

Figure 9-4. Coaching script with David's mother.

Continuing the coaching...

OT: "so you understand that there are several options that would calm David by having something on top of him; that is insightful of you." *(alternatives)*
Mom: "I have been worried about putting things in his crib; I don't want to get David hurt."
OT: "You are right to be careful. Because we know that blankets are safe, would you be willing to try using the quilt this week, so we can evaluate whether it helps David sleep?" *(action)*
Mom: "I will try it; I would like to talk on the phone in case it doesn't work."

Figure 9-5. Continued script with David's mother.

second visit. This is referred to as joint planning by Shelden and Rush (2008) and is a critical part of using a coaching framework with families.

Outcome

On the second home visit, the occupational therapist began the visit with re-visiting the joint plan from the first visit. David's mother had decided at the end of the first home visit that she would first like to try using the quilt for transitioning David to horizontal positions and for sleeping. Therefore, the OT started the visit by saying, "Tell me how using the quilt while transitioning David has worked the past few days." David's mother then explained to the OT the times it worked and the times it did not work. They further discussed and tried additional strategies for calming David.

The occupational therapist provided home visits twice weekly for the first 3 weeks and, on average, weekly until David was about 1 year old. The speech and language pathologist conducted two joint visits with the OT in the first few weeks to address David's feeding issues. The team then closely monitored David's and his family's progress in meeting the outcomes. Three months after services were begun, the entire early intervention team again reviewed the outcomes, and frequency and duration of services were modified accordingly. At 6 months, the team formally reviewed David's progress and again modified the outcomes.

The occupational therapist identified various strategies to support David's mother over this time. She stated that she had a difficult time remembering exactly how to position her hands on David in order to calm him. Using the camera on David's mother's cell phone, the therapist took pictures of David's mother holding him during home visits so that his mother could refer back to these pictures during the times between the home visits. This strategy was also used for feeding positions.

Over time, David began to stay calm for longer periods of time while awake, and the amount of time for feedings decreased to 30 minutes. He also began to sleep for longer periods of time at night in his own crib, which allowed his mother to get more sleep also. During this time, the OT helped David's mother find resources to complete her GED and part-time child care for David.

References

Crott, H. W., Giesel, M., & Hoffman, C. (1998). The process of inductive inference in groups: The use of positive and negative hypothesis and target testing in sequential rule-discovery tasks. *Journal of Personality and Social Psychology, 79*, 938-952.

Dunn, W. (1997). The impact of sensory processing abilities on the daily lives of young children and their families: A conceptual model. *Infants and Young Children, 9*(4), 23-35.

Dunn, W. (1990). A comparison of service provision models in school-based occupational therapy services: A pilot study. *Occupational Therapy Journal of Research, 10*(5), 300-320.

Dunn, W. (2009). Ecology of human performance model. In S. Dunbar (Ed.), *OT models for intervention with children and families*. Thorofare, NJ: SLACK Incorporated.

Dunn, W., & Brown, C. (1997). Factor analysis on the sensory profile from a national sample of children without disabilities. *American Journal of Occupational Therapy, 51*(7), 490-495.

Dunn, W., & Daniels, D. (2001). Initial development of the Infant Toddler Sensory Profile. *Journal of Early Intervention, 25*(1), 27-41.

Dunst, C. J., Brookfield, J., & Epstein, J. (1998). Family-centered early intervention and child, parent and family benefits: Final report. Asheville, NC: Orlena Hawks Puckett Institute.

Kandel, E. R., Schwartz, J. H., & Jessel, T. M., (2000). *Principles of neural science* (4th ed.). New York, NY: McGraw-Hill.

Mahoney, G. (2009). Relationship focused intervention (RFI): Enhancing the role of parents in children's developmental intervention. *International Journal of Early Childhood Special Education, 1*(1), 79-94.

Morris, S. E., & Klein, M. D. (2000). *Pre-feeding skills, A comprehensive resource for mealtime development* (2nd ed.). San Antonio, TX: Therapy Skills Builders.

Parks, S. (1992). *Hawaii Early Learning Profile*. Palo Alto, CA: VORT Corporation.

Raab, M., Swanson, J., Roper, N., & Dunst, C. J. (2006). Promoting parent and practitioner identification of interest-based everyday child learning opportunities. *CASEtools, 2*(6), 1-19.

Royeen, C. B., & Lane, S. J. (1991). Tactile processing and sensory defensiveness. In A. G. Fisher, E. A. Murray, & A. C. Bundy (Eds.), *Sensory integration theory and practice* (pp. 108-133). Philadelphia, PA: F. A. Davis Company.

Rush, D., & Shelden, M. (2008). Script for explaining an evidence based early intervention model. *Family, Infant and Preschool Program, 1*(3), 1-5.

Swanson, J., Raab, M., Roper, N., & Dunst, C. J. (2006). Promoting young children's participation in interest-based everyday learning activities. *CASEtools, 2*(5), 1-22. www.fippcase.org/casetools/casetools _vol2_no5.pdf.

Turbiville, V. P., Umbarger, G. T., Guthrie, A. C. (2000). Fathers' involvement in programs for young children. *Young Children, 55*(4), 74-79.

Vergara, E. (1993). *Foundations for practice in the neonatal intensive care unit and early intervention*. Rockville, MD: AOTA.

Wilson, L. L., & Mott, D. W. (2006). Asset-based context matrix: An assessment tool for developing contextually based child outcomes. *CASEtools, 2*(4), 1-12. www.fippcase.org/casetools/casetools _vol2_no4.pdf.

Ted

Winnie Dunn, PhD, OTR, FAOTA and Jane A. Cox, MS, OTR/L

Evaluation

Occupational Profile

Ted is a 32-month-old boy, who has been receiving occupational and physical therapy services through his local infant toddler network. Because he is approaching 36 months, he is being referred to the early childhood program at his local school district.

Part C of IDEA 2004 serves children 0 to 3 years. 90 days prior to turning 3, children receiving infant toddler services are referred to Part B of IDEA which is typically the local school district.

Part B of IDEA 2004 serves children 3 to 21 years.

History

Ted has a medical diagnosis of cerebral palsy. He was referred to the local infant toddler network by his pediatrician when he was 12 months of age. At Ted's 1-year well check, his mother talked with the pediatrician about concerns she had regarding Ted's lack of movement and poor head control. She talked about diaper changes being difficult because Ted's legs were tight, and she was having a hard time getting Ted to eat from a spoon. There were no other medical concerns present.

Cerebral Palsy (CP) is a medical diagnosis which is defined as having an alteration in muscle tone and movement. It is caused by damage to the brain either before, during or shortly after birth. CP is non-progressive. There are several different types of CP such as spastic, athetoid, ataxic and mixed.

The early childhood program at Ted's school district has scheduled an initial home visit to get acquainted with Ted and his family. As a part of the transition process, Ted will be evaluated by the early childhood team. Ted's family is concerned about his inability to play and interact with other children due to his lack of mobility. At home, Ted can sit on the floor with support and enjoys reaching for toys that have been placed within his reach. Ted is most successful when he is lying on his side because he can reach and grab toys more easily here. Ted's family currently uses a stroller to transport him in the community but they are worried that he will soon grow out of the stroller. Ted's mother expressed concern that none of the other 3-year-old boys in the neighborhood ride in strollers. Someone had mentioned to her the possibility of getting Ted an electric wheelchair, and she would like some more information about wheelchairs.

Sometimes Early Childhood teams want to get to know the child and family before they receive all the EI reports so they can get their own impressions. Other times, the EC team would go with the EI team on a regular visit to indicate their joint planning as Ted transitioned into school.

After talking with Ted's family, the Part B early childhood team decided to complete a Transdisciplinary Play-Based Assessment (TPBA-2) (Linder et al., 2008). The TPBA-2 is an adult-directed play-based assessment that provides structure for observing a child in a preschool classroom environment. Children are observed in four areas: sensorimotor, emotional and social, communication and language, and cognition—the observation team gathers qualitative information about what the child can do. Because being around other children is important to Ted's family, the team decides to conduct the assessment in one of the district's early childhood classrooms. Because the primary concerns for Ted are related to functional movement, the team decided that the occupational therapist would facilitate the assessment in the classroom.

Linder, T., Anthony, T.L., Bundy, A.C., Charlifue-Smith, R., Christian, J., Forrest Hancock, H., & Rooke, C. C. (2008). Trans-disciplinary play-based Assessment (TPBA2) (2nd ed.). *Baltimore. MD: Paul H. Brookes.*

Occupational Analysis

The team (i.e., the occupational therapist, physical therapist, speech pathologist, early childhood teacher) completed the TPBA-2 in the

The peer model is a child close in age to the child being assessed (Ted) and is present in order to see how Ted interacts with another child his age.

classroom with parents present as well as the parent facilitator and a peer model. Parents also offered additional information during a discussion period.

Ted was encouraged to explore and play within the classroom environment. Ted does best when he is sitting in a supported position either in an adapted seating device or with another person providing support behind him. Ted enjoys going after toys and is sometimes able to pick one up with his hands. Ted is trying to bring toys to his mouth but isn't quite able to get them up to his mouth. Ted has muscle spasticity in his arms and legs and tends to flex (bend) his arms and extend (straighten) his legs; his right side is more involved than his left side. Ted is very comfortable laying on the floor and has better use of his arms and hands when laying on his side. In fact, he was able to bring his mouth to a toy while lying on his side. Ted moves about the room by rolling. With help from another person, Ted can sit up, and then he needs support to maintain sitting. Ted has several primary reflexes (moro, flexor withdrawal, tonic labyrinth, asymmetrical, and symmetrical tonic neck reflexes) that are still present and interfere with his ability to move.

When placed in a well-supported sitting position, Ted is very expressive and bright-eyed. The team observed and his mother reported that Ted enjoys a variety of sensory experiences such as music, rhythmic movement, and colorful scenery. During snack time, Ted ate when being fed by another person. While he is not able to feed himself, he eats from a spoon and drinks from a cup. His mom reported that they had been working on helping Ted to hold a cup himself to drink.

Ted's mom provides all of his care at this point, although Ted indicates when he is soiled and needs changing. Ted is a very happy child who enjoys the activity of the classroom setting. He was very engaging and motivated to get a toy of interest or the attention of another person.

Throughout the play-based assessment, open dialogue and communication are occurring with Ted's parents. It is important to ask the right questions and actively listen to the answers. Many times parents have figured out ways of doing things that are beneficial and should be carried on in the classroom setting. In this situation the family is considered equal members of the team.

Because Ted's primary means for moving is to roll, he has not had many experiences that require him to stand. His mom would like him to be able to stand so that he can interact eye-to-eye with his peers. It is also important for the development of the joints in his hip, legs, and feet that he stand even if it is with the support of another person (for short periods of time) or a standing frame (for longer periods of time).

The week following the evaluation, the team met again to develop an IEP for Ted. At the IEP meeting, which included his primary early intervention provider, the team decided that Ted would need supportive seating and standing as a first step to facilitating play and socialization and to continue gaining use of his hands for play and drinking from a cup. Ted's parents also wanted him to be around other children and the team agreed. Ted would attend early childhood classroom 3 mornings a week.

What would some intermediate goals be for Ted? What adaptations might we employ to create opportunities for him to practice?

For example, we might use a cup with built-up handles on both sides so Ted could grab the cup more easily.

The team decided upon the following annual goals:

- Target Outcome 1—In 36 weeks, Ted will independently drink from a cup with a lid during snack time.
- Target Outcome 2—In 36 weeks, Ted will actively participate in a table-top classroom art project alongside his peers.

Ted will receive occupational therapy, physical therapy, and speech therapy once a week. All services will be provided in the context of Ted's preschool classroom. All therapists will also be in contact with the family to provide support for family concerns as they arise as well.

Intervention

The first step to addressing Ted's goals is for Ted to have a well-supported seating system. When children such as Ted have good support in sitting, they can use their arms and hands for playing and eating. The occupational therapist recommended that Ted go to a seating clinic at a local teaching hospital to be evaluated for a possible wheelchair. While waiting to get a wheelchair, the occupational therapist found a Rifton chair (Rifton Equipment, Rifton, NY) that the school district owned so Ted could begin immediately to have a supporting sitting plan for use in the classroom. The physical therapist brought a standing frame to Ted's classroom. She recommended that Ted stand in it for 20 minutes a day to facilitate weight bearing through his legs, which is necessary for healthy joint development of the hips, knees, and feet. Ted's teacher decided that music group was a good time for Ted to be standing because she had the other children stand during music as well.

A Rifton chair is a chair which is adjustable and has a variety of attachments to provide the specific support that Ted requires. Rifton is one brand, there are others as well.

A standing frame is a device that positions a child into a supported standing position. There are straps on the frame so the children are safe when using the frame.

The next thing that the occupational therapist recommended was the use of switch toys. Switch toys would give Ted an opportunity to practice controlling his arm and hand movements while activating a switch that, in turn, activates the toy to move, play music, etc. The OT sent a switch home for Ted to use, and his mom experimented with different toys and household items like a fan and the TV.

The classroom teacher and the OT met regularly to collaborate and discuss what was going well for Ted and what needed to be tweaked.

As Ted became accustomed to sitting in an upright supported position, he began to have better control of his arms. With help from his classroom teacher, Ted began to use toys and utensils that had built-up handles, making them easier to grip.

Outcome

Ted got an electric wheelchair about 6 months after he started preschool. Everyone worked with him to learn how to drive his new wheelchair. With proper support of his new wheelchair, Ted was beginning to drink from a cup that had two handles. Ted adjusted well to the classroom setting and really seemed to enjoy being around the other children. His classmates did a great job of bringing materials to him or helping him at snack time. As Ted gained more skills, the speech therapist approached Ted's family about exploring augmentative communication.

Augmented communication refers to any device that makes it easier [or possible] for a person to communicate with others. Simple devices are picture boards that children can point to indicate their needs. More complex devices are programmed with a computer to speak or create words or phrases. Some have individually sized keyboards to take advantage of the person's range of motion or are slanted to make the components easier to see.

The occupational therapist communicated with Ted's mom periodically. Mom asked if there was anything that would help with sitting at the dinner table because he was getting too big for the high chair and his wheelchair was too short for the dinner table. The OT provided some literature regarding adaptive seating for the home and coached the parents about what critical features would be most helpful for Ted, including flexibility for when Ted grows.

Reference

Linder, T., Anthony, T. L., Bundy, A. C., Charlifue-Smith, R., Christian, J., Forrest Hancock, H., & Rooke, C. C. (2008). *Trans-disciplinary play-based assessment* (TPBA2) (2nd ed.). Baltimore, MD: Paul H. Brookes.

James

Winnie Dunn, PhD, OTR, FAOTA and Jane A. Cox, MS, OTR/L

Evaluation

Occupational Profile

James and his parents were referred to a local early education agency program that serves children 3 to 5 years of age. James' parents are concerned about his development, specifically play, eating, and talking. James' parents report that James is difficult to understand when talking and does not play the way that other children his age play. James eats slowly, sometimes chokes or gags on his food, and is a messy eater (i.e., he cannot keep food in his mouth while trying to chew and swallow). James' mother found out about preschool screenings from the public service announcements on the radio and scheduled one for James. James' parents want him to be able to eat without choking or gagging and to be able to talk and play with other children his age.

History

James' mother had a normal pregnancy with a long but not significant labor. James was a large baby (over 10 pounds) and post-term by 1 to 2 weeks. James' early developmental milestones were delayed. He sat at 1 year, pulled to stand at 16 months, and walked at 22 months. James' mother noted frequent choking and gagging problems when she fed him solid foods. The parents managed these concerns by thinning foods, making smaller bites, and taking extra time during feeding. The parents described James as a rather clumsy child who is motivated to try anything and persists until he can accomplish the tasks.

The therapist interviewed James' mother to obtain basic information and found that James doesn't play the way other children his age play. They say he has difficulty moving around his environment and interacting with toys. His parents describe him as a clumsy child. James' mother also reports that it is difficult to understand James when he is talking. James' parents have figured out ways to support him during particularly challenging activities. For example, they discovered that James eats better when they cut his food into small bite-sized pieces and when they give him thicker liquids to drink. The therapist decides to recommend further assessment to determine the underlying causes contributing to challenges with play and eating and to make sure the speech pathologist gets involved to address talking concerns.

It is important to listen to the family's story because we learn what adaptive methods they have figured out on their own. This provides an opportunity to acknowledge the family's insights and explain why their ideas are great ones for James.

Analysis of Occupational Performance

The early childhood case manager sat down with James' parents and discussed the process of comprehensive evaluation. Because James is having trouble with eating, talking, and playing, the director talked to his parents about including occupational therapy, speech therapy, and early childhood special education in the assessment.

REMEMBER

The assessment plan is a **family-centered assessment** that focuses on the immediate concerns of the family, which for James' parents are playing, eating, and talking. As a result, the assessment plan does not include all possible areas of assessment (e.g., James' parents do not indicate concerns with personal hygiene skills; therefore they will not be addressed at this time).

The team met to plan the assessment and decided that the early childhood teacher would facilitate a play-based assessment (Linder et al., 2008). The occupational therapist would serve as the parent facilitator, and the speech-language pathologist would videotape the assessment. This allowed the team members to obtain information about James at the same time without duplicating assessment items. It is also considered a holistic approach that allows team members to observe the child in the natural environment. In addition to the play-based assessment, the team will conduct an Interest-Based Everyday Activity Checklist (Swanson, Raab, Roper, & Dunst, 2006). The occupational therapist and the speech-language pathologist will observe James while he is eating. The occupational therapist will ask the family to complete a Sensory Profile to determine whether sensory processing patterns are supporting or interfering with any of these daily activities.

The occupational therapist and speech-language pathologist on James' team often collaborate to assess and provide intervention when children have oral motor issues that interfere with eating and talking. The therapists in this situation were primarily concerned with the variability and functional use of James' suck, swallow, and breathe synchrony. Frequently, children who have low normal muscle tone demonstrate difficulty coordinating the use of various body components, such as are required to make a seal, suck, swallow, and then breathe between events. Poor oral motor synchrony can compromise development of orchestrated movements for eating and talking, but can also be a sign of more general difficulties with movement organization and planning. The therapists will also need to be attentive to these possibilities during the play-based assessment.

Linder, T., Anthony, T.L., Bundy, A.C., Charlifue-Smith, R., Christian, J., Forrest Hancock, H., & Rooke, C. C. (2008). Trans-disciplinary play-based assessment *(TPBA2) (2nd ed.). Baltimore, MD: Paul H. Brookes.*

Swanson, J., Raab, M., Roper, N., & Dunst, C. J. (2006). Promoting young children's participation in interest-based everyday learning activities. CASEtools, 2(5), *1-22. Available at www.fippcase.org/casetools/casetools_vol2_no5.pdf*

This assessment identifies everyday interests, and so provides us with possible activities and settings within which we can build interventions that are relevant to children and families.

Remember, even though we consider these performance skills as we try to understand the child's situation, we remain focused on the child's participation. In James' case, this is eating and talking.

Findings and Interpretations

The team combined data from all of their assessment methods to gain insight about James. One area that the occupational therapist wants to examine carefully is James' movements during play. James does not run and play like other children his age, making safety a possible concern. It is common for parents to seek help during this age period because their child has become more mobile and frequently falls more than other children of the same age. Children like James can have many more scrapes, cuts, bruises, and sometimes broken bones, because of their inability to plan and organize their movements within and around the environment. Because the occupational therapist heard some of these themes during history taking, she wants to observe carefully during the play-based assessment.

Figure 9-6 is an excerpt from their summary report about their specific assessment methods.

You will notice here that the therapist is framing her report in positive terms. By telling precisely what James CAN do, we also make it clear what is challenging for him, e.g., variable surfaces.

As you will see later, James has typical sensory processing, so we will need to come up with alternative hypotheses for these behaviors.

The therapist is creating an alternative hypothesis here.

Dunn, W. (1999). Sensory Profile. *San Antonio, TX: Therapy Skill Builders, The Psychological Corporation.*

It was a reasonable hypothesis to consider that sensory processing might be interfering with eating and/or talking because of the important role that sensation plays in and around the mouth. However, in James' case, it turns out that sensory processing is not a contributing factor. The therapists need to look elsewhere and not use sensory processing strategies for interventions because of these findings.

Report Excerpt: Findings From Specific Assessments

Transdisciplinary Play-Based Assessment (TPBA-2, Linder et al., 2008)

James enjoys moving around and exploring his environment. When the ground is clear and level, James moves slowly around his environment with a wide base of support (i.e., feet wide apart) and a high guard (i.e., hands above shoulders). When James has to navigate around furniture or toys on the floor, he is unsteady and often trips and/or falls. This is indicative of poor motor planning and balance.

While playing with toys either on the floor or sitting at a table, James enjoys playing with building blocks and puzzle pieces. James uses a fisted whole-hand grasp (rather than using his thumb and fingers) to pick up and manipulate the blocks and puzzle pieces. When building with blocks or attempting to put a puzzle together, James is not always sure of the best way to orient the puzzle pieces to get them to fit in the puzzle. He is beginning to use a crayon or marker and was able to imitate a horizontal and vertical line.

James wears glasses to correct for farsighted vision. He also occasionally wears a patch over one eye to correct for strabismus (cross-eyedness). These factors could be contributing to challenges James is experiencing with play.

James may not be getting accurate sensory feedback from his hands or eyes that would allow him to know where his body is in space in relation to his ability to interact with his environment to participate in play and other daily life activities. The occupational therapist also noted that James is unstable when moving around; his muscles may be weak, which seems to interfere with his ability move and play efficiently.

Eating

We offered James a snack consisting of crackers, cheese, applesauce, and juice in a cup. James drank juice from the cup, spilling some of it down the front of him. He enjoyed the crackers and cheese, chewing the food in an awkward manner. Some of the cracker came out of his mouth while eating, and some of it was pocketed in his cheeks after snack time was over. When eating applesauce from a spoon, James partially closed his lips around the spoon in order to get the food off of the spoon.

The occupational therapist and the speech-language pathologist determined that while eating, the food stayed in the middle of James' mouth, reducing opportunities for chewing. James holds his tongue still and uses an up-and-down chewing motion (rather than a rotary chewing action needed for efficient means for breaking up food and moving it around the mouth). James choked on the cracker twice during the session when trying to swallow.

While eating, James' breathing was irregular and lacked coordination needed for safe and efficient swallowing. When talking, James has a breathy quality to his words as well.

James' challenges with coordinating his movements for chewing and swallowing food efficiently and safely and his awkward breathing patterns suggest motor planning difficulties (i.e., the inability to plan and execute new and unfamiliar motor movements).

Sensory Profile (Dunn, 1999)

James has typical sensory processing as compared to other children his age. His mother reports some sensitivity to textures in food and clothing but it does not interfere with his daily life participation.

Interest-Based Everyday Activity Checklist (Swanson, Raab, Roper, & Dunst, 2006)

James' parents completed the Late Preschool Interest-Based Everyday Activity Checklist. The checklist indicates that, as a family, they enjoy going out into the community to parks and playgrounds. James enjoys imaginary play with cars and trucks. He likes to build with bristle blocks, play with puzzles, ride on toys/wagons, play in dirt or mud, and watch sports on TV with his dad. Family activities in which James' family participate is going to church most Sunday mornings and visiting extended family for birthday celebrations.

Figure 9-6. Excerpts from James' reports.

Intervention

Following the assessment, the team met with the family to discuss findings and establish the IEP. The team was careful to talk in a strengths-based manner and to avoid the use of jargon as it is not useful in establishing a working relationship with the family. Sometimes, team members forget, so other team members must be vigilant with each other on the family's behalf. For example, during James' IEP meeting, the speech-language pathologist reports her assessment information and uses the term "dyspraxia" without explanation. So, the early childhood education teacher asks the speech-language pathologist to explain dyspraxia to her and the rest of the team. This releases the family from either staying confused or having to ask. Many families do not feel comfortable asking the "professionals" to explain what they are saying. The teacher's strategy enables the parents to understand the information being shared with them without them having to ask themselves. Team members discussed their findings by describing James' participation in areas of concern identified by the parents in the assessment plan (i.e., eating, talking, and playing).

Jargon can be confusing and intimidating and creates a barrier to families, particularly if they are entering the system for the first time.

In James' case, the team verified that he was in need of and eligible for early childhood special education services. Additionally, the occupational therapist would play a key role on James' interdisciplinary service provision team, with several areas targeted for intervention:

Remember: The team includes professionals AND family members.

- Improved participation in play activities
  - With similar age peers
  - To manipulate age-appropriate toys
- Successful eating strategies
- Effective interactions (talking) with peers

In practice, the team would prioritize the identified needs for participation. For now, we will illustrate some examples using the IEP language; you can create intervention plans for James on other areas if you like. We are going to focus on play for the examples.

James will play with peers.

Goal 1

To increase opportunities for play with peers, James will arrive at a new learning center at the same time as peers three of four times within 36 weeks.

Although we might understand that arriving at the learning center provides James with more opportunities to play with his peers, others that read the plan might not make this connection. By stating explicitly the relationship between the activities, settings and our team's goals, everyone understands why we have selected this particular strategy.

Some states would require more precision than this. For example, they might require a specific time (e.g., 30 seconds). In this example, we would expect the other children to get more efficient across the school year, and would expect this of James as well, so we are providing a flexible measurement to reflect all the children's growth. We want James to be in sync with his peers as they learn, so having one time target might not be appropriate for the entire year.

This is a term used in IDEA to remind us to write short term steps to reaching the long term goal.

Benchmarks

- To increase opportunities for play with peers, James will arrive at a new learning center within 1 minute of peers 2 of 4 times by 9 weeks.
- To increase opportunities for play with peers, James will arrive at a new learning center within 1 minute of peers 3 of 4 times by 18 weeks.
- To increase opportunities for play with peers, James will arrive at a new learning center within 30 seconds of peers 3 of 4 times by 27 weeks.
- To increase opportunities for play with peers, James will arrive at a new learning center at the same time as peers 3 of 4 times within 36 weeks.

Using movement with heavy work in activities that require planning a sequence of steps will promote better performance and more interest and motivation for the activity. As James receives the input during active movement, his brain will be able to establish more mature body maps for use in planning motor behaviors.

These activities are useful for all children James' age and also provide opportunities for social interaction.

Each of these options allows increased feedback from small postural movements that occur while James is sitting. However, by practicing these postural shifts during table-top activities, James must incorporate postural control into his performance schema. If the therapist only practiced postural control in an isolated therapy setting (e.g., on a therapy ball), she would not be taking responsibility for making sure that this background skill would be available to support participation in everyday life.

Watch for changes in this; as there is a growing trend to look at strengths, there is also a trend to change access to supports. It may become obsolete that children must have a diagnosis to "qualify' for supports in the community. For example, there has been a "regular education initiative' to integrate all children into classrooms in their neighborhoods. Stay ahead of the trends to continue being a Best Practice therapist!

Intervention Implementation

The OT collaborated with the classroom teacher and the family to determine when naturally occurring opportunities for play occur. The preschool teacher provided a schedule of a typical day in her classroom; Table 9-2 shows some ideas they generated when looking at the schedule.

Because James enjoys intense movement experiences, the OT was able to work with the classroom teacher to create play that involves movement with heavy work within the context of her classroom and activities that were already in place. For example, one of the classroom centers contains games that include bean bags, weighted balls, a child-sized indoor basketball hoop, hula hoops, and mats.

The OT also provided a therapy ball and an inflated seat cushion for use during circle time and table-top centers. Because these items are popular with most children, the OT provided two balls and three seat cushions to be available for other children as well as James.

Recommendation/Referral to Other Professionals

Because this is the first time James has been evaluated, a referral to a neurologist may be appropriate given the motor planning, persistent primitive reflexes, and developmental delays that interfere with James' ability to play, eat, and talk. It may be helpful for James to be seen by a pediatric neurologist to either confirm or rule out other CNS disorders, because James' movement organization problem is so pervasive.

It is possible that James has mild cerebral palsy. A pediatric neurology consultation could help to confirm or deny this possibility for the parents. This diagnosis will not significantly alter the program planning strategies for the team, because their observations of his performance will form the basis for intervention. A specific diagnosis is sometimes very important to families; sometimes, a specific diagnosis makes programs or community resources available to a family. For example, if James has a mild form of cerebral palsy, his family will have access to the resources of United Cerebral Palsy or the state program for children with special health-care needs. A differential diagnosis is also useful in those cases where a family trend may be present or when the disorder may have new or different manifestations as the child grows. In some cases, the occupational therapist may accompany the family and child to the appointment with a specialist when seeking a diagnosis or guidance on intervention. The occupational therapist can be a filter or interpreter of the physician information. Many families are quite intimidated

Table 9-2.

Sample Preschool Schedule With Ideas for Supporting James Within the Curriculum

Classroom Schedule	Examples of Therapeutic Opportunities for Play
8:10-8:25 Child-directed play while others are arriving	Suggest activities for James that encourage his movement practice, such as moving toy boxes around the room
8:25-8:45 Circle time with the good morning song and calendar time	Encourage James to sit on the cushion
8:45-9:15 Centers	Always assign James to the center with movement with heavy work play items
9:15-9:35 Outdocr recess	Encourage James to pull other children in the wagons, climb on the jungle gym
9:35-9:50 Bathroom: toileting and washing hands	Assign James to hold the classroom and bathroom doors for other students so he gets the "heavy work" of holding the doors
9:50-10:05 Snack time	
10:05-10:35 Specials (music, art, or PE)	(Explore these curricula with these teachers to identify ways to support James)
10:35-10:55 Child-directed play within classroom	
10:55-11:10 Story time and goodbye song	Collaborate with teacher to identify movement songs and stories that can be acted out
11:10-11:20 Line up, get coats, backpacks, etc., go home	Assign James to get coats and backpacks for other children who are slower to get ready

by these experiences with the medical community, and it is often helpful for the therapist to ask questions the family might be too overwhelmed or intimidated to ask and then respond to the family's questions after the appointment.

Outcome

Because James was interested in exploring, the therapeutic enhancements of the preschool program were very helpful for him. When it was time for James to transition into public school, the family had involved James in tumbling and swimming activities outside of school. With consultation from the occupational therapist, the first grade teacher, physical education teacher, and music teacher were able to provide a successful environment for James. The occupational therapist routinely met with each subsequent set of teachers to support James' transition each year.

References

Dunn, W. (1999). *Sensory profile.* San Antonio, TX: Therapy Skill Builders, The Psychological Corporation.

Linder, T., Anthony, T. L., Bundy, A. C., Charlifue-Smith, R., Christian, J., Forrest Hancock, H., & Rooke, C. C. (2008). *Trans-disciplinary play-based assessment* (TPBA2) (2nd ed.). Baltimore, MD: Paul H. Brookes.

Swanson, J., Raab, M., Roper, N., & Dunst, C. J. (2006). Promoting young children's participation in interest-based everyday learning activities. *CASEtools,* 2(5), 1-22. Available at www.fippcase.org/casetools/casetools_vol2_no5.pdf.

Peter

Winnie Dunn, PhD, OTR, FAOTA and Becky Nicholson, MEd, OTR

Evaluation

Occupational Profile

Peter is a 6-year-old boy attending regular kindergarten. His teacher has concerns regarding his ability to participate in and benefit from learning activities similar to other children in her class. She refers Peter to the building team, and the team initiates a process called RtI (Response to Intervention). Specific concerns include difficulty completing school work, following directions, and recess (Figure 9-7).

RtI... "integrates assessment and intervention within a multi-level prevention system to maximize student achievement and to reduce behavior problems. With RtI, schools identify students at risk for poor learning outcomes, monitor student progress, provide evidence-based interventions and adjust the intensity and nature of those interventions depending on a student's responsiveness, and identify students with learning disabilities or other disabilities."

(Retrieved on March 4, 2010 from www.rti4success.org/.)

If you need to review RtI, review that section in Chapter 7.

Following the first team meeting, the school psychologist observed Peter in the classroom and collaborated with the classroom teacher to make some modifications in an attempt to improve Peter's ability to follow directions. The psychologist recommended modifying instructions during transitions and allowing Peter more time. During RtI, Peter did not make adequate improvements, so the team recommended a comprehensive evaluation to understand Peter's educational needs in more depth.

History

Peter is the older of two boys. The pregnancy, labor, and delivery were unremarkable. His mother described Peter as an alert and active baby with a mind of his own. Mom had no concerns about his development, because he achieved major milestones within expected ages. Peter had attended a church-sponsored preschool 2 mornings each week since the age of 4. The preschool teacher mentioned and the mother noticed when she was a parent helper in the preschool that Peter had difficulty following directions, staying on task, and participating in fine and gross motor activities. Both the teacher and the mother felt that by the time Peter reached the more structured kindergarten program, he would be more mature and would respond to this increased structure.

Peter does best in familiar environments with familiar routines. He also does well with child-directed activities (i.e., activities that he has self-selected). For example, Peter's favorite activities include playing with familiar toys at home, such as cars and trucks. Peter enjoys curling up in front of the TV with his favorite blanket wrapped tightly around his body. Challenging

Referral Process

Peter's teacher spoke with the parents at parent-teacher conferences regarding her concerns. The parents were also concerned about Peter's readiness for learning, particularly when he goes on to first grade. Because of Peter's struggles in kindergarten, his teacher brought up his difficulties at the collaborative team meetings held each month. These collaborative team meetings are an opportunity for regular education teachers, special education teachers, related service personnel, and administrators to discuss individual children who may be having difficulties. In this particular school, the principal hires a substitute teacher who assumes duties for each of the regular education teachers for about 45 minutes at a time. This enables the regular education teacher to discuss her concerns about the children in her classroom with a team of professionals.

Figure 9-7. Referral process for Peter.

times of the day for Peter are when there are many people in close proximity, or there are unexpected changes in his schedule.

Both the parents and the classroom teacher observed that Peter often chooses to hang back before and during transitions to new activities and that these were particularly difficult times for him. Peter sometimes cries for no apparent reason. For example, he has cried while riding the bus to and from school, while playing on the playground, and sometimes while in the community with his family at places like the mall or at a restaurant. He occasionally has mild temper outbursts during transitions, free play on the playground, and once on the bus. Parents noted these behaviors are more significant at home when there is a sudden change in plans of the normal routine.

Information from both parents, as well as the classroom teacher, helped define the kind of sensory input and situations that lead to poor coping, over-arousal, and "fight or flight" behaviors. It appeared that unexpected light touch, moderate to intense background noise, unpredictable movement of children in his vicinity, as well as unfamiliar situations were most likely to negatively affect his ability to maintain attention to tasks and remain in control of his own behavior. The team asked the occupational therapist to follow up on these observations.

As the conversation progressed, it became apparent that his family has understood his sensitivity to certain situations and has approached his behavior in different ways. Peter's mother has taken responsibility for protecting Peter from situations that he perceives as threatening, whereas Peter's father has believed that Peter needs to "act right" in all situations and that Peter's mother is "too soft" on Peter. The classroom teacher has been reluctant to implement strategies, such as allowing Peter more time to make transitions or allowing him to redefine or not participate in some directed activities, as she feels this would show favoritism and/or would be unequal treatment that the other children would see as unfair.

Occupational Analysis

Information from the occupational profile led to some early hypotheses about Peter's situation. The occupational therapist decided to follow-up on early developing hypotheses by first observing Peter in the classroom during transition times, during a table-top art activity, and on the playground.

This is an interesting case, because we see the adults responding differently to Peter. From a coping frame of reference, we would have to consider the coping strategies of each important person in Peter's life before we would know how to proceed with planning. For example, teachers sometimes feel that making accommodations for an individual student would be seen as unfair by the other students. This is especially true for students who do not have an obvious physical disability but may be perceived as just "misbehaving" or being "non-compliant." The occupational therapist can play an important role in explaining the nature of sensory processing difficulties and how they affect a student's behavior and learning. The therapist could also provide an in-class lesson for the other students regarding how different people respond differently to sensory input. Once the therapist shares this information and teachers and students understand, they become more able to recognize Peter's behaviors as coping responses related to his processing ability; then they can have alternative ways to support him to be more adaptive.

Both the classroom teacher and the parents provided information that suggested possible sensory sensitivities and motor planning problems. It is common for early motor milestones, such as walking, to occur within the normal age expectations. Children with motor planning problems can sometimes use motor skills in free-play situations. But as the child has to problem-solve using his movement abilities, his performance breaks down.

Many times children such as Peter are bright enough to manipulate situations to minimize their use of motor planning and to cope with their situation the best they can. Peter recognizes what needs to happen, and so uses his cognitive abilities to tell others what to do. This leads family members and other care providers to believe that the child can do things that he may not be able to do. However, the child is unable to use those same skills when they are required in directed learning or play situations that require organization and planning on the spot.

It is not uncommon that a classroom teacher and a parent would each rate a child differently on the Sensory Profile and the Sensory Profile School Companion. This is to be expected because the assessments are an evaluation of the child in context. The context for home and school are often understandably different. In Peter's case, the findings from both of these assessments provide a common point of discussion for the parent and teacher. They were able to discuss situations and experiences that both support and disrupt Peter's ability to participate in his home and school environment.

The certified occupational therapy assistant (COTA) would assist in this assessment by doing the observation on the playground. The OTR would also consult with Peter's teacher regarding observations. The occupational therapist decided after completing her observations that she would ask the teacher to complete the School Function Assessment (SFA). The SFA will provide information regarding Peter's performance in physical and cognitive tasks throughout his school day.

The occupational therapist also asks Peter's parents to complete a Sensory Profile and Peter's teacher to complete the School Companion to the Sensory Profile. Together, these assessment tools will provide the team with information regarding how Peter interprets sensory information from his environment both at home and at school.

The COTA assists the OTR in assessing a student after the COTA has demonstrated competency on whatever portion of the assessment she will be doing. The OTR and COTA must partner in the development of the COTA's competency in completing portions of the assessment. The OTR is legally responsible for all aspects of the occupational therapy process. In this OTR/COTA partnership, the OTR and COTA have biannually watched videotapes of children together to discuss what they observe and record. This process enables them to maintain consistency in their data collection.

The psychologist decided that a coping inventory (Zeitlin, 1985) would provide additional insights about Peter's behavior. The coping inventory revealed that Peter has difficulty "coping with internal resources," especially when situations require Peter to manage his own reactions in busy environments. He also has challenges when "coping with the environment" when situations are unexpected or when social interaction is necessary to engage appropriately. For example, Peter occasionally strikes out at people when they invade his space. Sometimes, he will crawl under the table to avoid contact with others.

The School Function Assessment is a measure of children's performance during life tasks at school. The teacher reported that Peter has difficulty with recreational movement, manipulation with movement, and using materials. He struggles more than other children to complete tasks and is not always happy with his own performance. He has difficulty with behavior regulation and social interaction categories; the teacher reported that she frequently mediates interactions between Peter and his peers.

The teacher's report on the SFA confirms Peter's difficulties with task performance, particularly tasks that require manipulation and movement. As is common with children who have motor planning difficulties, Peter does not negotiate social situations effectively, perhaps because social situations for first graders frequently involve sensory motor-based playing.

Findings on the Sensory Profile (completed by Peter's parents) and the Sensory Profile School Companion (completed by Peter's teacher) indicate that Peter is sensitive to touch and movement. He likes to maintain space between himself and others and prefers to watch others engage in a classroom or recess activity before attempting it himself. At home, when Peter is able to make his own choices about what and how he wants to do something, he is not as sensitive to the environment. Peter also does best when he has additional time or no time restrictions in which to engage in and participate in activities of his choosing.

A summary of the assessment information suggests strengths in some aspects of school performance. For example, Peter manages well in situations that have structure and support from adults as long as he has some power to make decisions about what he will do (e.g., play with particular toys). He seems to be interested in activity and enjoys self-directed play. He observes situations first before jumping in to participate with other children. Peter is hypersensitive to touch and movement; he also struggles to organize and execute motor movements (motor planning) during classroom work and play.

You will notice that we talked about Peter's strength of hanging back, rather than focusing on him not interacting with peers. Taking a strengths perspective sets a better tone for planning.

Since hypersensitivity was an unfamiliar term to the parents, the occupational therapist took extra time during the interpretation to define the term and describe the impact of sensory defensiveness on Peter's behavior.

Intervention

The team meeting included the parents, all members of the evaluation team, the school principal, and the kindergarten teacher.

As described earlier, Peter does best in self-selected activities. When structure and adult directions are imposed on Peter, he begins to struggle more. Cognition and language are areas of strength for Peter, and he seems to use his cognitive and language skills to compensate for sensory-motor challenges. Peter also has more challenges with social skills needed in the academic environment. The team members determined that Peter was eligible for services and would benefit from regular education in the first grade with special education and occupational therapy support.

In some cases, team members may send a copy of their evaluation results to the meeting with another team member as it may not be possible to attend every meeting. In other cases, the occupational therapist may collaborate with other team members to develop one report in which there is an integrated interpretation provided by all team members. While it is preferable to have all team members present, sometimes having fewer professionals is more conducive to parent participation. Having a large number of people present can be overwhelming to the parents.

One area that had the potential to be disruptive to the entire school day was the bus ride, so the team decided to address this issue early in their planning.

Target Outcome

Peter will ride the bus to school each day and be ready for learning in his first-grade classroom. Right now, Peter is hitting and screaming on the bus, and so he is unsettled when he gets to school. The bus driver is wondering whether Peter can continue to ride the bus, so the team wants to get a plan in place so Peter and the bus driver can have a successful transition from home to school.

Benchmark

Peter will earn only neutral and positive reports from the bus driver for an entire week.

The teacher and occupational therapist designed a progress monitoring plan for Peter's rides on the school bus to prevent him from getting kicked off the bus (Table 9-3). The therapist and teacher approached the bus driver to design an intervention. They decide to assign Peter a front seat, to minimize the amount of space he has to negotiate getting to his seat, and to decrease the amount of inadvertent bumping and shoving that he would have to cope with during the trip. The bus driver agreed that this would be a manageable plan.

After beginning the bus intervention, the teacher and therapist worked on plans for the lunchroom. Initially, they decided that sitting at the end of a table in the corner of the lunchroom would reduce the amount of bumping Peter would have to manage. They also had Peter lead the class into the lunchroom so he could get his lunch and get seated as other children were filing into the lunch room.

The family requested more information on strategies they could employ at home. Bath time was always a challenge, so they discussed why this

Remember, light touch activates arousal mechanisms; Peter does not need more arousal.

Table 9-3.

Progress Monitoring Plan for Peter and His Bus Ride

Process	Peter's plan
Behavior	Each day, when it is time for Peter to ride the bus to school, he becomes very upset. Peter hits, screams, and fights with others, often getting out of his seat. The bus driver is worried about the safety of the children (including Peter).
Goal	Peter will ride the bus with a calm, nonintrusive behavior that results in neutral or positive reports from the bus driver.
Hypothesis	Peter has sensory sensitivity that interferes with his ability to ride the bus. When others brush up against Peter, he becomes very upset and sometimes acts out by screaming and hitting.
Intervention	Collaborate with the bus driver to arrange for Peter to have a front seat on the bus. This will minimize the distance Peter has to travel while managing his backpack and finding a seat. Collaborate with family and school for Peter to have two sets of school supplies, one at home and one at school so he does not have to carry a backpack that gets in the way.
Measurement/ Data Collection	The OT will provide the bus driver with three cards: a red (rough day for Peter), yellow (bus ride went okay), and green (Peter had a great day on the bus). Each morning when the bus arrives at school, the driver will give Peter a card indicating how the ride went that day. Peter will give the card to his teacher after getting off the bus.
Decision-Making Plan	The teacher and OT will monitor Peter's progress on the bus. When Peter has 5 consecutive days in which he earns all yellow and green cards, then the goal will be considered met, and the plan can be revised.

Touch pressure input is more calming; there is no activation of arousal mechanisms, so Peter can get input and stay calmer.

activity was difficult for Peter and created strategies for managing this time. For example, rubbing Peter lightly with a towel would upset him, due to his sensitivity for light touch. A better strategy would be to show Peter how to press the towel firmly into his skin to dry him after his bath or change to another fabric for drying (towels have lots of texture, and the threads "move" on the skin). Other strategies were developed as the parents identified problem situations.

Because unexpected situations were more challenging for Peter, the team decided they needed to create opportunities for him to practice handling new and unfamiliar situations throughout his school day. For example, one experience involved coaching Peter through field day at school. Field day provides many opportunities to try a variety of physical activities with a lot a sensory input. Peter was allowed to watch the other children participate and then choose which activities he wanted to try first. The occupational therapist joined the class during story time once a week to provide intervention, because the teacher incorporated movement into this part of each day. Many of the strategies the therapist used were slowly incorporated into Peter's classroom day as the teacher began to understand what Peter needed; having the therapist in the classroom providing intervention was very helpful in this process. The occupational therapist also collaborated with the physical education teacher to support Peter as they explored new movement activities.

Once the teachers and family understood Peter's behaviors and their meaning in relation to his attempts to cope with situations, they all began to come up with ideas. They would share their ideas at the quarterly meetings they held to review Peter's program and identify the next steps for Peter. Eventually, Peter began to participate in idea generation and was able to ask for changes when he needed them to remain calm and in control of himself. Peter had access to a interactive video game system at home in which he was able to play and experiment in a safe and non-judging environment with new and unfamiliar movements. Peter was particularly fond of video chess, which capitalizes on the cognitive challenge without requiring quick or precise motor movements, and so Peter was successful and developed a new set of friends from this activity.

Although the therapist has a professional responsibility to inform families about identified needs, it is also important to delineate for them school-related needs from other needs that they may choose to act upon using family resources. For example, the issue of family counseling came up during a discussion with the mother, due to her frustration managing Peter's outbursts and the different parenting styles between the mother and father. The occupational therapist noted their struggles to cope with Peter, and reminded herself to suggest a referral to a local pediatric psychologist with whom she had worked on a similar case. She would suggest this to the team as an outside referral.

Outcomes

Peter's parents requested information and suggestions for outside-of-school activities, so the occupational therapist talked about the benefits of activities such as swimming or martial arts. While these services are not educationally relevant and are not required in order for Peter to benefit from school, they are activities that can be beneficial for children like Peter. They can include swimming, gymnastics, martial arts, and art programs, or may include a referral to an occupational therapy program in another agency. Care must also be taken to identify these nonschool-related occupational therapy needs; it is not the school district's responsibility to pay for services that are not educationally related.

Reference

Zeitlin, S. (1985). *Coping inventory*. Bensenville, IL: Scholastic Testing Services Inc.

Derek

Winnie Dunn, PhD, OTR, FAOTA and Becky Nicholson, MEd, OTR

Occupational Profile

Derek is 10 years old and has been receiving special education services since his third birthday, when he was diagnosed as having autism. Derek has been enrolled in a self-contained special education classroom since kindergarten, with limited inclusion in the regular education classroom. For the new school year, Derek is being moved to his home school where he will be included in a regular fourth-grade classroom with same-aged peers. Derek's current academic curriculum includes second-grade reading level and third-grade math skills. He has required one-to-one assistance to complete academic tasks.

Autism has a number of characteristics, including unique sensory processing patterns. Derek's prior school had not examined how these sensory issues might be affecting his participation in school-related activities. The previous educational team chose a developmental and cognitive approach to intervention. The occupational therapist was providing standard practice when addressing Derek's difficulties with fine motor and writing skills. By expanding the scope of the assessment process to include sensory processing influence and participation in the school setting, the occupational therapist provides critical information to the educational team.

Derek lives with his mother and older sister. Derek's father sees him occasionally, as he finds Derek's behaviors difficult to deal with. Derek's mom describes him as a child who has a good memory, can recite information, and enjoys building and drawing. She also describes Derek as socially isolated; he has difficulty communicating and engaging with his peers as well as adults, has difficulty with any change or transition, and has limited foods that he will eat.

Derek's mother wants Derek to have friends and likes the idea of him being at their neighborhood school with his sister, but she is quite concerned about Derek being included in the fourth-grade classroom. She is particularly concerned about how Derek will get along with other students and how students will react to and get along with Derek. She also expressed concern about Derek's difficulty with schedule changes and his limited diet choices. Derek's parents are changing their ideas about what they want for Derek's school experience. It appears that everyone was more focused on his academic performance early on, but now the parents seem more focused on socialization and daily life.

The information from Derek's current IEP, as well as information from Derek's mother, suggests that Derek's patterns of responding to sensory events may be interfering with his ability to interact with peers appropriately, to participate in school activities appropriately, to make changes in the schedule, and to eat a varied diet. The team, including Derek's mother, decide that if some of these sensory factors could be sorted out and understood, Derek would have a more successful and positive experience in fourth grade.

The fourth-grade teacher was quite concerned about how Derek would do in her classroom, although she was receptive to having Derek as a student. The team from his prior school recommended a paraprofessional for the fourth-grade classroom to assist the teacher as the team supports her to implement Derek's IEP.

Paraprofessionals are frequently assigned to regular education when a particular classroom needs additional adults to manage the routines. This is particularly true when a student with special needs is part of the class. However, it is inappropriate for the paraprofessional to "hover' around the student with special needs. This strategy runs the risk of the student becoming dependent on another adult, which is counter-productive to the purposes of inclusion.

Rather, the paraprofessional should be engaging in activities to support the teacher throughout the day, focusing on all the students, and all the instructional activities. The extra help creates "room' in the teacher's schedule so the teacher can provide appropriate guidance to students, including students with special needs like Derek.

Analysis of Occupational Performance

In preparation for the transition to his home school, the teacher, paraprofessional, and occupational therapist from the previous school completed the School Function Assessment to give the receiving team information about Derek's participation in his previous school. In addition, the classroom teacher completed the Sensory Profile School Companion to provide information about Derek's sensory processing patterns in school. Over the summer, the mother completed the Sensory Profile Caregiver Questionnaire to give the team information about sensory processing issues in the home environment. Once Derek begins attending the fourth grade in his home school, the school psychologist will do additional classroom observations, the speech-language pathologist will do both classroom observation and direct one-on-one assessment, and the regular classroom teacher will determine where Derek is functioning in the curriculum.

During skilled observations, Derek played parallel to his peers, interacting infrequently. If peers attempted to enter or change Derek's play, he became upset and sometimes screamed, flapped his hands, or struck out at the peer. He frequently lined up small objects or stacked blocks to make an elevator. He also preferred to draw elevators on paper. He frequently hums to himself when engaged in a self-directed activity. During isolated play, he appears to be oblivious to voices and sounds around him.

Derek clearly prefers interaction with adults. He seems to notice the adults moving around the room more readily than he notices peers, unless the peers are interfering with his current activities. When playing alone, he checks on where the teachers are and sometimes repositions himself so he can see them while he is playing or working.

Derek communicates in a variety of ways, including gestures and nonverbal communication, as well as some phrases that are repetitive in nature. At times, adults provide a verbal cue to facilitate Derek to use his words when he wants or needs something. The teachers and therapists also report that Derek has difficulty with situations that are unpredictable, such as on field trips or days on which there are 'special programs." They report that Derek had increased screaming or hitting on these days.

On the School Function Assessment (SFA), Derek performed like other peers in cognitive performance tasks, but had difficulty with peer interactions and behavioral responses. This indicates his need for control over situations. Although the findings indicate that Derek needs more assistance (i.e., someone helping him) during tasks, he rejects another person trying to show him how to do something, particularly when they try to guide him through the task. This is consistent with other observations that Derek does not like to have his hands messy or for others to touch his hands, which limits the teachers' ability to provide physical prompting during new tasks. He also needed more assistance when there were unpredictable situations in the classroom. The teacher also reported that Derek had difficulty making transitions to new tasks, demonstrating perseveration (i.e., repeating the same behavior over and over when it is no longer useful) behaviors at these times.

Additional scores on the SFA indicate that Derek requires more assistance than typical children on many physical and cognitive tasks. However, the team has not put any adaptations in place that might increase his independence. When a child presents scores on the SFA that indicate he or she is not able to participate in activities without significant adult assistance and no adaptations have been implemented, the team should focus efforts on developing possible adaptations (Figures 9-8, 9-9, and 9-10 contain excerpts from the SFA).

For example, the paraprofessional continues to help Derek with hygiene, so he did not increase his independence. It is important that the team problem solve ways to provide accommodations that will increase his personal independence, rather than relying on physical assistance from the paraprofessional.

On the Sensory Profile, Derek's scores were variable, with some in the typical range, and others below the typical response range (Figures 9-11 and 9-12). He has an avoiding pattern overall and has more challenges with touch and sound (see Figure 9-9). He also has difficulty with oral sensory processing (i.e., textures, tastes, and temperatures in the mouth area). Derek prefers to drink 6 to 8 drink boxes each day and eat a minimal amount of solid foods. The solid foods he prefers are macaroni and cheese and french fries.

The Sensory Profile Supplement (2006) provides guidelines for interpretation of the Sensory Profile scores.

Derek's sensory processing abilities are consistent with the 'sensation Avoiding" category (see Dunn, 1997, 2006). Many of Derek's behaviors seem to be the result of Derek needing to control or avoid potentially unfamiliar sensory input, particularly touch and sound. However, there are also some indications of "Low Registration," as Derek sometimes appears oblivious to auditory input and generates his own sounds. If these behaviors are interpreted from a neuroscience viewpoint, "checking out" may be Derek's way of managing incoming auditory input to maintain an appropriate level of arousal (Figure 9-13).

Review the summary score form from the SFA and the score sheets from the two versions of the Sensory Profile. The figure provided is the item map

The team can consider why Derek has some areas that are OK while others are not, and target areas for accommodations to increase Derek's participation throughout the day.

For example, "Behavior Regulation" needs further consideration. Look at the Item Maps and the details of the Behavior Regulation scores to obtain more insights about exactly what you could adapt to support Derek's participation (look at the next 2 figures for Derek's scores).

School Function Assessment *Summary Score Form*

Name: Derek Date:

	Total Raw Score	Criterion Score	Standard Error	Criterion Cut-off Score K-3	Criterion Cut-off Score 4-6
Part I Participation					
Regular Classroom + 5 Settings	23	58	4	100	100
Special Education Classroom + 5 Settings				100	100
Part II Task Supports					
Physical Tasks—Assistance	28	61	5	100	100
Physical Tasks—Adaptations	36	100	16	100	100
Cognitive/Behavioral Tasks—Assistance	22	47	5	77	92
Cognitive/Behavioral Tasks—Adaptations	36	100	17	91	100
Up/Down Stairs—Assistance	4				
Up/Down Stairs—Adaptations	4				
Written Work—Assistance	3				
Written Work—Adaptations	4				
Computer and Equipment Use—Assistance	4				
Computer and Equipment Use—Adaptations	4				
Part III Activity Performance					
Travel	76	100	10	100	100
Maintaining and Changing Positions	48	100	16	100	100
Recreational Movement	40	73	6	83	100
Manipulation With Movement	59	75	5	93	100
Using Materials	72	59	3	83	100
Setup and Cleanup	65	70	4	87	100
Eating and Drinking	56	100	15	100	100
Hygiene	41	52	3	92	100
Clothing Management	61	62	3	93	100
Up/Down Stairs	24	100	10	100	100
Written Work	38	61	4	73	94
Computer and Equipment Use	32	100	15	65	100
Functional Communication	36	50	3	91	100
Memory and Understanding	40	100	13	79	100
Following Social Conventions	27	43	4	73	92
Compliance With Adult Directives and School Rules	50	65	4	76	82
Task Behavior/Completion	47	80	3	72	81
Positive Interaction	39	48	3	81	83
Behavior Regulation	24	39	4	74	78
Personal Care Awareness	25	61	4	92	100
Safety	36	69	7	91	100

Functional Profile

Setting	Classroom Reg. Spec.	Playground/ Recess	Transportation	Bathroom/ Toileting	Transitions	Mealtime/ Snack Time
Rating	3	4	5	3	3	5

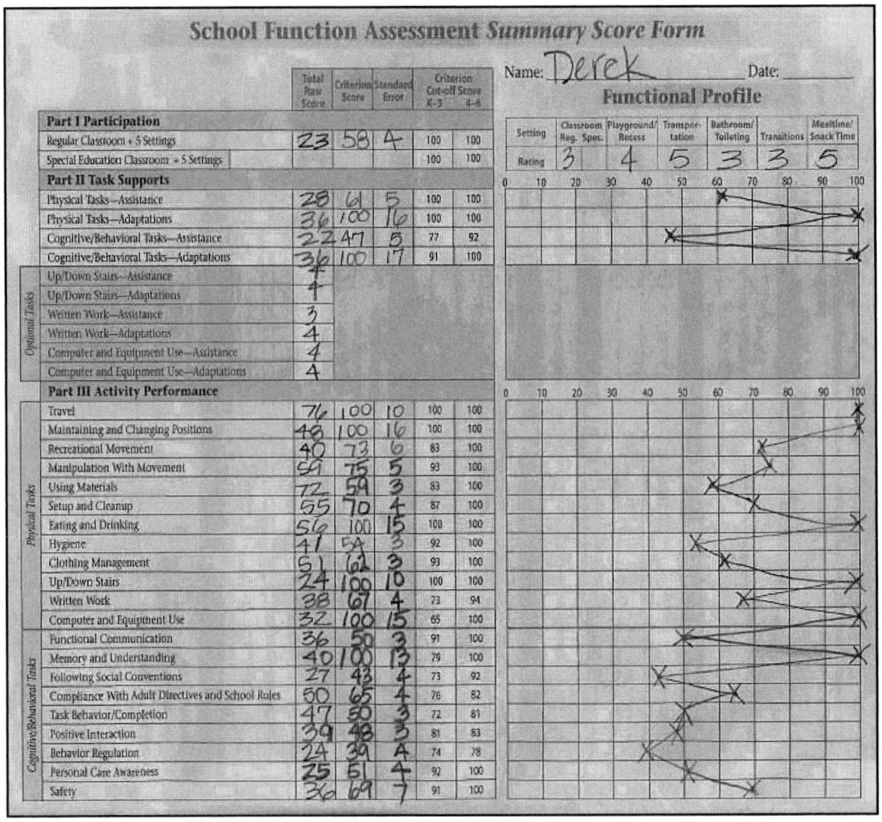

Figure 9-8. Derek's SFA summary score form.

We are not surprised that Derek has more difficulty with changes in routines when compared to other students; however, this standardized documentation provides a way to mark changes as your interventions take effect.

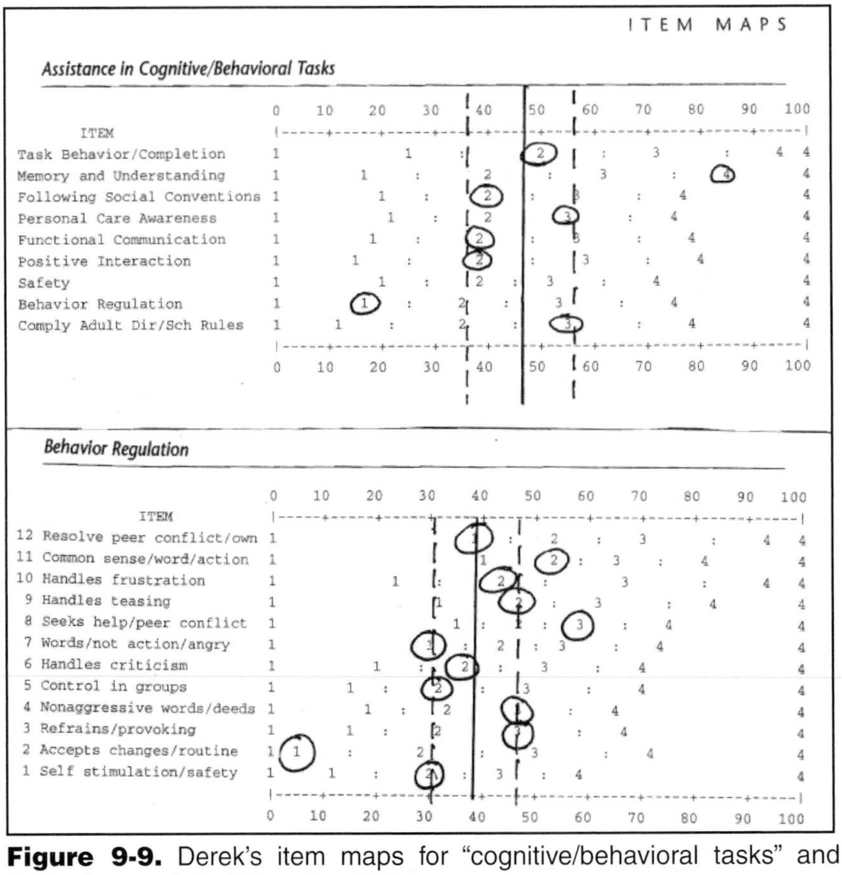

Figure 9-9. Derek's item maps for "cognitive/behavioral tasks" and "behavior regulation" from the SFA.

Behavior Regulation

1. Displays appropriate restraint regarding self-stimulation (e.g., refrains from head banging, hand flapping). 1 2 3 4
2. Accepts unexpected changes in routine. 1 2 3 4
3. Refrains from provoking others. 1 2 3 4
4. Uses nonaggressive words and actions. 1 2 3 4
5. Maintains behavioral control in large groups of students (e.g., cafeteria, assemblies). 1 2 3 4
6. Hears constructive criticism without losing temper. 1 2 3 4
7. Uses words rather than physical actions to respond when provoked or angry at others. . . 1 2 3 4
8. Seeks adult assistance, if necessary, when experiencing peer conflict, especially conflicts involving violence. 1 2 3 4
9. Responds to/handles teasing in a constructive way. 1 2 3 4
10. Handles frustration when experiencing difficulties with school tasks/activities. 1 2 3 4
11. Shows common sense in words and actions around bullies, gangs, or strangers. 1 2 3 4
12. Resolves ordinary peer conflicts or problems adequately on his/her own without requesting teacher assistance. 1 2 3 4

Respondent's Initials | **Behavior Regulation Raw Score** 24

Figure 9-10. Derek's scores on "Behavior Regulation" on the SFA.

Quadrant Summary

Instructions: For each quadrant, transfer the Quadrant Raw Score Totals from the Quadrant Grid to the corresponding Quadrant Raw Score Total box. Plot these totals by marking an X in the appropriate classification column (Typical Performance, Probable Difference, Definite Difference).

Quadrant	Quadrant Raw Score Total	← Less Than Others: Much Less Than Others — Definite Difference	← Less Than Others: Less Than Others — Probable Difference	Similar to Others — Typical Performance	More Than Others →: More Than Others — Probable Difference	More Than Others →: Much More Than Others — Definite Difference
1. Registration	56 /75	**	75 — 73	72 — 64	63 — 59	58 X 15
2. Seeking	88 /130	**	130 — 124	123 — 103	102 — 92	91 X 26
3. Sensitivity	56 /100	**	100 — 95	94 — 81	80 — 73	72 X 20
4. Avoiding	90 /145	145 — 141	140 — 134	133 — 113	112 — 103	102 X 29

**There is no Definite Difference/Much Less Than Others score for this quadrant.

The Normal Curve and the *Sensory Profile Supplement* Classification System

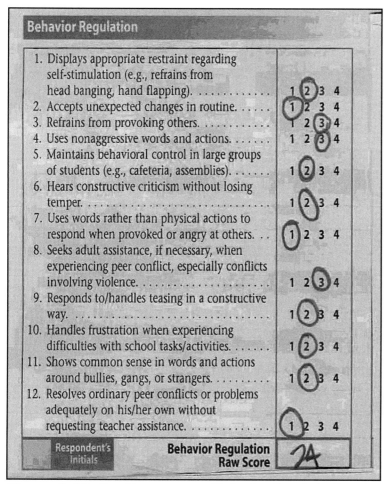

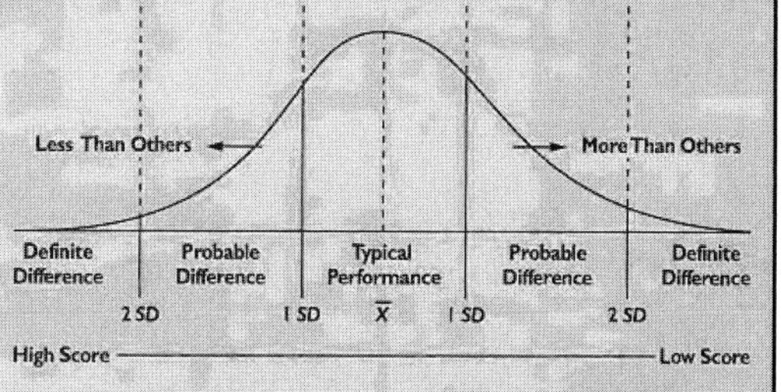

Scores 1 standard deviation or more from the mean are expressed as "More Than Others" or "Less Than Others." Scores 2 standard deviations or more from the mean are expressed as "Much More Than Others" or "Much Less Than Others."

Figure 9-11. Derek's sensory profile quadrant scores.

Here we see that Derek might need support for using words to express himself in stressful situations (No. 7).

You will notice that the teacher sees Derek as "similar to others" on Registration and Seeking, while the parents have rated Derek "much more than others" on these same quadrant scores. Both parents and the teacher agree about Derek's Sensitivity and Avoiding scores being "much more than others."

This difference between home and school points out how important context is as we consider the meaning of children's behaviors. There are different settings and expectations at home and school, so we are not surprised by differences in scores across these settings.

It is important to point out to parents and teachers that we are not comparing their scores to see who is "right', but rather, we use the similarities and differences to identify what might already be a successful strategy at home or school that we can expand to support Derek in all settings. Perhaps at school, Derek's ability to detect is similar to the other children's patterns because he has a lot more cues to remind him what to do. Parents also bathe and dress Derek, an area of need that the teacher has less information about. Brokering the information about context and participation gives us another tool to support Derek.

Quadrant Summary

Instructions: Transfer each Quadrant Raw Score Total from the Quadrant Grid to the first column below. Plot these totals by marking an X in the appropriate classification column (e.g., Typical Performance, Probable Difference, Definite Difference).

	← Less Than Others			More Than Others →	
	Much Less Than Others	Less Than Others	Similar to Others	More Than Others	Much More Than Others
Quadrant Raw Score Total	Definite Difference	Probable Difference	Typical Performance	Probable Difference	Definite Difference
1. Registration 66 /85	**	85	84 ---X--- 64	63 ------ 53	52 ------ 17
2. Seeking 48 /60	**	*	60 ---X--- 43	42 ------ 34	33 ------ 12
3. Sensitivity 19 /80	80 ------ 79	78 ------ 69	68 ------ 51	50 ------ 41	40 ---X--- 16
4. Avoiding 30 /85	**	*	85 ------ 70	69 ------ 61	60 ---X--- 17

**There is no Definite Difference/Much Less Than Others score for this quadrant.
*There is no Probable Difference/Less Than Others score for this quadrant.

Figure 9-12. Derek's school companion quadrant scores.

Figure 9-13. Interpretation of SFA and Sensory Profile on Derek.

Interpretation using information from the Sensory Profile and the School Function Assessment

The occupational therapist analyzed the findings from these two assessments to identify patterns of sensory processing that may be interfering with his performance in school-related activities. For example, Derek does not perform tasks such as obtaining soap or drying hands. The team knew from the Sensory Profile information that Derek avoids touch in many situations not just during art activities. They began to see a pattern of Derek having difficulty performing school activities that had a touch component that he would avoid. Understanding Derek's sensitivity to touch is also critical in developing social skills. For example, it will be important that the team makes sure that the children with whom Derek interacts understand that hugging or giving high fives will be upsetting to Derek because of his sensitivity to touch, not because he doesn't like them. Derek needs to have alternative ways to interact with the kids, such as giving a thumbs up or waving. When the occupational therapist considered performance across a variety of school activities, the team began to develop adaptations to a variety of activities so that Derek might be more independent.

from the behavior regulation section of the SFA. Derek presents scores in this area that are significantly different from typical children. His performance in this area consistently interferes with his ability to participate in the school environment. Now, look at the individual items in this section. The ratings indicate that Derek is unable to accept changes in routine. Using the information from the Sensory Profile, we know that Derek is highly alert to visual information in his environment. The team needs to use Derek's highly developed visual processing to provide support through the use of a visual schedule so that Derek will be better prepared for changes in his daily routine. Review the other items listed, and consider additional sensory strategies that may support Derek's performance.

This team is taking a broader view of Derek's performance needs at school, including socialization and communication as critical areas of emphasis, rather than only addressing the curricular educational needs to learn (e.g., math, reading, writing). This is also occurring because the parents are ready to expand their view of Derek's needs in life.

Program Planning

Derek's team (which consisted of the occupational therapist, special education teacher, regular education teacher, school psychologist, and speech-language pathologist) decided to focus on increasing interactions with peers in controlled situations as well as increasing Derek's ability to communicate, because this is a core skill for socialization at his age. The team also decided to honor Derek's need to control sensory input (i.e., sensation avoiding) as they constructed their plans so that Derek would remain available to learn (i.e., he would not burst out in response to unfamiliar input).

Target Outcome 1

Derek will work with two peers to complete an art project in the same time frame as peers. The team is going to gradually increase the time and number of successful projects as the year proceeds. They decided they would discuss the criteria as they go, because different projects require different attention, skills, etc.

Intervention Approach

The team decided to include students from Derek's fourth-grade classroom in the intervention. In addition, they discussed the sensory supports they would make available to Derek in order to honor his need to control sensory input throughout the day.

Intervention Procedures

Derek's mother gave permission to implement the Circle of Friends approach, which helped identify students in Derek's classroom who would be willing to assist in Derek's program. The teacher and students discussed activities that the students thought Derek could participate in successfully. The teacher and paraprofessional selected two students to actively engage with Derek on a consistent basis. The teacher and paraprofessional trained these students to give Derek feedback when he was making inappropriate noises in the classroom. For example, they would tell Derek that "the noises you are making make it hard to get work done. You need to go to the library." They also learned to ask Derek if they could join his play and then proceed to copy what Derek was doing with similar materials. This gained Derek's interest and honored his need for familiarity, which increased Derek's ability to be more participatory with the other students.

The team also discussed how to rearrange the classroom in service to Derek's needs. The teacher seated Derek at the far end of the aisle (to reduce random contact with objects and other children passing by) in a pod of four desks facing one another. One of the peers who had agreed to assist Derek sat next to him. The quiet area was directly to Derek's right, making it more available to him when he needed it.

The occupational therapist on a team such as this must also see the role of occupational therapy in this broader view and offer expertise to all aspects of this program. It is common for students with autism to respond differently to sensory events in daily life, and this is an area of expertise for occupational therapy. This viewpoint offers the team a way to approach Derek's socialization and communication needs in a completely different manner, while also giving the parents some ways to understand Derek's behavior as a coping strategy (i.e., he is keeping new stimuli from occurring by fleeing situations or by acting out to limit participation). In a program such as this one, the team must be vigilant about collecting data so they can adjust the program based on Derek's responses. Remember, the team's goal is for Derek to socialize, not to "improve sensory processing."

It is important to measure what you actually want Derek to do. We know that right now he is striking out, hand flapping, and screaming; these will interfere with his ability to complete the art project in a timely manner. So instead of writing the goal with all these negative behaviors in is (e.g., "without screaming"), we write the goal about the desired participation, knowing that for him to participate, he will need to reduce the unacceptable behaviors.

References/ resources:

www.circleofriends.org/

www.txautism.net/docs/Guide/Interventions/CircleFriends.pdf

Barrett, W., & Randall, L. (2004). Investigating the Circle of Friends approach: Adaptations and implications for practice. Educational Psychology in Practice, 20, 353-368.

Frederickson, N., & Turner, J. (2003). Utilizing the classroom peer group to address children's social needs: An evaluation of the Circle of Friends intervention approach. The Journal of Special Education, 36, 234-245.

Stacking books provides input to support postural control and organize body scheme information because the weight of the books activates the proprioceptive receptors, which contribute to one's sense of self (see Chapter 6).

The team identified "getaway places" both in the classroom and in other parts of the school building. If Derek needed to control his own sensory input, he was allowed to go to the "quiet" area of the classroom where students would go to read. This area included a claw foot bathtub with pillows in it and bean bag chairs, enabling students to construct an environment that supported their bodies and provided the amount of sensory input that was comfortable (e.g., how many pillows piled underneath and on top of you, laying on the bean bags, or sitting on them). In addition, Derek was allowed to go to the library to re-stack books when he needed to stand and move.

The team also discussed the appropriate use of the paraprofessional in the classroom. They knew that an adult hovering over Derek would not facilitate peer interactions, so they planned for the paraprofessional to move around in the classroom to assist any of the students who needed help. She did not sit next to Derek unless the task was not suitable for a peer to help him. This was critical for Derek's socialization; if he had an adult hovering all the time, students would not have an interest or need to interact with Derek and vice versa.

The occupational therapist provided handouts (see Chapter 6) for team members, including the regular education teacher, regarding the impact of sensory processing patterns on performance and suggested ways to structure other activities to support children like Derek.

Derek's collaborative team initially met each week to plan Derek's program and make modifications. After 6 weeks, they agreed that they had worked out all the inconsistencies and could touch base monthly.

Outcome

Derek's tantrums and screaming decreased over the first few months. Derek's interaction with the two targeted peers increased, and Derek accepted directions, assistance, and even began initiating interactions with each of them. The next step would be to include several more peers in a structured manner in Derek's program.

With guidance from the teacher at first, and then independently, Derek used the "quiet" area of the classroom frequently and eventually was able to return to his desk after spending brief periods in the quiet area. Derek was becoming aware of his own internal signals and acting on his own behalf to get needs met. This is a critical skill for transition to middle school.

These activities engage the touch pressure/proprioceptive systems, which provide organizing input to the nervous system and do not send collateral input to the reticular formation which can generate additional arousal (Dunn, 1998). Studies suggest that providing this type of input during school supports students to be more productive at school (see Chapter 3 and Dunn 2009).

The team decided to increase the organizing sensory features of his school routines. They provided a weighted blanket for Derek to lay across his legs while seated at his desk and added weight to his writing utensils. They asked him to wear a backpack with heavy books in it when transitioning among rooms and activities and designated him to be the "carrier" when getting trays of milk from the cafeteria. All of these interventions supported Derek to participate while receiving discriminatory sensory input (i.e., input that does *not* activate the arousal systems and generate a "fight or flight" response).

The occupational therapist provided Derek's mother with information about interventions that worked for Derek in the classroom and how she could adapt these in the home environment.

Over a period of several months, Derek became more interactive with other students, as well as with his sister at home. The family found that Derek could interact with others via e-mail, and he has two pen pals this way. During e-mail interactions, Derek did not have to worry about extrasensory experiences interfering with his socialization; he frequently piled books on his lap during these sessions, an adaptation of the blanket from school.

References

Coster, W., T. Deeney, T., Haltiwanger, J. & Haley, S. M. (1998). *School function assessment, user's manual.* San Antonio, TX: Therapy Skill Builders.

Dunn, W. (1997). The impact of sensory processing abilities on the daily lives of young children and families: A conceptual model. *Infants and Young Children, 9*(4), 23-35.

Dunn, W. (1998). Implementing neuroscience principles to support habilitation and recovery. In C. Christiansen & C. Baum (Eds.), *Occupational therapy: Achieving human performance needs in daily living.* Thorofare, NJ: SLACK Incorporated.

Dunn, W. (2006). *Sensory profile supplement.* San Antonio, TX: The Psychological Corporation.

Dunn, W. (2009). Ecology of human performance model. In S. Dunbar (Ed.), *OT models for intervention with children and families.* Thorofare, NJ: SLACK Incorporated.

Cameron

Winnie Dunn, PhD, OTR, FAOTA and Becky Nicholson, MEd, OTR

Evaluation

Occupational Profile

Referral

Cameron's initial referral to special services occurred as a toddler, and he has been receiving related services since that time. He is currently making the transition to middle school, where he will be changing classes and teachers hourly. He will have to maneuver around a new building and will want to participate in school-related extracurricular activities.

History

Cameron is the oldest of four children. He was born 3 months prematurely and had anoxia at birth that resulted in spastic quadriplegia. His parents noted that at age 1 he was not sitting up. They took him to a neurologist who diagnosed Cameron with cerebral palsy. They enrolled Cameron in an early intervention program where he received occupational, physical, and speech-language therapy until he was 5 years old. Beginning in kindergarten, Cameron attended the local elementary school in regular education with paraprofessional support, as well as occupational and physical therapy and adaptive physical education as related services. Cameron uses a power wheelchair for mobility and a laptop computer for written assignments.

This is not a new referral, but an ongoing case. Whenever a student with special needs transitions to a new environment, the demands and supports also change. In this case, the occupational and physical therapists are instrumental in assessing the environment demands of the new environment and recommending modifications.

It is important to inspect environmental modifications in buildings. Although they might appear to meet the standards, there can be subtle things that interfere with everyday use. For example, a bathroom door might be wide enough, but may open into the bathroom without enough space for clearance when a person is in a wheelchair. A door might be too heavy for a person to open from a sitting position. Check things out WITH the person to be sure!

Occupational Analysis

The occupational therapist obtained a copy of this school district's ADA plan for accessibility for each of its buildings including the middle school. The occupational and physical therapist used an Accessibility Checklist to help identify potential problem areas Cameron might encounter during this transition to a new building and new program. The therapist was particularly concerned about activities of daily living skills, including toileting, eating, and dressing for physical education class. In addition, the parents wanted to ensure that socialization opportunities were not overlooked and that any modifications needed for those activities were also addressed. Other questions centered around how independent Cameron could be in this new environment and what task trade-offs would be necessary in order for him to be successful at the middle school level.

(e.g., eclkc.ohs.acf.hhs.gov/hslc/ecdh/Disabilities/Program%20Planning/Accessibility/disabl_pub_00006pdf_081905.html; or search "accessibility" to find other options)

Assessment Plan

The preliminary plan was for the occupational and physical therapist to walk through the middle school building with the elementary school principal from Cameron's current school, the middle school principal, the building maintenance supervisor, Cameron, a friend of his choice, and Cameron's parents. The occupational and physical therapist made a list of areas of the building or certain programs that might be particularly difficult for Cameron to access. They determined the accessibility of the cafeteria, restroom, locker room, library, track, office, locker area, gymnasium, and hall areas with doors.

The teams also decided to have a meeting with the sending and receiving staff members from the elementary and middle schools so they could discuss curricular modifications that had been useful and would be possible in this new setting.

Socialization during middle school is a critical part of student development. This team is making sure that Cameron can stay with his peers for the transition times, which is when they talk and "hang out" together. We can inadvertently isolate a student like Cameron by being insensitive to these needs.

For example, a team might say "Let's let Cameron leave class early so he has time to get to the new location, or to use the bathroom." This strategy removes his opportunity to socialize which may be very important to Cameron.

Teenagers are also very sensitive to adult supervision. They are trying to emancipate, so having an aide help the student in the lunch room may also be intrusive. It may be better to engage one of Cameron's peers to help him open containers, etc., just like they would if they were in the community together.

Findings and Interpretation

The middle school building is a one-story building with virtually no steps (one exception is one step up into some of the outside entrances). One entrance did not have a step, but Cameron was unable to enter the building independently as there were no automatic door openers on any of the outside entrances. Once inside the building, Cameron could easily access the office, the library, the common areas, and the gymnasium. The boy's restroom was not accessible, as the entrance into it was not wide enough for Cameron's wheelchair. The seventh grade wing of the building had double fire doors dividing it from the rest of the building that are required by fire code to be kept closed. Cameron was unable to open the heavy doors by pushing against them with his wheelchair.

Once inside this wing, Cameron could reach the padlock on the upper locker but he was unable to rotate the padlock in order to open it. The hallways in this wing are quite narrow with double lockers on both sides, resulting in a very crowded hall when students change classes. The students sit at large round tables in the language arts class that Cameron easily maneuvered up to and fit underneath. The algebra class had chairs with attached desks that were packed tightly into the classroom, making it impossible for Cameron to enter past the doorway. This was also the case in his other core classes.

The gymnasium was accessible to Cameron but, due to the old style, there was no seating on the floor level. The bleachers started right outside the perimeter of the basketball court, making it difficult for Cameron to sit safely on the gym floor. There were no ramps or lifts up to the bleacher level. Cameron could also not access his physical education class when they went outside, as there was a step down onto the track. Cameron was interested in attending sporting events as well as being a photographer for the school newspaper or yearbook. The bleachers were not accessible to him.

This team conducted the assessment of the next environment for Cameron in the spring of the year prior to his entrance into middle school so the district would have adequate time to make modifications. The family, district administrators, and therapists sat down and made a specific plan for Cameron, including where classes would be scheduled (so time issues could be addressed as well).

This assessment time also enabled the members to discuss what situations might require extra staff support for Cameron to be successful in this educational environment. Cameron and his parents also met the middle school principal and became familiar with the building and programs.

Program Planning

The team used the information from the assessment of the middle school for Cameron's IEP meeting. The district agreed to make the building and programs accessible to Cameron. Cameron's parents were part of this team and helped in making decisions for how modifications could best be made for Cameron.

They made the following decisions and actions:

1. The outside entrance closest to the office had an automatic door opener installed that Cameron could operate. This was the one entrance that did not have an outside step up and was the one the students used most frequently.
2. The restroom in the wing for Cameron's classes was large, so they installed a stall that met ADA standards without compromising other uses.
3. Automatic door openers for the double doors to the 7th grade wing were installed, and it was agreed to work on installing these in the other wings in subsequent years.
4. The family agreed to locate a digital lock for Cameron's locker.
5. The team discussed the narrow halls at great length. The teachers were clear that the "crowdedness" served a very important socialization function and so wanted to enable Cameron to participate in this activity, even though to adults it was chaotic. The team decided to develop a progress monitoring plan for this activity and see how Cameron managed without physical changes.
6. The counselors agreed to limit the number of children in classes with too many desks (and the teachers were happy), so that Cameron and other children could get around successfully; the administration hired an additional teacher for the 7th grade team to accommodate the shift in scheduling and used a room in the 8th grade wing for this activity.
7. The administration contacted a construction company that specialized in modifying existing bleachers to meet the ADA requirements.

The administration obtained an estimate for one new set of bleachers at one end of the gym and agreed to replace additional bleachers as improvements in the gym were implemented. In addition, the administration modified the bleachers to include wheelchair seating on all sides until larger renovations had been completed. (For additional information, see www.bleacherseating.com/specifications.html.)

8. The same construction company and the occupational therapist collaborated to design a ramp that provided accessibility to the field and the bleachers around the track. Cameron would then be able to access the field and bleachers for physical education class. This also provided Cameron close access to the field for sporting events and would enable him to photograph sporting events from the best perspective.
9. The occupational therapist located a camera mount with an articulating arm that could be mounted on Cameron's wheelchair. In addition, the school purchased a remote control switch for the school camera so that Cameron could operate the camera independently.
10. The team decided to have the district purchase "Dragon Naturally Speaking" (New World Creations, Wellington, Florida, www.speechtechnology.com/dragon/whatsnew10.html) so that he has speech-recognition software on his laptop. This technology enables Cameron to search the Web, create voice commands for other software, and transcribe his words into typed text. As Cameron grows older, these tools will be invaluable for his school work, socialization, and vocational exploration.

Intervention Planning

As you can see from this case, not all children require the same type of approach, and sometimes a more "institutional" approach is in everyone's best interest. Cameron already knew the cognitive, language, and other learning strategies for himself, and his condition is stable, but he needed the environment to be more user-friendly to support him being there. This is a great role for occupational therapy in schools—to support these transitions.

Outcome

The district had to scramble to complete the plans by the start of school, and Cameron and his family visited the school several times during the summer so that Cameron could practice getting around. Their strategy was that if it was all very familiar to him, the disruptions would be less upsetting to Cameron's overall functioning. They also went to school during the various enrollment periods so there would be more traffic, and this additional challenge seemed to excite Cameron. The teachers and Cameron collected data on his timeliness in the halls when changing classes and found that he was late like many other children at first, but that he was able to socially broker his needs in the hall to get to his next class. This helped Cameron get immersed very quickly, and he was one of the first children everyone knew at school. The speech-language pathologist and occupational therapist came to school to program some "cool" phrases into his computer for those times when he could not produce language fast enough for the needs of the situation; everyone loved this. Cameron was in the journalism club and was a photojournalist for the school newspaper. In the first semester of school,

Cameron had a featured article that included both text created from his special voice-operated software and photographs he had taken of the football players and fans on a Friday game day.

Sarah

Winnie Dunn, PhD, OTR, FAOTA and Becky Nicholson, MEd, OTR

Occupational Profile

Sarah is a 16-year-old student who was a passenger in a vehicle involved in an accident in May of the previous school year. She sustained an injury to the left parietal region. Sarah has been an inpatient at an area rehabilitation hospital through the summer and is returning to school on a limited basis at the start of the school year. The occupational therapist working in the rehabilitation setting had developed a program to assist school-aged children with traumatic brain injury (TBI) in transitioning back into the school setting. An integral part of the rehabilitation plan was to collaborate with professionals in the school setting to provide ongoing support and create the continuum of services needed between the clinical and community-based setting. The rehabilitation team got permission from the family to have two-way communication with Sarah's school to facilitate the transition.

The high school's special education team and the rehabilitation team collaborated to identify Sarah's areas of strengths and needs in order to develop a program that focused on enabling Sarah to participate in the activities she found meaningful.

History

Sarah has been a regular education student who was just completing her sophomore year in high school. She was a member of the high school color guard and the spirit club. Sarah was a passenger in a car driven by another high school student when the driver lost control of the car on a gravel road and hit another vehicle head on. Neither girl was wearing her seat belt. Sarah was thrown from the car and sustained serious head injuries. The driver sustained internal injuries, was hospitalized, and was released after 1 week. Sarah is the only child in her two-parent family. Sarah's father is an accountant, and her mother is a homemaker. Both parents are quite involved with Sarah, although Sarah's mother is the primary care provider.

Occupational Analysis

A student who has sustained a serious head injury needs to have coordinated services between the medical and educational settings. Because Sarah has sustained a serious head injury with resulting difficulties in both cognitive and motor areas, the school-based therapist will want to observe Sarah in the rehab setting prior to school starting and gain as much information as possible from Sarah's medical team.

The referral and history suggest that Sarah will only be able to fully participate in the school environment with modifications and assistance. It will be important to conduct ongoing assessment of Sarah's abilities, as she

Students with TBI may have emotional or affective difficulties, memory difficulties, attention problems, and perceptual and motor problems. Any of these may affect the student's ability to complete simple tasks, such as following directions and completing simple self-care tasks. Physical sequelae of TBI could include reduced stamina, seizures, headaches, and hearing and vision losses (e.g., Savage, Depompei, Tyler, & Lash, 2005). Cognitive problems of TBI could include memory, intellectual functioning, attention and concentration, language, and academic functioning.

A student's ability to adjust to TBI is often influenced by any affective problems, personality disturbances, behavior problems, pre-injury personality traits, the family's ability to cope, the sense of guilt over the injury circumstances, or denial of illness (Ylvisaker et al., 2001). In addition peers, teachers, and family must learn about the new characteristics and challenges before them; it is often helpful to offer them reading materials about TBI so that they can feel a sense of control over their own coping with the changes that will occur. Most states have a brain injury association that provides materials and support for families and service providers.

The Ylvisaker et al. (2001) article provides guidance about educating students with TBI, and is an excellent reference for your library.

is still in a recovery phase from her head injury. Because she will have both rehabilitation services and school-based services as she transitions back to school, it is important to understand the ways to integrate occupation-based practices into the school. Table 9-4 provides an illustration of a best practice, integrated approach to supporting Sarah.

Assessment Plan

The occupational and speech-language therapist will visit the rehab center where Sarah is receiving daily outpatient occupational, physical, and speech-language therapy. They will also visit with Sarah and her mom and observe therapy sessions with the various disciplines. In addition, the professionals decide to hold a joint team meeting in which Sarah's entire rehab team, as well as the team from the high school, meet to discuss Sarah's strengths and needs and plan for her transition back to high school.

The school's state Department of Education was operating a TBI state grant designed to assist school districts in understanding about TBIs of their students and assist teams in planning for these students. The team also consulted with these experts to obtain additional information and training for the school team.

Findings and Interpretations

The team used a combination of record review, observation, and interview prior to Sarah returning to school to collect data. The rehab team reported that Sarah has right hemiparesis with limitations in all movements of her right upper extremity. Sarah has limitations in all shoulder, elbow, wrist, and hand movements. She has right-side neglect and does not use her arm or hand unless prompted. She also has limited sensory awareness of her right upper extremity. Sarah is able to get dressed and undressed, complete most of her own self-grooming with minimal assistance, and feed herself with utensils (although overall, she is slower than her peers). Sarah walks with a slight limp, but is functionally walking on different surfaces and up and down stairs. She has mild disorientation with directions and spatial relations. Sarah has gained good comprehension and expression skills.

Sarah's goals are to get back to school full-time, drive again, attend extracurricular activities, and spend time with her friends. This includes participating in color guard again. She would also like to be able to use her right arm and hand better so that she looks more "normal." When asked about post-high school goals, Sarah said she plans on attending a local community college or vocational school but does not know what she wants to study.

Considering what Sarah would like to accomplish is extremely important; Sarah is old enough to speak for herself and has the power to participate in or sabotage the team's plans. This is true with all children for whom therapists provide services, but because Sarah is an adolescent, it is extremely important that she feels a part of the process. The therapist must consider this even more when designing a program for an adolescent who does not want to 'stand out" (or in Sarah's words, "look like a freak"). The therapist must place as much emphasis on Sarah's mental health needs as on her physical needs.

Table 9-4.

Illustration of Best Practice Approaches to Integrate Sarah Into Her School Program

What It Does Look Like (in School Practice)	What It Doesn't Look Like (in School Practice)
Goals are written that reflect Sarah's priorities. Sarah wants to be able to drive and be a member of the color guard.	Goals are written that reflect remediation of an underlying skill.
Sarah guides the therapist as they make adjustments in her intervention process.	The therapist's expert opinion determines the need for adjustments in intervention process.
The interventions are directed at activities that naturally occur throughout the school day.	Intervention routines are developed by the therapist that require isolated practice and do not have connections to her daily routine.
The therapist recognizes they will need creative solutions to overcome issues that are interfering with achieving her goals. So, for Sarah, participating in the color guard will mean that the therapist will have to assist the school personnel to adjust expectations and develop creative ways for Sarah to participate.	The therapist convinces Sarah to compromise on her goals in order to accommodate limitations imposed by other people or the situation.
Sarah chooses the intervention methods.	Intervention methods are selected by the therapist, and implementation of the procedures are prescribed by the therapist
Sarah's social community (i.e., family, friends, agencies) understands her goals and has necessary information and resources to support her participation.	No one outside the client is involved in the intervention process.

Of course it is important to keep Sarah's rehabilitation needs in mind when planning her school program. However, school-based practice requires that we integrate her needs into the routines of her school day. It is not appropriate to create a "rehab clinic' situation in the school.

These comparisons illustrate the differences between a standard rehab approach and a best practice approach within the school. Since we are working in the school with Sarah, we need to take that perspective when planning her program.

Program Planning

The team planned a number of activities designed to enable Sarah to be as successful as possible in her school program. Several of these activities included the following:

1. Continue contact with the rehab center where Sarah is receiving outpatient therapy and with Sarah's parents about the interaction of school and rehab center's plans. The school-based therapists and the hospital-based therapists arranged to talk weekly about Sarah's program. This allowed for the school-based therapist to convey information regarding Sarah's ability to function in the school environment to the hospital-based therapist. This arrangement also allowed

Savage, DePompei, Tyler, and Lash (2005) outline 5 guidelines for education teams when supporting a student with head injury:

1. *Develop individualized programs for each student*
2. *Include flexibility into the plans and schedules*
3. *Measure success in small increments*
4. *Communicate with families about plans and progress*
5. *Develop a system for long-term monitoring*

Please refer to this article for more detailed suggestions.

for consistency across therapists and environments. By keeping the parents informed about this communication method, everyone understood the integrated plans that were being implemented on Sarah's behalf (reflecting #4—Communicating with the family).

2. The school team arranged Sarah's class schedule so that she attends afternoon classes and can attend her outpatient therapy sessions in the morning during the initial transition period. This would allow Sarah to be at school over the lunch hour and for three classes in the afternoon, which would also allow her to attend after-school extra-curricular activities. After 2 months, rehabilitation therapy sessions were less frequent, affording Sarah the chance to begin her driving class and color guard practice (reflecting #2—Flexibility in planning).
3. The collaborative teams set a goal to transition Sarah to school-based therapy over the next 6 months. The occupational therapist would continue to work on increasing Sarah's functional capabilities to use both arms in bilateral activities (e.g., during required Family Living skills class), while at the same time working on modifications to support her participation (e.g., adaptive cooking tools in Family Living). The rehabilitation therapist had been working on Sarah's upper extremity strength and coordination to support her participation in the Family Living class. The resource room teacher agreed to take responsibility for overseeing Sarah's educational plans in each class as she moved to the next school year (reflecting #5—Long-term planning).
4. The occupational therapist consults with the Family Living teacher to make sure Sarah learns the precautions she needs to incorporate into her routines because of lack of sensitivity in her right arm and hand (reflecting #1—Individualized planning).
5. Sarah will begin attending color guard practice and participating in practices to the extent she is able. With the consent of the sponsor and other color guard members, the therapist will attend these practices to observe, get ideas for how Sarah can practice, and make modifications so Sarah can participate in some routines (reflecting #3—Measure success in small increments).
6. The occupational therapist at the rehabilitation program will communicate with the driver's education teacher at school to identify adaptations to support Sarah as she learns to drive (e.g., using driving simulations, teaching knowledge and safety skill development). The driver's education teacher meets with parents regarding insurance requirements and driving practice parameters; the rehabilitation therapist plans to meet with parents to discuss adaptations for their family car (reflecting all of the Savage, Depompei, Tyler, & Lash, 2005, criteria).

Target Outcome

Sarah will march with the color guard in the Spring community parade (April).

Intervention Approach

Create an adapted flag pole (e.g., lighter material, a holder for both hands) so Sarah can practice with the color guard team.

Explore opportunities for Sarah to use other tools during color guard routines (e.g., ribbons, pom poms).

Collaborate with color guard choreographer to shorten the distance Sarah must travel during routines.

Intervention Procedures

Color guard practices were a viable means of providing both therapeutic intervention for Sarah's need to move, developing better spatial relationships, and re-integrating Sarah into a small supportive peer group. Practices were held 3 days each week: 1 day during band class and 2 other days after school. Color guard uses long plastic poles with flags on one end to develop routines to music. Sarah had been instrumental in starting color guard at the school and had co-developed many of the initial routines. The therapist looked at the movements necessary to hold and move the poles and the speed and strength required. The therapist then modified some movements with the help of the rest of the color guard team so that Sarah could participate in at least one routine.

Outcome

Sarah initially just attended and observed at the color guard practices with the therapist. The other girls consulted with Sarah on the routines they were developing and solicited any suggestions she could make. By the second week, Sarah was attempting to move the pole by holding it with her right hand and moving the pole with her left hand. This provided therapeutic activity for Sarah that was motivating for her. The occupational therapist also designed a glove attached to the pole so Sarah could hold the pole with both hands. The team developed new "moves" that Sarah could also complete. By the first of November, Sarah partially participated in a color guard performance at the half time of a football game.

Sarah began attending school full-time the second semester and reduced outpatient rehabilitation to once a week. She continued in physical education class to provide continuing movement activities in her school day. The occupational therapist and the physical education teacher worked on an individual program for Sarah during this period.

As a senior student, Sarah participated in a job shadowing program through the high school to help introduce her to a variety of careers that she might consider (Table 9-4).

The color guard activities provide an authentic context for addressing person factors that might be interfering with Sarah's everyday life. Because the rehabilitation therapist and the school therapist are keeping in touch, they can use the color guard performance as a benchmark for measuring therapeutic progress in context. For example, the rehabilitation therapist is working on bilateral integration, strength, and balance—which we can evaluate during color guard.

When occupational therapists are implementing best practices, they understand how to imbed the person factor needs in the person's chosen daily life activities. The therapist might have a difficult time convincing Sarah to complete her exercises for her arms, but Sarah is very interested in re-joining the color guard. The routines contain the same movements and endurance requirements that a more clinical therapy regime would contain. By using the high interest activity, both the therapist and Sarah have a better chance at a successful outcome (both for color guard participation and for rehabilitation).

References

Savage, R., Depompei, R., Tyler, J., & Lash, M. (2005) Paediatric traumatic brain injury: A review of pertinent issues. *Pediatric Rehabilitation, 8*(2), 92-103.

Ylvisaker, M., Todis, B., Glang, A., Urbanczyk, B., Franklin, C., DePompei, R., Feeney, T., Maxwell, N., Pearson, S., & Tyler, J. (2001). Educating students with TBI: Themes and recommendations. *Journal of Head Trauma Rehabilitation, 16*(1), 76-93.

TAMMY

WINNIE DUNN, PHD, OTR, FAOTA AND JANE A. COX, MS, OTR/L

Occupational Profile

Tammy is now in the fall semester of her last year of high school. She anticipates graduating with her classmates in the spring. Tammy began participating in special education instruction as a first-grade student, and supports continued across her school career. Now that she is in her final year of high school, part of the transition planning process includes contact with the State Division for Vocational Rehabilitation. Tammy talks to her parents, teachers, and friends about having a job after high school but her ideas about the kind of work she might do seems to change. Through her life skills class, she has had the opportunity to explore a number of work environments but gets confused about the possibilities. Tammy also hears others talk about going to college and expresses an interest in going to the local community college. Without a specific plan that includes ongoing and timely intervention, Tammy would likely spend unproductive time at home or in a work setting that does not match her interests or abilities. These two options were unacceptable to Tammy and her family. Tammy's parents are not sure whether college is a reasonable option for Tammy, but they mostly want her to be happy and as self-sufficient as possible.

Tammy's case illustrates her "transition" from student to a productive adult worker role. Her transition program began at age 16, when the transition coordinator employed by the special education cooperative along with Tammy's IEP team started planning for Tammy's post-secondary transition. It is important that this transition be timely and smooth. Without a timely referral and attention to Tammy's transition needs, it is likely that a significant delay or gap in services would have occurred and possibly resulted in Tammy losing valuable skills and confidence.

History

Tammy has had both a medical diagnosis and an educational eligibility identification of mental retardation. She originally received special education services as a preschooler under the category of "developmental delay." When she entered elementary school, the team identified additional educational needs; further testing revealed cognitive delays classified as "mental retardation."

Currently, professionals and families are reevaluating what terms are appropriate for intellectual disabilities (e.g., Hoffman & Field, 2005). As we understand more about individual differences in children, we see that there are other factors that also contribute significantly to a child's abilities. Taking a strengths approach, we look for the child's interests and abilities in a broader framework, so cognitive level is merely one aspect of a comprehensive picture. With Tammy's age, we see how historic patterns occurred, and how, as the system changes, we make adjustments accordingly.

Go to www.aamr.org (American Association of Intellectual and Developmental Disabilities) if you want to know more about these changes.

Her high school education included basic academics, some school- and home-based training in independent living activities, and vocational preparation activities that included community-based instruction. During her last year of high school, Tammy spent a half-day every day in a work position at a local restaurant.

Tammy lives with her parents, who are very supportive and desire to see Tammy assume a worker role in the community. They also express anxiety about Tammy traveling independently in the community. Tammy's home is on the public bus route that provided access to needed transportation, although Tammy does not know how to use the bus system independently. Tammy's family assumes responsibility for food preparation, shopping, and house maintenance. Tammy assists with house cleaning; she has had some incoordination and judgment limitations when handling cleaning equipment and materials. This interferes with her ability to perform independently in this area. Tammy performs self-care activities independently, with occasional reminders from her mother. Tammy's recreational activities are almost always family-centered and family-initiated.

When Tammy was 16 years old, her team at the time developed a transition plan (Table 9-5).

Table 9-5.

Tammy's Transition Plan

Initial Transition Plan for Tammy, Age: 16

Self-advocacy *(Go to www.sackonline.org for more information on self advocacy.)*	Personal Advocacy: To speak up for myself and let others know what I think. Solving problems and making decisions. I need help with banking. I need to know how to get around town. System Advocacy: I want to volunteer in the community. (Family) We need to understand what supports Tammy needs to be independent.
Work factors	Tammy has a strong desire to work so that she may earn money. Tammy has been exposed to a variety of occupations throughout her schooling working part-time in supported employment situations.
Living skills	Tammy lives with her family. She is able to care for her basic needs with supervision and occasionally guidance from a family member. Currently, there is no immediate plan for Tammy to change her current living situation.
Leisure	Tammy spends her leisure time participating in activities with her family. Tammy also enjoys swimming and has participated in Special Olympics swimming on and off over the years. During unstructured leisure time, Tammy enjoys looking at fashion magazines and watching TV shows such as "What Not to Wear" and "How Do I Look."

This plan got the team on the right track, thinking about long-term outcomes with Tammy. They can frame their high school activities in relation to this initial transition plan and then adjust as needed.

Analysis of Occupational Performance

The current education team includes Tammy, her parents, and teachers; they have a long history with Tammy, which enables them to plan her transition to adulthood more easily. They decide to review her history at school, at work, with friends, with family, and with community activities to obtain additional details for planning. The team decided to use the Canadian Occupational Performance Measure (COPM) to gather additional information from Tammy and her parents. The COPM is an outcome-based assessment in which people/caregivers identify the five most important issues in areas of self-care, productivity, and leisure. Parents rate performance and satisfaction on a scale from 1 to 10. Goals for intervention are based on the problems identified by the parents. After intervention, parents again rate performance and satisfaction on the previously identified issues. The difference (change score) between the initial and post-intervention scores indicate whether outcomes are met. A change score of two or more is considered clinically significant (Law, Baptiste, Carswell, McColl, Polatajko, & Pollock, 2005; Law, Polatajko, Pollock, McColl, Carswell, & Baptiste, 1994) (Figure 9-14).

Because employment was a primary concern, they also discuss inviting community employment personnel (which includes an occupational therapist) to join in the assessment and planning processes. School personnel and Tammy's parents also felt that she would need significant help finding, learning about, and retaining a job, thus requiring the referral for supported employment services. Although Tammy could not identify specific

Supported employment is defined in federal statute as a highly individualized approach for assisting individuals with significant disabilities to obtain and maintain employment. Supported employment includes three essential components:

1. *Paid work.*
2. *Employment in integrated community settings.*
3. *The availability of on-going support and training as needed to assure job retention or subsequent job placement.*

Supported employment frequently operates through the Vocational Rehabilitation system within states. Some community developmental disability organizations also provide these types of supports, so be sure to investigate in your area. For example, in Kansas, Social and Rehabilitation Services (SRS) oversees this process.

COPM Findings

Tammy's parents with input from Tammy identified paid employment and personal care as occupational performance priorities. Tammy wanted to have a job and be able to get to her job independently. Tammy's parents wanted her to get ready for work by herself.

Figure 9-14. Tammy's COPM priorities.

job-related interests, she expresses a strong desire to work and earn money. Tammy's dependence on her parents for transportation, along with her difficulty with judgment and handling materials in a coordinated manner, required further investigation.

Last, some of the team members provided information from their observations of Tammy in her natural environments, which included supported work settings through her school programming. They reported Tammy's strengths as well as areas of need. Tammy was highly skilled in many areas and was able to learn new skills effectively (e.g., identifying the correct bus, placing an order in a restaurant, crossing streets safely) when given the opportunity to follow a model and to practice. Tammy learned quickly in the authentic community environment that required a specific skill (e.g., a store, restaurant, city bus, bank).

She was unable to readily generalize across learning environments or situations. Tammy appeared to enjoy spending time in the community with people other than her family; however, she lacked confidence to do this without some sort of support and assistance. In the self-care area, Tammy required cueing from her mother to shower and wash her hair on a regular basis. She also had some difficulty selecting matching clothes from her closet. Tammy carries a food tray in the lunch room, walks around campus over a variety of surfaces, runs to catch the bus, climbs the stairs of the bus, and finds a seat while the bus is moving. Tammy has more difficulty in situations that require situational problem-solving. For example, Tammy started walking across a newly mopped floor and slipped; she did not recognize the need to walk around the wet area. However, with explicit instruction and demonstration, she was able to learn to walk around (compensation) the wet area even if this took her out of her way.

When a functional situational assessment process is used, it is important for the therapist to observe and record skills and needs within the context. We cannot assume, for example, that an individual's ability to safely cross a street with a crossing light means that he or she can also cross safely at an unmarked intersection. A functional assessment allows the team to focus on an individual's strengths (vs. weaknesses) in a variety of relevant situations. Family members generally understand and can actively contribute to such an assessment process that builds cooperation, a sense of shared planning, and problem-solving.

Based on extensive observations and interviews used to assess Tammy's work-related interests and needs, the team identified the critical conditions for Tammy to work successfully. Tammy would require a job where supervision was always available and a setting where co-workers would be able to redirect or instruct Tammy when she ran into difficulty. It was clear based on the assessment, that Tammy would do best working with other people where she could have frequent contact with other co-workers. Assessment of Tammy's ability to learn new tasks (e.g., riding the public bus) led the team to recommend that she have on-the-job "coaching" available in order to learn a job (i.e., explicit demonstration, practice, and feedback). The team felt that an employer would not be able to assume total responsibility for training Tammy given her unique learning needs.

The assessment process also allowed team members to identify Tammy's job-related interests. After spending time at a local restaurant, Tammy expressed that she would like to "help" with a salad bar and to "wash" tables. She also stated that she liked the uniforms worn by restaurant workers, perhaps reflecting her fashion interests.

Intervention

The supported employment service team focused primary attention on the performance area of work. Because getting ready in the morning would also affect employment success, the team planned for the occupational therapist to coach mom and Tammy to identify an effective morning routine.

Target Outcomes

1. Tammy will work in a paid position for 6 months.
2. Tammy will get herself ready for work each day prior to leaving home.

Community-based programs use a team-oriented effort to plan programs and, therefore, reflect the individual situated within the appropriate environment. The contribution that the occupational therapist makes on the team is unique and vital, but is incorporated into natural life tasks along with the contributions of the other team members. Community-based programs demonstrate this important principle very well and, therefore, provide a model for all program planning across the lifespan.

Intervention Approach

The employment specialist will provide coaching so Tammy can identify options, interview, and obtain employment.

An occupational therapist will provide coaching to design adaptations with cues for the "getting ready" routine.

The job coach will plan on-the-job training and support with needed modifications or adaptations.

Mom will support Tammy to get to the bus for transport to and from job site.

Intervention Procedures (Examples)

The following intervention sequence will be implemented:

1. Analyze the work environment and specific job tasks to identify opportunities (e.g., a supportive co-worker, color coding on salad bar ingredients) and barriers (e.g., typical business use of many written notices and written instructions for workers) for Tammy.
2. Observe Tammy doing the work activities, collect data on work task performance, and adapt environment or teaching methods to allow Tammy to succeed.
3. Meet with employer and co-workers to discuss job adaptations needed, and provide support and direction regarding interaction with Tammy.
4. Meet with parents and Tammy to provide coaching for home routines, so that the parents can reduce their involvement in her morning routine and enable Tammy to have her own consequences (e.g., be late for work if not ready).

Outcomes

Tammy receives supported employment services from the Community Developmental Disability Organization. This supported employment program designs and provides individualized community-based services that lead to paid employment.

Occupational therapists are critical members of the team and use their skills in functional assessment, environmental, and job analysis, as well as adaptation to maximize opportunities for employment success. Tammy's service environments are the environments she uses on a regular basis and include her home, the city bus system, and her job. Utilization of natural community environments promotes meaningful learning and retention of skills and behaviors. Enabling Tammy to operate in a variety of natural environments allows the team to reduce the impact of problem-solving, while greatly increasing the efficiency of her success as a worker.

Tammy, with the help of the supported employment service team, obtained a paid job at a local pizza restaurant. She required extensive on-the-job training by a job coach for the first few months of employment. Additionally, the job coach provided explicit training in the use of the public transportation system until Tammy was able to demonstrate independent and consistent use. Tammy's parents were very supportive in prompting Tammy to shower regularly and launder her uniform. They also prompted Tammy to get ready each morning and to catch the bus at the appropriate time. After several months of direct support by the occupational therapist and the job coach, Tammy demonstrated competence traveling and necessitated only occasional follow-up from the supported employment team. Her co-workers and employer assumed responsibility for daily support and training and reported tremendous satisfaction with Tammy's performance. The supported employment team gradually became consultants to the employer, but remained available on an as-needed basis.

References

Hoffman, A., & Field, S. (2005). *Steps to self-determination: A curriculum to help adolescents learn to achieve their goals.* Dallas, TX: Pro-ed.

Law, M., Baptiste, S., Carswell, A., McColl, M., Polatajko, H., & Pollock, N., (2005). *Canadian Occupational Performance Measure.* Ottawa, Ontario: Canadian Association of Occupational Therapy.

Law, M., Polatajko, H., Pollock, N., McColl, M., Carswell, A., & Baptiste, S. (1994). Pilot testing of the COPM: Clinical and measurement issues. *Canadian Journal of Occupational Therapy, 61*(4), 191-197.

Web Sites

Think College! College Options for People with Intellectual Disabilities. www.thinkcollege.net.

Self Advocate Coalition of Kansas. www.sackonline.org/uploads/Microsoft_PowerPoint_-_What_is_Self_Advocacy_2.0_On.pdf.

PROVIDING SERVICES TO WESTWOOD CHARTER SCHOOL

WINNIE DUNN, PHD, OTR, FAOTA

Charter schools have specific educational missions. The Westwood Charter School, which will serve as our example of population-based services, provides an alternative learning experience for students in grades 9 to 12 from a rural county who are either educationally disadvantaged or at high-risk for dropping out of school. This school has this mission:

> *to provide an authentic, nurturing, and academically challenging learning environment for high school students which is connected to the world outside of school, is meaningful for students, and promotes their positive sense of community and enthusiasm for learning."*

This school was developed in response to a longitudinal study of dropout rates in participating LEAs that revealed 120 students in a 7-year period left high school prior to graduation. The previous year's students included 6 who were parents, 2 who were living on their own, 6 who were involved in the legal system, and 5 who were in custody of the welfare agency or were assigned to a social worker.

The principal of Westwood Charter School had formerly been an administrator and a teacher in the neighboring school district, and he had worked with occupational therapists on his teams before coming to Westwood. He discussed the member requirements of the professional teams for this new school with his board of directors, and they decided that an occupational therapist would be a useful addition to the staff.

Determining Needs

The occupational therapist's initial strategies included interviewing the administrative and teaching staff, reviewing the longitudinal study that led to the formation of Westwood Charter School, reviewing the records of the previous year's students, and discussing the mission and vision of Westwood Charter School with the staff.

During the interviews, the occupational therapist considered what factors might be at play to support or interfere with either the students' or the staff's ability to carry out the mission of Westwood Charter School. The occupational therapist determined that the students enrolled in Westwood Charter School were having life challenges that revealed the relationships among the students' capacities, their contexts, and what was expected of them in school and in the community. She found two main areas to concentrate her attention.

Remembering the mission of the school ensures that she remain relevant to this specialized context.

1. Some students were having difficulty with their worker and student roles. Difficulties seemed to have related several factors:
   a. Some students have limited social awareness and skills for their worker and student roles.
   b. Some students were struggling to understand their particular work cultures and its demands.
   c. Some students seemed to need skills training for the work tasks themselves (e.g., study skills for student role, task performance expertise for the work role).

   d. Some students seemed to be unable to relate their own actions to the consequences in particular contexts and, therefore, did not take responsibility for outcomes.
2. Some students were having difficulty establishing and maintaining social relationships (including family, peers) to support them in their roles as student, family member, and friend.
   a. Some students seemed to lack awareness of social demands and cues.
   b. Some students expressed lack of confidence in their ability to develop and maintain relationships.
   c. Some students seemed to have difficulty creating a sense of autonomy (i.e., feeling effective as an individual who can take control of one's own life).

The occupational therapist checked back with the staff regarding these impressions. The Westwood staff agreed that these were key issues to address in their curriculum and with individual students. They felt that these were the issues that interfered with the students' success and satisfaction with their lives and that many of the negative situations that arose had their roots in these dilemmas.

Identifying Factors That Were Supporting or Interfering With Participation

Once the occupational therapist had a clear overall understanding of the needs, she could use her unique occupational perspective to characterize supports and barriers to performance within the Westwood Charter School system.

Supports for Participation Within the Westwood Charter School

A particularly strong support for the students' performance is the staff at Westwood Charter School. They are very willing to receive and integrate new information and suggestions, and seem clear about the mission of their school to support the students to have a successful and satisfying life.

The curriculum is also a support for planning. Charter schools in general have great flexibility to be innovative and design non-traditional curricula. The Westwood Charter School is structured around the development of individual learning plans that assist student performance and achievement in core academic areas, Internet and other learning technologies, and out-of-school/field-based learning experiences, including service-learning.

Academic goals of the Westwood Charter School include reading, writing, communication, and mathematical problem-solving. They have reported improvement in both narrative and expository reading comprehension and mathematical problem-solving. Westwood Charter School also has nonacademic goals for its students. These include promoting students' positive sense of community and promoting students' sense of resilience. These academic and non-academic goals set the stage for effective intervention planning on the areas of need.

The faculty designed a set of standards for enhancing students' overall critical thinking skills across the curriculum. Some of these standards include making informed decisions by examining options and anticipating consequences of actions, transferring learning from one context to another, working effectively in groups to accomplish a goal, identifying personal interests and goals and pursuing them, and recognizing the influence of diverse cultural perspectives on human thought and behavior. These goals and standards provide many opportunities for an occupational therapy perspective and intervention strategies.

Potential Barriers to Participation at Westwood Charter School

The Westwood students have multiple risk factors that create barriers to their success, including being teen parents, being removed from their biological family home, being involved with the legal system, failing in a traditional educational placement, and/or having learning and behavioral difficulties and attention problems. In addition, these students have a sense of failure and generally lack motivation and a sense of responsibility for their own actions. Reports from the admissions records indicate that many of their psychosocial issues have not been identified or explored.

The occupational therapist also noted that classroom arrangements feel and look chaotic. There are no "quiet" areas to reduce sensory stimuli to enhance student learning. Some students wear headphones to listen to music while working on the computers but often have the volume up so high that their music interferes with other students' learning. Lights are bright everywhere, both students and staff are talking most of the time, and the traffic flow between areas seems disruptive to other students' learning. The occupational therapist notes that she will explore environmental re-design to accommodate a wider range of sensory processing needs while working.

Designing the Intervention Program

The occupational therapist decided to organize the intervention plan using the Ecology of Human Performance framework because it provides both a method for characterizing the occupational therapy perspective on person/task/environment interaction as critical to performance and a structure for organizing the intervention options for the staff.

Intervention Plan

The occupational therapist met with the school administrator to discuss general plans, then met with the whole staff to cover general information, and finally met with the respective teams to collaborate on specific ideas for effective interventions for each team's students. This strategy provided the occupational therapist with an opportunity to explain the overall occupational therapy perspective and then apply those concepts to specific problems. This strategy also set the stage for more effective use of her skills and expertise in the future.

During the meeting with the administrator, they discussed the possibility of resource allocation to enable the occupational therapist to provide peer coaching for staff to improve their teaching effectiveness and design options for the student to have community experiences. Because the administrator was anxious for the community to view the school as a positive community resource, he decided that this might be a good use of resources initially and wanted to make sure that staff knew that he would support using money to include the occupational therapist in their implementation processes.

The staff meeting provided an opportunity for coaching and dialogue. The occupational therapist discussed her perspectives on supporting and designing successful performance options and illustrated her perspective by using a case from the school (a student everyone was familiar with).

Characterizing the Occupational Therapy Perspective

Tom's Identified Priorities for Participation

1. Tom wants to be an effective worker.
2. Tom wants to have friends.

The therapist interviewed Tom and his teachers and watched him during the school day. Tom seems motivated, but undirected about what kind of work might suit him. He makes attempts to interact with peers, but is not always successful. The staff composed a team that would work with Tom and the occupational therapist to address these two priorities. This one example provided the therapist a way to illustrate her process and to begin helping a particular student immediately. Her goal was that the team would begin to advocate for her services regarding other students as they understood how she could be helpful.

The occupational therapist provided guidance in several areas as described in the following examples.

1. Exploring employment options in the community through job shadowing and use of job coaches. The occupational therapist assisted with task analyzing the jobs and matching the tasks required with Tom's, and then other students', abilities.

   (i.e., application of Alter and Prevent interventions)

2. Assessing the educational environments to identify the sensory features that either increase or decrease the students' ability to complete work. Tom was distracted by others bumping into him, and so this provided a way for the occupational therapist to explain the impact of this sensory experience on his behavior. The occupational therapist then provided consultation to the other classroom teachers and administrator regarding rearranging the physical environment to provide low lighting and sound-absorbing partitions with large floor cushions and comfortable chairs in one area of the classroom.

   (i.e., application of Modify/Adapt intervention)

3. Providing sensory processing information for students and staff so that each person could become more aware of his or her own sensory preferences and dislikes. The therapist used the Adolescent/Adult Sensory Profile (AASP) as a staff training tool; staff completed the tool, and they discussed their patterns in the group. Then, staff administered the AASP with their students as well.

   (i.e., application of Establish/Restore intervention because they were learning a new skill; when they used this knowledge to make adjustments, this would be Adapt)

4. Designing community-based activities to increase the students' positive sense of community as well as positive feelings about themselves. The occupational therapist collaborated with Early Head Start (EHS) and Head Start to arrange volunteer experiences for students after they had a positive experience with Tom. The charter school students read to students at Head Start on a regular basis and assisted the EHS provider on home visits by playing with the siblings of the EHS child while the EHS provider visited with the parent(s). Additional activities included pairing up charter school students who have behavior and motivation difficulties with early elementary

   (i.e., application of Create, Prevent, and Alter interventions)

students with similar difficulties as learning buddies, as well as cooking a weekly meal for a community congregate meal site. This included planning the meal, purchasing the groceries, cooking and serving the meal, and cleaning up.

She also planned a trip to visit the NICU to learn about the complications of prematurity as they relate to teenage pregnancies, lack of prenatal care, and the effects of drug and alcohol use on babies.

(i.e., application of Establish/Restore, Adapt, and/or Prevent interventions)

5. Offering creative outlets to explore the students' self-concept and self-expression. The occupational therapist designed activities to encourage students to be more expressive about their feelings and themselves. An example of one activity was using mannequin heads that the students were able to decorate with various materials to represent how they see themselves or how they think others see them. This activity was followed up with discussion and feedback.

(i.e., application of Establish/Restore, Adapt, Create, and Prevent interventions)

Conducting Program Evaluation

The staff used the program evaluation protocol for their whole school to evaluate the overall effectiveness of the occupational therapy services. This protocol includes methods for evaluating both the overall outcomes and the specific activities. The students and staff identified criteria for success of activities prior to beginning and then were able to complete an evaluation of each suggested activity or modification using these criteria. An example of criteria for the first activity is the percentage of students who are successful part-time employees:

- Have been employed consistently at the same job.
- Received acceptable performance evaluation from their employer.
- Interviewed with unsuccessful students to identify mismatch issues.
- Have job satisfaction (self-reported).

The occupational therapist and school administrator met quarterly to review the occupational therapy utilization for the last quarter. They used several sources of information during these reviews, including billing records (which included time and types of activities), feedback forms from teams and other staff, satisfaction information from community partners, data from student performance, and records about the patterns and nature of usage (e.g., which teams used the occupational therapist in what ways during the quarter). They discussed more effective methods for using these services and drafted a plan for the next quarter at each meeting.

The overall evaluation criteria for the Westwood Charter School included measures of academic progress as well as measures of non-academic performance, such as attendance records, parent satisfaction survey, student and teacher reflections, student drawings, School Climate Survey, Social Skills Rating System (SSRS), and The Adolescent Resiliency Attitudes Scale (ARAS). The administrator had an advisory team that reviewed these materials for presenting to the board. When occupational therapy services became part of their discussion, the occupational therapist would either attend the meetings or provide the needed information. Once a year, the occupational therapist provided an analysis of the overall contribution of her services to the school's current outcomes, as well as suggestions for the future.

Resources

Kansas Public Charter Schools Grant Application submitted by USD 341 Oskaloosa (1998-99).

Williams, J. (1999). Interview. (Personal communication regarding development of the intervention planning).

Summary

We hope you have enjoyed studying all of our cases; remember the lessons for your own practice and have a great time being a best practice occupational therapist!

Financial Disclosures

Jane A. Cox, MS, OTR/L has no financial or proprietary interest in the materials presented herein.

Winnie Dunn, PhD, OTR, FAOTA is an author of the Sensory Profiles, which are referenced in this text. Pearson Inc. owns the copyright for these tools; Dr. Dunn receives a royalty for these products.

Becky Nicholson, MEd, OTR has no financial or proprietary interest in the materials presented herein.

Ellen Pope, MEd, OTR has no financial or proprietary interest in the materials presented herein.

Louann Rinner, MS, OTR has no financial or proprietary interest in the materials presented herein.

INDEX

Wait...There's More!

SLACK Incorporated's Health Care Books and Journals offers a wide selection of books in the field of Occupational Therapy. We are dedicated to providing important works that educate, inform an improve the knowledge of our customers. Don't miss out on our other informative titles that will enhance your collection.

Bringing Evidence into Everyday Practice: Practical Strategies for Healthcare Professionals

Winnie Dunn PhD, OTR/L, FAOTA

376 pp., Soft Cover, 2008, ISBN 13 978-1-55642-821-0, Order# 38129, $48.95

Bringing Evidence into Everyday Practice: Practical Strategies for Healthcare Professionals is a unique workbook that offers students and professionals efficient strategies for translating evidence into everyday practices.

Dr. Winnie Dunn has designed this text to be used as a step-by-step resource for students and professionals on how to understand and use evidence available in research and how to build solid decision-making patterns that will support professional practice.

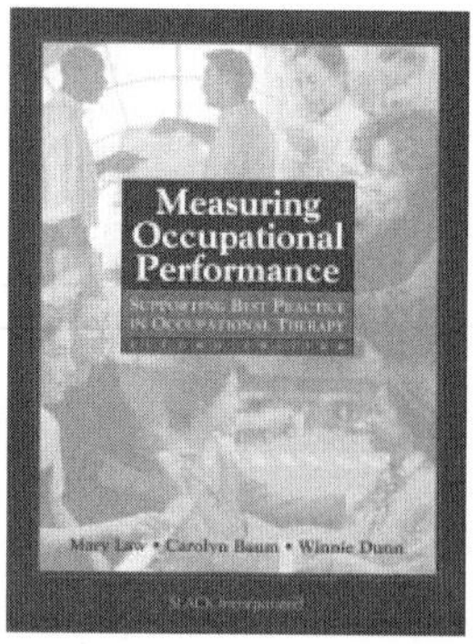

Measuring Occupational Performance: Supporting Best Practice in Occupational Therapy, Second Edition

Mary Law PhD, OT Reg. (Ont.), FCAOT; Carolyn M. Baum PhD, OTR/C, FAOTA; Winnie Dunn PhD, OTR, FAOTA

440 pp., Hard Cover, 2005, ISBN 13 978-1-55642-683-4, Order# 36836, $60.95

Measuring Occupational Performance, Second Edition provides easily accessible, up-to-date information for all occupational performance measures, including a systematic, detailed focus on measures important for evidence-based occupational therapy. Measurement issues and practices are discussed, and a decision-making framework is provided to guide the choice of assessment tools. This timely work helps to simplify a complex subject, and is a must-have for both occupational therapy students and practitioners.

Please visit **www.slackbooks.com** to order any of the above titles!

24 Hours a Day...7 Days a Week!

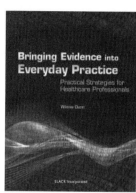

Attention Industry Partners!

Whether you are interested in buying multiple copies of a book, chapter reprints, or looking for something new and different — we are able to accommodate your needs.

MULTIPLE COPIES

At attractive discounts starting for purchases as low as 25 copies for a single title, SLACK Incorporated will be able to meet all of your needs.

CHAPTER REPRINTS

SLACK Incorporated is able to offer the chapters you want in a format that will lead to success. Bound with an attractive cover, use the chapters that are a fit specifically for your company. Available for quantities of 100 or more.

CUSTOMIZE

SLACK Incorporated is able to create a specialized custom version of any of our products specifically for your company.

Please contact the Marketing Communications Director for further details on multiple copy purchases, chapter reprints or custom printing at 1-800-257-8290 or 1-856-848-1000.

**Please note all conditions are subject to change.*

SLACK® INCORPORATED

Health Care Books and Journals • 6900 Grove Road • Thorofare, NJ 08086

1-800-257-8290

Fax: **1-856-848-6091**

E-mail: **orders@slackinc.com**

CODE: 328

www.slackbooks.com